Community and Public Health Nursing

Community and Public Health Nursing

5TH EDITION

Edited by

David Sines

Professor of Community Health Care Nursing, Pro Vice Chancellor, Faculty of Society and Health, Buckinghamshire New University, Uxbridge, Middlesex, UK

Sharon Aldridge-Bent

Senior Lecturer, Community Health Care Nursing, Faculty of Society and Health, Buckinghamshire New University, High Wycombe, UK

Agnes Fanning

Head of Academic Department, Primary Care and Public Health, Faculty of Society and Health, Buckinghamshire New University, High Wycombe, UK

Penny Farrelly

Senior Lecturer, Faculty of Society and Health, Buckinghamshire New University, High Wycombe, UK

Kate Potter

Senior Lecturer and Course Leader Specialist Community Public Health Nursing, Faculty of Society and Health, Buckinghamshire New University, High Wycombe, UK

Jane Wright

Senior Lecturer, Specialist Community Public Health Nursing, Faculty of Society and Health, Buckinghamshire New University, High Wycombe, UK

WILEY Blackwell

This edition first published 2013 © 2013 by John Wiley & Sons, Ltd
© 1995, 2001 by Blackwell Science Ltd for first and second editions
© 2005 by Blackwell Publishing Ltd for third edition

Registered Office
John Wiley & Sons, Ltd, The Atrium, Southern Gate, Chichester, West Sussex, PO19 8SQ, UK

Editorial Offices
9600 Garsington Road, Oxford, OX4 2DQ, UK
The Atrium, Southern Gate, Chichester, West Sussex, PO19 8SQ, UK
111 River Street, Hoboken, NJ 07030-5774, USA

For details of our global editorial offices, for customer services and for information about how to apply for permission to reuse the copyright material in this book please see our website at www.wiley.com/wiley-blackwell

Library of Congress Cataloging-in-Publication Data

Community health care nursing (Sines)
    Community and public health nursing / edited by David Sines, Sharon Aldridge-Bent, Agnes Fanning, Penny Farrelly, Kate Potter, and Jane Wright. – 5th edition.
        p. ; cm.
    Preceded by: Community health care nursing / edited by David Sines, Mary Saunders, Janice Forbes-Burford. 4th ed. 2009.
    Includes bibliographical references and index.
    ISBN 978-1-118-39694-0 (paper)
    I. Sines, David, editor of compilation. II. Title.
    [DNLM: 1. Community Health Nursing–Great Britain. 2. Public Health Nursing–Great Britain. 3. Primary Health Care–Great Britain. WY 106]
    RT98
    610.73'43–dc23
                                                    2013026529

A catalogue record for this book is available from the British Library.

Wiley also publishes its books in a variety of electronic formats. Some content that appears in print may not be available in electronic books.

Cover image: iStockphoto.com/A-Digit.
Cover design: Sarah Dickinson

Set in 10/13pt Trump Mediaeval by SPi Publisher Services, Pondicherry, India
Printed and bound in Malaysia by Vivar Printing Sdn Bhd

1   2013

Contents

Notes on Contributors   xii

1 **The Context of Primary Healthcare Nursing**   **1**
  The changing context of service provision   1
  The changing face of the community healthcare workforce   4
  The primary care vision for the next decade   8
  The impact of primary care policy changes on the role
    of the primary care nurse   14
  The scope of primary care nursing practice within the
    context of a changing workforce   15
  Conclusion   19

2 **Community Development and Building Capacity**   **22**
  Introduction   22
  The current context for community development practice   23
  Defining the terms   24
    Defining community   24
    Defining social capital   25
    Defining empowerment   26
    Defining capacity building   27
    Defining community development   27
    Defining community engagement   28
  The role of community health professionals   29
  Conclusion   34

3 **Multi-Sector Working and Self-Management, Community Health Care**   **37**
  Introduction   37
  Context for multi-sector working in the United Kingdom   38
  Key drivers for multi-agency working   41
  Examples of multi-sector working and self-management initiatives   43
  Dementia   44
  Obesity   45
  Asthma   47
  Concluding reflections   48

4 **Moving Care Closer to Home**   **53**
  Hospital provision: A brief history of the last 50 years   53
  Health care: What does it mean?   58
    Selective definitions of health   58
    Universal definitions of health   59

Caring and nursing: Where are we now?   61
Nursing at the interface between paid and unpaid care   63
Public health and care closer to home   65
Conclusion   68

**5   Evidence-Based Practice and Translational Research Applied
to Primary Health Care**   **71**
Introduction   71
Evidence-based practice   72
Designing the study   73
Translational research   73
   Overview   73
Experiments, randomised controlled trials and quasi-experiments   74
Health impact assessments   75
   Surveys   76
   Case studies   77
Different methodologies and methods give you new insights   77
Participatory approaches for community research   78
   Participatory appraisal   78
Data collection methods   79
Data management, analysis and interpretation   79
   A multi-method evaluation of a clinical educational innovation   80
   Example of PA   81
General research issues   81
   Validity, reliability and generalisability   81
Presentation and dissemination   82
The internet or world wide web (www)   83
Research proposals   83
Ethical issues   84
IRAS   85
The NHS research passport   85
   Ethics committees   86
Conclusion   87
Acknowledgments   88
Further reading   88
   Journals   88
   Ethics   89
   Funding   89
   Statutory body   89

6   Integrating the Children's Public Health Workforce   **91**
Introduction   91
Health indicators   92
The policy context   95
The role of the specialist community public health nurse   97
The HCP   97

Delivering the HCP 101
Pregnancy and the first 5 years of life 101
   The recommended schedule: pregnancy (Universal Services) 101
   The recommended schedule: pregnancy progressive services
     (Universal Plus and Universal Partnership Plus) 102
   The recommended schedule: birth to 6 months (Universal) 102
   The recommended schedule: birth to 6 months (progressive services)
     (Universal Plus and Universal Partnership Plus) 102
   Recommended schedule: 6 months to 1 year (Universal) 103
   Recommended schedule: 6 months to 1 year (progressive services)
     (Universal Plus and Universal Partnership Plus) 103
   Recommended schedule: 1–5 years (Universal Services) 103
   Recommended schedule: 1–5 years (progressive services)
     (Universal Plus and Universal Partnership Plus) 103
   The recommended schedule: 5–11 years (Universal Services) 104
   The recommended schedule: 5–11 years (progressive services)
     (Universal Plus and Universal Partnership Plus) 104
   Recommended schedule from 11 to 16 years (Universal Services) 105
   Recommended schedule from 11 to 16 years: progressive services
     (Universal Plus and Universal Partnership Plus) 106
   Recommended schedule: 16–19 years (Universal Services) 106
   Recommended schedule: 16–19 years (progressive services)
     (Universal Plus and Universal Partnership Plus) 107
The practitioner's role in safeguarding and child protection 108
The practitioner role in improving emotional health and well-being 109
Conclusion: future development and challenges for practice 110

7 Community Children's Nursing **113**
Introduction 113
Early days 114
The NHS 115
NHS at home: Community children's nursing services 118
Children with acute and short-term conditions 119
Children with LTCs 123
Children with disabilities and complex conditions, including
   those requiring continuing care and neonates 125
Technology dependence 127
Continuing care 128
Neonates 128
Children with life-limiting and life-threatening illness, including
   those requiring palliative and end-of-life care 128
Conclusion 130

8 Public Health Nursing (Adult): A Vision for Community Nurses **135**
Introduction 135
The vision for health reform: the policy context 138

The public health outcomes framework (2012)   140
   Improving the determinants of health   140
   Health improvements   141
   Health protection   141
   Healthcare public health and preventing
     premature mortality   142
Health promotion versus public health   143
An upstream approach   145
Health protection   145
Community nursing and public health   146
Conclusions: the future   149

9   Caring for the Adult in the Home Setting   151
End of life   152
The policy context   152
Managing LTCs in the community   154
Case Study based upon complexities of patient
  care in the home setting   155
Maximising health and well-being: helping
  people to stay independent   158
Working with people to provide a positive experience of care 158
Adult safeguarding   159
Measuring impact of service through patient feedback   160
Delivering high-quality care and measuring impact   160
Building and strengthening leadership   161
Ensuring we have the right staff, with the right skills in
  the right place   161
Technology   164
Informal carers   164
Supporting positive staff experience   165
Conclusion   166

10 General Practice Nursing in Context   169
Introduction   169
Origins   170
The advent of contemporary general practice nursing   172
Practice nursing roles and functions   174
Core skills for the GPN   174
Education   175
   Scheduled care   176
   Unscheduled care   178
Chronic disease management   179
Asthma management   180
Hypertension   180
The future   181

11   Occupational Health Nursing   **184**
OHNs as specialist practitioners   184
Historical perspective   185
Provision of OH services in the United Kingdom   189
The changing nature of UK workplaces   191
Changing work patterns   192
Workplace practices   193
The domains of OH nursing practice   193
The professional domain   194
The environmental domain   197
The educational domain of practice   197
Public health strategies   198
Specialist community public health nursing: Part 3 of the register
  maintained by the NMC   198

12   Caring for the Person with Mental Health Needs in the Community   **201**
Introduction   201
Background: Why bother with community mental health nursing?   202
Clinical profile: John   203
Recovery: Conceptual explanation   203
Development of therapeutic relationship   205
Assessment of needs   206
Instilling hope   207
Promoting life beyond distress   208
Promoting connectedness   209
Promoting personal responsibility   209
Principles of community mental health nursing   210
  Examining experience with service users   210
  Linking experiences   210
  Acknowledging service users' wishes   211
  Working together   211
  Therapeutic presence   211
  Risk assessment and management   212
Conclusion   213

13   Caring for the Person with Learning Disabilities in the Community   **216**
Introduction   216
People with learning disabilities   217
The number of people who have learning disabilities   218
Service principles in learning disability services   220
Moving forward   224
The health of people with learning disabilities   226
  Physical health   227
  Mental health   228
What community nurses for people with learning disabilities do?   230

The future role of community nursing services for people
  with learning disabilities   233
Conclusion   236

14   Leadership: Measuring the Effectiveness of Care Delivery   241
Introduction   241
Influences on leadership   242
Government policies   245
Front-line staff   247
Spend some time looking at these four scenarios   251
Measuring the effectiveness of delivery   253
Conclusion   254

15   Social Innovation and Enterprise   257
Introduction   257
What is social innovation?   258
Research on social innovation   259
Characteristics of a social innovator   260
Social innovation and community health   261
Commissioning   263
Approaches to social innovation   264
Social innovation as a concept   265
Conclusion   268

16   Adult Vulnerability in the Community   271
Introduction   271
Adult safeguarding   271
Definitions of abuse of adults   272
Legal framework of adult safeguarding   274
Mental Capacity Act 2005   274
Recent adult safeguarding guidance   275
Domestic violence   276
The prevalence of domestic violence in the United Kingdom   277
Effects of domestic violence   277
Contextual issues   278
Substance and alcohol misuse   279
Conclusion   281

17   End-of-life Care   285
Whole systems approach   286
Assessment: The foundation to providing good care   288
Symptom management   289
Beyond the management of physical symptoms   290
Advance care planning   290
  Advance statement/Preferred priorities for care   291

Advanced decisions to refuse treatment (ADRT)   292
Assisted suicide   292
Do not attempt resuscitation orders   293
Care in the last days of life   294
Models of interdisciplinary working: The road to successful
   end-of-life care   295
Community nurses: The lynchpins of successful end-of-life
   care in the community   295
Death of a child   296
Dementia   297
Care of the bereaved   298
Conclusion   299
Case study   300

**18   Interprofessional Learning and Teaching for Collaborative
    Practice Community   305**
Introduction   305
Inter-professional education and collaborative practice   305
Learning theory   308
Teaching and learning in practice   314
Responsibilities for teaching and learning of all members of the team   315
   Team leader   315
   Community practice teacher   316
   Mentor   316
   Associate mentor   316
   Learner   316
   Sign-off mentor   317
   Mastering mentorship   317
Adult safeguarding: an example   318
Conclusion   318

19   User Involvement, Self-Management and Compliance   322
The modern PPI system   323
The rationale for greater user involvement   324
The patient as co-producer   332
Co-production cannot be realised without support   334
Conclusion   335
Acknowledgement   336

Index   338

Notes on Contributors

Sue Axe
Faculty of Society and Health
Buckinghamshire New University
Uxbridge
UK

Owen Barr
Faculty of Life Sciences
University of Ulster Magee
Londonderry
Northern Ireland
UK

Sharon Aldridge Bent
Faculty of Society and Health
Buckinghamshire New University
High Wycombe
UK

Zoe Berry
Faculty of Society and Health
Buckinghamshire New University
Uxbridge
UK

Michelle Boot
Faculty of Society and Health
Buckinghamshire New University
Uxbridge
UK

Jenni Burton
Faculty of Society and Health
Buckinghamshire New University
High Wycombe
UK

Ruth Clemow
Faculty of Society and Health
Buckinghamshire New University
Uxbridge
UK

Agnes Fanning
Faculty of Society and Health
Buckinghamshire New University
High Wycombe
UK

Penny Farrelly
Faculty of Society and Health
Buckinghamshire New University
High Wycombe
UK

Anne Harriss
Faculty of Health and Social Sciences
London South Bank University
London
UK

Kate Potter
Faculty of Society and Health
Buckinghamshire New University
High Wycombe
UK

Susan Procter
Faculty of Society and Health
Buckinghamshire New University
Uxbridge
UK

Margaret Rioga
Faculty of Society and Health
Buckinghamshire New University
High Wycombe
UK

Peter Sandy
Faculty of Society and Health
Buckinghamshire New University
High Wycombe
UK

Jason Schaub
Faculty of Society and Health
Buckinghamshire New University
High Wycombe
UK

David Sines
Faculty of Society and Health
Buckinghamshire New University
Uxbridge
UK

Mark Whiting
Nurse Consultant
West Herts PCT, Peace Children's Centre
Watford
UK

Jane Wills
Faculty of Health and Social Care
London South Bank University
London
UK

Jane Wright
Faculty of Society and Health
Buckinghamshire New University
High Wycombe
UK

Maryam Zonouzi
Peer Exchange
London
UK

1

The Context of Primary Healthcare Nursing

David Sines

Faculty of Society and Health, Buckinghamshire New University, Uxbridge, Middlesex, UK

The changing context of service provision

The population of the United Kingdom is projected to increase by 4.9 million from an estimated 62.3 million in 2010 to 67.2 million over the 10-year period to 2020. Projected natural increase (more births than deaths) will account for 56% of the projected increase over the next decade, resulting in an overall UK population increase to 73.2 million over the 25-year period to mid-2035. The population is also projected to continue ageing with the average (median) age rising from 39.7 years in 2010 to 39.9 years in 2020 and 42.2 by 2035 (Office for National Statistics 2011).

The key drivers for population growth within the United Kingdom relate to greater life expectancy and migration, particularly from Eastern Europe (migration being expected to account for 68% of population growth during this period). Over the 25-year period to 2035, the number of children aged under 16 is also projected to increase from 11.6 million in 2010 to 13.3 million in 2026 before decreasing slightly to 13.0 million in 2035, whilst the population is projected to become older gradually, with the average (median) age rising from 39.7 years in 2010 to 39.9 years in 2020 and 42.2 years by 2035. As the population ages, the numbers in the oldest age groups will increase the fastest. In 2010, there were 1.4 million people in the United Kingdom aged 85 and over; this number is projected to increase to 1.9 million by 2020 and to 3.5 million by 2035, more than doubling over 25 years (Office for National Statistics 2011). The age of the working population will also increase during this period,

Community and Public Health Nursing, Fifth Edition. Edited by David Sines,
Sharon Aldridge-Bent, Agnes Fanning, Penny Farrelly, Kate Potter and Jane Wright.
© 2013 John Wiley & Sons, Ltd. Published 2013 by John Wiley & Sons, Ltd.

demonstrating unforeseen lifestyle patterns, which in turn will impact on those people of state pensionable age.

According to Mathers and Loncar (2006), the ten leading causes of death by 2030 will be ischaemic heart disease, cerebrovascular disease, upper respiratory tract and lung cancers, diabetes mellitus and chronic obstructive pulmonary disease (COPD). Within the top ten leading causes of death will also rank dementias, unipolar depressive disorders, alcohol use disorders, stomach and colon cancers and osteoarthritis. The combination of longer-term physical disorders and psychosocial challenges will demonstrate the importance of integrated service provision and workforce capability and capacity to respond to presenting co-morbidities. Other worldwide challenges relating to infectious diseases, such as HIV and tuberculosis, will provide additional pressures on our healthcare systems.

So how do society and its associated health and social systems respond to such challenges? In the first place, it can be assumed that societal change moulds the institutions that are created to respond to the needs of the population. Demands change over time, and in so doing, socio-demographic factors drive the process of change that in turn requires the National Health Service (NHS) to adapt its operational base. Examples of such changes relate to the needs of an increasingly demanding and complex population, a reduction in the number of available informal carers, advances in scientific knowledge and technological innovation and a heightened awareness of ethical challenges (such as gene therapy, stem cell research, embryology and euthanasia). In addition, the 2010 Coalition Government's quest to locate healthcare delivery as 'close to home' as possible has placed greater priority on primary and community service developments.

Such changes were enshrined within the context of the Government's inaugural healthcare White Paper 'Equity and Excellence: Liberating the NHS' DH (2010a). The 2010 White Paper placed much emphasis on sharing decision making between clinicians and patients, leading to their empowerment and ultimate engagement in sharing responsibility for their own care:

> Too often patients are required to fit around services, rather than services around patients.

This is a key component of the Government's 'Big Society' mandate, encouraging a move to self-care and a reduction in dependency on State-sponsored healthcare delivery.

The resultant 'care closer to home' initiative has been influenced by a range of external forces, driven by government pressure to drive down NHS costs and to reduce dependency on hospital admission (DH 2008a, b). Such changes however come at a price in their own right, and if the NHS is to succeed in responding effectively to the demands of the new community care culture organisation, then it will have to be prepared to face the demands of a changing environment of care practice and delivery (Buchan 2008).

Care closer to home has been defined by Nancarrow *et al.* (2006) as 'shifting all resources and expertise to primary care trusts'. This somewhat simplistic definition was adopted throughout the NHS 5 years ago and became the foundation for healthcare reform in the United Kingdom (Ham 2011). For example, NHS London announced in September 2008 that it would develop a new community-focused workforce plan for the city by 2013 (Workforce for London – NHS London 2007). The Health Authority advised that it wanted to see a 50% shift of hospital-based activity into community and primary care. This ambitious plan included a 10% reduction in inpatient bed admissions and a 41% increase in outpatient attendances in community healthcare service facilities. In order to achieve this, the workforce was challenged with the need to work more flexibly alongside patients, across care pathways in a variety of settings closer to home (DH 2008a, b). The workforce strategy that accompanied the SHA plan (NHS London 2010) advised that 15 000 healthcare workers would need to be trained or retrained to work in the community. More specifically the community nursing workforce would need to expand from 22% of the total nursing population in London to 40%. This presents a major challenge for the NHS and its educational providers (Buchan 2008) and represents three decades of investment in community-focused health service reform.

Other influencing factors were emphasised by Professor Stephen Field (DH 2012) in his healthcare 'Listening Exercise' for the Coalition Government (as a prelude to the implementation of the 2012 Health and Social Care Act). He identified the importance of promoting self-care and in encouraging patient and user involvement in healthcare prediction and co-treatment and service design. In his report he noted the major challenges facing the health of the population regarding obesity, smoking and alcohol/ substance abuse, all of which place a heavy burden on the state healthcare system and contribute to the incidence of dual diagnoses and longer-term, complex healthcare conditions.

The expectations of higher service response from the health service and its professional workforce also continue to rise, particularly as service users engage more fully in the determination of the shape and scope of local healthcare provision. The Government received a final report from Professor Steve Field (DH 2012) that advised the Secretary of State for Health to continue to position care closer to home and to accelerate the transfer of care from large acute hospitals to the community through a new process of 'clinical commissioning', to be led by general practitioners (GPs) (through new Clinical Commissioning Groups). The Government accepted these proposals and has now advised that NHS employees should be involved in the design and commissioning of new services, supported by new workforce training arrangements to prepare them for the transition. These changes will undoubtedly herald the way for a major transformation of the NHS workforce as it prepares to support care closer to home and reduces dependency on secondary care hospital-based services.

There are some risks attached to this shift in emphasis however since the concept of GP-led clinical commissioning (the new vehicle through which services will be commissioned) is untested and untried. Similar issues relate the nature, structure and deployment of the existing non-medical workforce in the NHS (Buchan 2008). Indeed, many practitioners remain defensive and tribalistic and tend to divide labour on the basis of historical or traditional trend rather than on the basis of actual customer or market need (Cipd 2010). A relationship also exists between professional groups and the State (Nancarrow *et al.* 2006), and in this regard the reshaping of the nursing workforce (with emphasis on community care) might provide an example of how government policy is driving change in how the professionals train and work.

Whatever the rationale for change, the impact of change, stimulated by a growing demand for flexible, high-quality services provided within local communities, will inevitably remould the NHS of the future. Resources are already being moved to the community at a rapid rate, and health service commissioners and providers are now required to demonstrate that the care they purchase and deliver is effective and responsive to consumer need. Field (DH 2012) has also written of the important role that members of the public are now making to the governance of the NHS, mainly through 'Ownership' of NHS Foundation Trusts and through engagement with Expert Patient programmes. NHS Trusts in turn are now responding more purposefully and seriously to user and patient expectations and are required to publish action plans in response to local and national patient satisfaction surveys and to demonstrate compliance with local service user requirements and feedback. Associated with the rise in consumerism and user engagement is a marked improvement in the capacity and capability of the NHS to respond to user complaints and to enhance governance procedures. Even more challenging to the NHS, however, is the increased number of litigation cases presented by patients, seeking recompense for less than satisfactory care experiences. It is perhaps therefore unsurprising that it is in the primary and community care sectors that change has been most rapid, demanding the creation of innovative workforce solutions and service reconfigurations.

The changing face of the community healthcare workforce

In this chapter, we have noted that more healthcare provision needs to be delivered through primary and community-based care with public involvement in health improvement in order to enable a shift away from over-reliance on acute care. This will help the healthcare service to evolve to meet the increasing challenges of an ageing population and an increased need for case management of those with long-term conditions in a way that allows patients to retain and regain an active role in society.

The NHS reviews of the last decade (Wanless 2004), the 'Prime Minister's Commission on Nursing and Midwifery' (DH 2010b) and the Royal College of Nursing (2011) have all recognised the need to upgrade the role of community nursing in order to respond to government policy. The Royal College of Nursing expresses agreement for this view and have advised that '80% of the nursing workforce will be working with local people to improve their health, rather than working in the hospital fixing the preventable, resulting in the safe reduction of a large number of hospital beds'. Changes in

Government policy will enable this to happen over the next decade, providing opportunities for the production of a competent, capable and confident workforce of community nurses and health visitors. Key changes in the new healthcare system [following the enactment of the Health and Social Care Act (Parliament 2012a)] will include:

A shift of power over health budgets to patients and GPs. The Government will allow patients the 'choice of any qualified provider' following a policy of 'no decision about me without me'. Patients will be supported whether they want a service from a hospital, from a GP, from a community health service or from a voluntary provider. This shift in policy towards patient choice has the potential to drive and reward innovation evidenced within community health services.

Promotion of a mixed economy of service provision, including an increased role for local authorities and voluntary and independent sector care provision; social enterprises will also be encouraged, in line with the Government's vision of the 'Big Society'.

Greater opportunity for clinicians and front-line staff to develop, design and deliver services that are responsive to the needs of local people and their GP commissioners.

Freedom for practitioners to innovate and to provide services and outcomes that improve the health and social capital of their local neighbourhoods.

In order to realise these aims, we argue in this book that:

1. There will be a continued demand to expand the community nursing and health visiting workforce and their role in delivering health provision over the coming decade.
2. The nature of community nursing and health visiting will change as a result with community practitioners taking on a greater role as expert clinicians, leaders, innovators and entrepreneurs.
3. There will be a major need to transform the delivery of care so that there is greater emphasis on public health and management of long-term conditions in the community as dependence on the acute sector is reduced.
4. Community practitioners will need to acquire additional skills in evidence-based practice and to create a community service with leadership, innovation and entrepreneurship as central skills. Emphasis will also need to be placed on enhancing patient safety (and safeguarding), on improving clinical effectiveness and on working productively and efficiently. Such skills will be needed to modernise the service.
5. The number of nurses working in the community who have specialist/advanced community nursing qualifications (health visitors and district nurses) will need to increase significantly over the next 5–10 years.
6. Key features of our contemporary society suggest that a much greater focus on health promotion and public health is required since people are living longer and healthier lives and are better informed about their needs and expectations of the health service with particular regard to promoting self-management.

7. Increasing emphasis will be placed on increasing social inclusion and valuing diversity for socially excluded groups, that is, those least likely to access healthcare, and on the reduction of health and social care inequalities experienced by significant groups within our population (geographical diversity will also demand local adaptation of national healthcare solutions, particularly within the context of devolved government to the four countries of the United Kingdom).

8. Practitioners will require greater competence and capability to work with assistive technology in areas such as tele-health, tele-care and tele-medicine; consumers and practitioners are also becoming increasingly dependent on e-based information systems and smartphone usage.

In order to ensure that the workforce is appropriately skilled and aligned to the needs of the new healthcare delivery system, the Government produced a consultation paper on education and training in the NHS – 'Developing the Healthcare Workforce' (DH 2010a) (The full paper is available at http://www.dh.gov.uk/en/Consultations/ Liveconsultations/DH_122590).

As a result of this paper, a national statutory body was created to determine the nature, structure and focus of the healthcare workforce in England (and its educational commissioning requirements) – Health Education England. This new statutory board will provide national oversight and support to Public Health England and all healthcare providers on workforce planning and the commissioning of education and training.

It is intended that the new system will fit with the Government's requirement to develop care closer to home and will be supported by a series of Local Education and Training Boards, so that employers have greater autonomy and accountability for planning and developing the workforce, alongside greater ownership of the quality of education and training by the professions.

These new arrangements will allow for:

- Robust workforce planning to ensure sufficient numbers of appropriately skilled healthcare staff in the right areas.
- A flexible workforce that can respond to the needs of local demand.
- Continuous improvement in the quality of education and training of staff aspiring for excellence and innovation for high-quality care.
- Transparency across provider funding to ensure value for money and demonstrate the quality of education and training.
- The creation of a diverse workforce that has access to fair education and training as well as opportunities to progress.
- Clearer definition of roles and responsibilities for commissioning and delivery of education.

Government healthcare reform has confirmed the significant role that primary care and health promotion play in the reformed health economy and emphasised that our focus should be on health outcomes, on user engagement and in the design and implementation of healthy communities and lifestyles at school, at home and at work. These policies have also pledged to 'break down' organisational barriers and to forge stronger links with local authorities, thus placing the needs of the patient/client at the centre of the care process. In so doing, a new foundation has been laid upon which to unite the principles of seamless care delivery and in particular the provision of self-directed care/direct payment packages, based on case management principles (Parliament 2012a). In practice this will require the provision of new inter-sectoral solutions to ensure that care is delivered between health and social service agencies through the development of positive partnerships and integrated case assessments between statutory agencies, consumers, their representatives and the voluntary and independent sectors to provide a positive choice in the provision of services. Emphasis on primary care has been reaffirmed in that, wherever possible, care should be provided as close to the person's home as possible.

In July 2012, the Government published its long-awaited White Paper on Social Care (Parliament 2012b) in which it outlined its vision for the reform of care and social support. Changes heralded in the report include:

- Placing dignity and respect at the heart of a new code of conduct and minimum training standards for social care workers.
- Introducing new social care apprenticeships.
- Legislating to give people the right to a personalised budget and direct payments (in eligible circumstances).
- Applying and embedding the principle of personalised care across all services.
- Placing a duty on local authorities to join up care with health and housing where this delivers better care and promotes people's well-being.
- Developing plans to ensure everyone who has a care plan has a named professional with an overview of their needs and responsibility for responding to their needs.
- Ensuring that partners remove barriers to promote the widespread adoption of integrated care.
- Developing coordinated care for older people and improving access that people living at care homes have to the full range of primary and community health services.
- Enhancing and extending joint funding arrangements between the NHS and social care to support integrated care provision (and to ensure joined-up thinking between housing, social care and healthcare provision).
- The establishment of a new Leadership Forum for social care to lead service transformation (including new standards for registered managers).
- A requirement for local authorities and Clinical Commissioning Groups to work together on Health and Wellbeing Boards to determine how their investment is best used to support and promote innovation and integrated working between health and social care.
- Planning and delivering effective re-ablement services and intermediate care and post-discharge support that enables people to regain their independence.

The primary care vision for the next decade

At the heart of the Government's reformed healthcare strategy is the greater focus placed on the delivery of services in primary care, underpinned by a new relationship between healthcare professionals and patients/clients through the promotion of supported self-care management. Accompanying this philosophy of care is the recognition that many patients present with complex (longer-term) conditions, arising from co-morbidity (DH 2011).

Amongst the key reforms resulting from the enactment of the Health and Social Care Act 2012 are:

- The creation of an NHS that 'helps people to stay healthy' and to benefit from more effective treatment, informed by research- and evidence-based practice.
- Requirements for local Clinical Commissioning Groups to commission comprehensive well-being and prevention services, in partnership with local authorities, with the services offered personalised to meet the specific needs of their local populations.
- Greater engagement of voluntary organisations and social enterprises between the Government, private and third sector organisations on actions to improve health outcomes.
- The entry of a series of new non-statutory sector healthcare providers (mandated by the NHS Commissioning Board as 'Qualified Providers' of healthcare in England).
- Support for people to stay healthy at work.
- Support for GPs to help individuals and their families stay healthy.
- Extended choice of GP practice.
- Implementation of personal health and social care budgets.
- Care plans to ensure that everyone with a long-term condition has a personalised care plan.
- Introduction of a new right to choice as enshrined in the NHS Constitution.
- Guaranteed patient access to the most clinically and cost-effective drugs and treatments.
- Measures to ensure continuous improvement in the quality of primary and community care.
- The creation of new partnerships between the NHS, universities and industry through the creation of new Academic Health Science Networks.
- The provision of strengthened arrangements to ensure staff have consistent and equitable opportunities to update and develop their skills.

Health service reforms have also been underpinned by the commissioning of new community healthcare facilities and in outcome/standard setting accompanied by matching increased diversity of supply. This will be accompanied by greater ability to respond to the new diversity of demand in preventive and curative medicine – tackling the underlying causes of health inequalities as well as providing the best care.

Decreased tolerance of failing services will also be a core component of the Government's strategic healthcare plan with the NHS Commissioning Board introducing tougher measures to improve standards and to close down services in the case of poor standards. Foundation Trusts will be implemented fully across England by 2014, some of which will also be able to take over failing hospitals to turn around their performance. In the case of primary care, there will be greater diversity of supply and strengthening of the power of Clinical Commissioning Groups to ensure that GP or community healthcare services can be improved or replaced where they fail to respond to local patient/user demand.

Major advances in technology and bioengineering have also brought about significant changes in treatment patterns and modes of delivery. For example, with cutting-edge techniques – ranging from genetics to stem cell therapy – and life-saving drugs to prevent, alleviate or cure conditions like Alzheimer's disease, it is likely that many of today's diseases will succumb to either eradication or amelioration. Investment in the implementation of world-class research programmes will accompany the Government's healthcare investment plan, and new Academic Health Science Networks will be sponsored for implementation across England, working in partnership with Foundation Trusts, Clinical Commissioning Groups, industry and partner universities. These will facilitate the discovery of new technologies, which in turn will enable clinicians the ability to diagnose and intervene at the earliest possible opportunity.

Similarly new alliances will continue to be developed with our emergency care services (e.g. the Ambulance Service) to equip paramedical staff with the requisite skills to treat people suffering from heart attacks with life-saving drugs in their own homes or to provide emergency interventions for longer-term conditions outwith hospital specialist treatment units. For others attendance at specialist treatment centres will become the norm. One such example relates to some stroke patients who now receive immediate treatment with the latest clot-busting drugs in specialist stroke centres, thus extending their lives and enabling many people to lead independent lives. Other patients will benefit from attendance at new trauma centres.

There will also be improvements in the way in which the 16 million people in England who present with longer-term diseases, such as asthma, heart failure, diabetes or psychosocial challenges, manage their care. The people who care for these service users – the 'carers' – also require additional support and 'seamless' access to services. In some cases personal budgets and direct payments will be made available to enable individuals and their families to purchase responsive care packages directly. The use of personal health and social care budgets will underpin reforms of our health/social care system.

Many of the people who will benefit most from new care packages will present with 'lifestyle'-related diseases such as mental health, diabetes, cardiovascular disease, stroke and some cancers. In order to combat the rising trend in such conditions, the health service will work in close partnership with patients and carers to co-design and co-deliver effective preventative and direct treatment services, aimed at encouraging the population to take their own health 'seriously'. In order to achieve this objective, more patients will become engaged with their care by managing their own conditions, taking advantage of support offered by GPs and nurses in the home or on the high street and by exercising more control over their lives and care. Greater emphasis on what we eat and participation in sports and leisure activities will also be encouraged – presenting a significant challenge for the way in which primary care nurses discharge their role and responsibilities.

There will also be opportunities for the provision of extended screening services, for example, for colon cancer and for breast cancer. An increasing number of patients will also access NHS directly through the internet, smartphones and digital TV to improve their access to evidence-based information about their health. Others, through the use of personalised budgets, will take control of their care packages and manage their care plan directly, rather than having to rely on others. By so doing, a greater range of patients will become increasingly empowered, giving them a greater say in their care, particularly in the later years of their lives.

Such fundamental changes in healthcare policy and process will require primary services to adopt new flexible and responsive approaches and to develop new partnerships with the voluntary and private sectors where they can contribute and innovate. Greater synergy will also be required between acute and primary care and between health and social care. New and dynamic approaches to clinical commissioning will be needed to deliver such changes, focusing on patient choice, direct payments (DH 2011), quality provision and market contestability.

The enactment of this policy shift will reduce patient/client dependency on inpatient or long-stay residential care in favour of seeking the development of a range of options based on local need, which will be flexible enough to meet the demands of service provision required by local people in their neighbourhoods. Clinicians are therefore being encouraged to work in close partnership with their patients and clients with the aim of making them more accountable for their practice and interventions.

At a strategic level, the NHS Commissioning Board now requires all Foundation Trusts and Clinical Commissioning Groups to secure significant improvements in the way in which services are delivered to the population, emphasising the promotion of positive health and safety and the promotion of high-quality care in the community. In order to provide these services, healthcare providers must demonstrate that they offer a range of services for their clients and families as equal participants whenever decisions that will affect their lives are involved. Such principles now underpin the NHS philosophy and form the basis of the Government's 'reformed' health and social care strategy.

NHS providers must also determine the role that they are going to play, with local authority social service departments, in making their contribution to a range of comprehensive service developments for clients. The Health and Social Care Act 2012 also demands that planning agreements should be reached between health and social service departments that identify clearly which services will be provided by each agency and that identify the processes to be adopted in assessing the needs of individuals in their care. The principle of effective alliance building between the NHS and social services will be further encouraged by the creation and operation of Local Education and Training Boards in England. They (and supporting Government policies) will outline requirements for health and social care services to work together to encourage the joint design, training and education of staff from both agencies in order to provide a workforce with the necessary capacity, skills and diversity to meet the needs of the local population. Alliance building is crucial if user needs are to be met within the context of an increasingly pluralistic health and social care economy, characterised by self-care and user choice and involvement.

The principles outlined in this chapter also require each government department to demonstrate emphasis on public health as a central concept within their business plan – a cornerstone of 'joined-up government'. For the health service, charged with responsibility to enact national quality standards and health improvement plans for local communities (via the newly established Public Health England Board and by local Health and Wellbeing Boards), a fundamental review is required to assess local public health capacity and capability, across sector boundaries.

In the future, emphasis must also be placed on the promotion of health and alliance building between professionals and users of services. The focus of care is clearly placed within the community with an expectation that resources will be deployed to meet identified health and social care needs through the provision of integrated, peripatetic support from a range of professionals who will include doctors, community healthcare nurses, community specialist public health nurses, social workers, clinical psychologists, physiotherapists, speech therapists, radiographers and occupational therapists (supported by an efficient and appropriately funded intermediate/acute sector, inpatient service). The acute sector will complement the work of local primary healthcare workers who will continue to provide the first point of contact for clients and their families through the provision of effective intermediate and ambulatory treatment/assessment services. In turn such services will be supported by the implementation of primary care-led emergency care walk-in centres, extended GP practices and community-based diagnostic and treatment centres, thus providing a range of 'seamless' assessment, diagnostic and treatment services for their local communities.

The next decade will therefore be characterised by the development of highly focused primary care services that will respond to the needs of local practice populations. In this model, much of the activity currently carried out by the local acute hospital will be transferred to general local primary services, some of them provided directly by the NHS, others provided by independent or voluntary sector agencies. New community-based services will also be introduced to provide an integrated, eclectic range of health and social care services, including diagnostic and treatment services for the local population. Such local services will increasingly undertake minor and invasive surgery, routine diagnostic testing, support for cases requiring observation and most outpatient activity. Centralised or specialist hospital facilities will continue to deal with severely ill people with complex therapeutic needs and provide for major surgery. Older people and those with mental health needs or learning disabilities will also continue to be cared for (almost exclusively) in community care settings.

From a practical perspective, the way in which primary care services will be delivered in the future will be determined from both national and local demand perspectives. Nationally, key priorities have been determined annually by the Department of Health and outlined in an operating framework document (see, e.g. the Department of Health's Operating Framework for the NHS in England for 2012/2013, DH 2011). Examples of key operating principles include:

- Listening and responding to patients, the public and staff and improving patient outcomes and experience; making decisions as close to the patient as possible.
- Moving towards clinical ownership and leadership local targets whilst delivering on national priorities.
- Co-production – all parts of the system working together to shape and implement change.
- System alignment – achieving complex cultural changes whilst encouraging different parts of the system to work together in partnership.
- Sustaining a financial regime that supports service reform goals incentivises service improvement.
- An emphasis on partnership working between NHS organisations, local authorities and other partners to ensure local health needs are better understood and addressed.

Other priorities include the need for community services to:

- Build better access for patients, clients and carers and ensure ongoing improvements in patient experience of access by assuring that GP health centres and practices deliver effective and innovative services (including flexible evening and weekend appointments).
- Keep adults and children well with a key focus on heart disease and cancer whilst responding to the needs of children and the newborn (through the 'sure start' and 'healthy child programmes') and by providing excellent maternity services.
- Further reduce health inequalities and deliver evidence-based and cost-effective interventions across all care pathways.
- Ensure more choice in service selection and treatment response; elicit objective feedback on 'the patient experience' and respond accordingly; and encourage active user engagement with all aspects of care design, delivery, and quality measurement.
- Tackle lifestyle issues, such as obesity, teenage pregnancy and problems associated with smoking and alcohol usage.
- Close the gap in life expectancy between affluent and deprived areas of the population by improving the health and well-being of the population (through regular health checks, physical activity programmes and targeted health promotion and public health programmes – sponsored by local, cross-agency Health and Wellbeing Boards).

- Work closely with local authorities to provide integrated and co-located services, including joint commissioning, personalised services, integrated care management and personalised budgets.
- Redesign and implement care pathways that respond effectively to patient and service demand to support patients with longer-term conditions (and to encourage integrated working, self-care and the use of assistive technology).
- Continue to reduce the rate of hospital-acquired infection.
- Strengthen management, leadership and clinical excellence in the workforce to enhance both capacity and capability.
- Put in place and lead local information (e.g. the development and application of the next stage of digital technology) and management and technology plans to improve the health service infrastructure and patient/user experience.

A range of enabling strategies will also be put in place to support the implementation of these delivery plans, including the empowerment of patients, the provision of choice, reduction of service variability, the implementation of a new quality framework, investment in professional training, education and workforce development, commissioning and system reform (including world-class commissioning and clinical commissioning) and estate developments. At the heart of the plan is an explicit requirement to transform community services to drive greater service integration (and in so doing improve patient choice and access whilst also reducing acute admissions and lengths of stay) by 'bringing care closer to home'.

There is little doubt that the introduction of these new service delivery imperatives will provide the primary/community care nursing profession with a range of major challenges that must be addressed if the balance of care is to shift, according to government policy, to the community. One specific question must relate to the future education and training that will be required to equip practitioners with the necessary skills, knowledge and value base to be able to function effectively in the community. In reality, there is also likely to be a reallocation of tasks between nurses and others, including informal carers and other professionals (many of whom work currently in acute hospital settings and who will be required to transfer into new primary care settings as the context of care changes). Primary care nurses must therefore be prepared to develop and change, drawing upon the very best of their past experience and becoming increasingly reliant upon the production of research evidence to inform their future practice.

This section has proposed that the most effective way to meet the health needs of the local population is to focus primary healthcare services within the very heart of naturally occurring communities and neighbourhoods. In so doing (using the general practice population of the focus and locus for care), opportunities for the further improvement of multidisciplinary teamwork and improved communication systems with clients (and others) will be provided. In order to transact effective care, the potential role that primary care nurses can undertake to fulfil the new NHS mandate must be acknowledged.

The impact of primary care policy changes on the role of the primary care nurse

In 2010, the then Prime Minister published a major document entitled 'Front line care – Report by the Prime Minister's Commission of Nursing and Midwifery in England' (DH 2010b). This confirmed the role that community nurses and health visitors are expected to play within the context of a contemporary and 'modernised' healthcare service:

> Community Nurses can play a vital role in coordinating services, maximizing continuity of care during the entire care pathway, advising on individual service users' needs and encouraging self-management by helping service users negotiate their way through the sometimes bewildering variety of services and support agencies available (p. 71). Nurses should be supported by a health system that focuses strongly on health promotion for all, while identifying and targeting those most in need...promoting health and preventing illness and reducing health inequalities has long been central to nursing and midwifery roles, and is the foundation of health visiting (p. 66).

The policy drivers outlined in this chapter will have significant impact on the status of the primary care nurse/health visitor as the 'lynchpin' within the context of a multidisciplinary team of specialist healthcare practitioners. Their work has also been directed by the advent of consumerism that has placed new demands for new competencies amongst the workforce with an emphasis on therapeutic skills, case management (this concept will be discussed later in this text), clinical leadership, clinical decision-making and social enterprise skills. Further endorsement of the significance of the role that community and primary care nurses and health visitors will play within the reformed health services has been provided by the Prime Minister's review on Nursing and Midwifery (DH 2010b).

In summary, the community and primary care nurses must be able to respond to the health needs, health gain requirements and expressed demands of their clients and local population groups so as to:

- Stimulate healthy lifestyles and self-care opportunities.
- Design and deliver cost-effective and evidence-based treatment and care responses (including efficient and effective prescribing practice).
- Further educate families, informal carers, the community and other care workers.
- Solve or assist in the solution of both individual and community health problems.
- Orient their own as well as community efforts for health promotion and for the prevention of diseases, unnecessary suffering, disability and death.
- Lead, work within, and with, inter-professional teams and participate in the development and leadership of such teams.
- Participate in the enhancement and delivery of primary healthcare in a multidisciplinary care context.

- Co-design and co-deliver innovative and responsive packages of care in partnership with service users and their carers (particularly in the effective management of longer-term conditions) that are coordinated effectively across integrated care pathways.
- Contribute to the effective commissioning of new and innovative services that are designed to meet the needs of the local population.
- Create the requisite conditions to provide entrepreneurial services that respond to the actual needs of local service users and commissioners.

Finally, in this section, the importance of public health is emphasised as the province of all community practitioners who are normally engaged in:

- Monitoring and profiling the health of their community/practice area.
- Ensuring that public health issues are identified and reported to managers and commissioners.
- Monitoring health outcomes of their interventions.
- Improving the effectiveness of their activities.
- Developing local health strategies and building healthy alliances necessary to implement these.
- Developing and maintaining partnerships with clients, informal carers, other community members and other professionals.
- Collaborating with local authorities (and Clinical Commissioning Groups and Health and Wellbeing Boards) and other agencies to monitor and control health-related issues considered to be hazardous to the well-being of the community.
- Informing the public about public health issues and engaging in health promotion programmes.
- Ensuring that members of the community have access to appropriate public health advice and information in a range of accessible formats.

The scope of primary care nursing practice within the context of a changing workforce

One key enabler of the proposed healthcare reforms will be the workforce and its ability to prepare itself for the new world of work, characterised by inter-professional teamwork and inter-sectoral care practice that follows the 'patient experience' (e.g. seamless and transitional care provision between the acute and primary care sectors). Flexible and adaptable career (and associated educational) pathways will be needed to support the new workforce. One key example relates to the need to provide flexible career progression opportunities to enable nurses and allied health professional staff to move seamlessly between acute and primary care service settings and to reduce dependency on the actual care setting itself. Flexibility will also be needed to encourage staff to move between employers and between the healthcare, social care and voluntary/independent care sectors.

Current government policy provides considerable opportunities for the development of innovative care solutions within which nurses, often in partnership with social workers and other support staff, will be able to provide responsive services to clients in response to their identified needs. As agency boundaries break down further between primary, intermediate, secondary and tertiary care sectors, and professional skills transcend previously defended frontiers, service users will have freer access to nursing and health visiting skills. The way in which access is negotiated for nursing skills will, in the future, be through single case assessment, personalised budgets and case management and direct payment processes, which should make nursing skills more easily accessible to the general practice population. Their understanding of local patient and family needs (often acquired from many years of experience and proven competence in the delivery of care to their clients) has placed primary care nurses (and those acute sector nurses who are intending to transfer to the community) in an ideal position within the 'reformed' NHS to respond more flexibly to locally identified health and social care-related requirements.

In order to respond to the demands of the new flexible workforce, primary care services will need to create, implement, share and explore key issues in relation to the local distribution, sustainability and transferability of innovative 'new role' solutions in primary and intermediate care in order to inform the competencies, practice, education and learning requirements of such new roles. This will include:

- Agreeing actions arising from local and national discussion relating to the key practice, education/training and regulation issues that need to be addressed to enable sustainability and spread of new 'fit for purpose' primary care practitioners whose roles are designed to meet the demands of evolving and complex inter-professional health and social care work streams.
- Ensuring that universities and their associated partner trusts/social service departments engage in the design and implementation of new education programmes that are informed by the standards of practice that will be identified through the national changing workforce programmes and other 'modernisation' imperatives.
- Agreeing a framework for the development of competencies and associated regulation for new emergent roles in order to maximise opportunities for new ways of working within the NHS career framework (including the delegation of appropriate tasks and functions to trained support staff/assistant practitioners).
- Undertaking operational research and evaluation that is designed to measure the effectiveness and impact of such new roles and competencies.

If these aims are to be achieved, then there is a need to ensure that the primary, social and intermediate care workforce is not developed in isolation, but set within the context of national and local workforce requirements, supported by education frameworks developed in partnership with local practitioners. A new workforce will also need to be prepared to meet the diverse needs of the reformed community workforce, underpinned by a new cadre of advanced practitioners who will be able to assess, diagnose, treat patients and prescribe. Additionally, new associate or assistant practitioner roles will emerge to enhance the skill base of the support worker workforce. Such 'new ways of working' have highlighted the challenges that the introduction of new roles present to employees, employers, regulators and educationalists. One key lesson learned to date is that new roles must be well defined and underpinned by competence-based role descriptions, accompanied by customised educational programmes and supervisory arrangements that reflect:

- The development and implementation of a defined 'role map' for a new inter-professional and multi-agency workforce.
- The introduction of these new roles underpinned by a short-, medium- and long-term strategic plan in order to ensure flexibility, transferability and sustainability and to encourage recruitment and retention of staff working in these new evolving roles.
- Key policy drivers impacting on service provision (particularly in relation to the management of longer-term conditions, personalised care, integrated case assessment, care/case management, unscheduled emergency care/out-of-hours provision and specialist care provision), which require expediency in the introduction of these roles.
- Local workforce delivery plans in order to facilitate the ability to change workforce profiles; current and future workforce profiles should focus on matching local need with national policy.
- Flexible commissioning arrangements for education programmes in and across strategic health/social care economies.
- The provision of effective educational provision through the creation of 'fit for purpose' learning/knowledge transfer environments in primary care and community service settings.

In addition, proficient primary care practitioners will need to ensure that:

1. They provide essential services to their local communities. These services are needed by a range of care groups with differing needs delivered in a variety of settings. Whatever the title, employer or setting, there are, amongst others, core functions that our staff will need to provide: first contact, expert continuing care and the delivery of effective prevention/public health programmes.
2. Their services are based on robust assessment of needs of individuals and populations and the skills required to meet those needs. These functions should be provided across all age and social groups according to need and designed around the journey that the patient/client takes. In order to safeguard vulnerable people, the local population requires high-quality generalist as well as specialist service responses.

3. Patients, clients, carers and communities are involved and engaged actively in service changes and provided with greater choice – services will therefore need to respond to the people who use and fund them.
4. A significant number of primary care practitioners are supported to assume advanced and specialist roles across a range of core functions, but in particular to:
   - Improve access to general practice services, as the role of nurses and health visitors in assessing, diagnosing and managing conditions (previously seen to be the remit of GPs) is increasingly recognised.
   - Provide more secondary care in the community (including care of people with longer-term conditions and ambulatory and palliative care needs).
   - Lead and deliver priority public health interventions.
   - Acquire and apply expert skills in clinical leadership, informed by a thorough understanding of service commissioning.
5. They engage in partnership with the wider health and social care team. As such, there will be more generic working with practitioners working across settings, providing a wider range of care to individuals, families and communities. Support workers and qualified staff will become more integrated within the primary/social care workforce.
6. They become more understanding of the commonality of roles across health and social care and hospitals and primary/community care with more joint posts and less anxiety about protecting professional roles when responding to patient and community needs.
7. Front-line practitioners have greater freedom to innovate and make decisions about services and the care that they provide. This will need to be matched with greater accountability for individual professional judgment and the use of best available evidence to inform their practice.
8. Effective leadership is evidenced if our services are to take on new roles, work differently and deliver the NHS plan improvements for patients, clients and communities. This will demand greater understanding of team development and the management capability to use human and financial resources creatively and to assess and manage risks accordingly within the parameters of 'safe and effective practice'.

The workforce of the future will also prepare and deploy a range of competent assistant practitioners who will work in direct support of the professionally qualified primary care team. New roles are now emerging to support assistant practitioners to acquire a range of competencies that have been designed to enable them to respond to the needs of the local health/social care economy.

As the scope of primary healthcare widens, opportunities for appropriately skilled and experienced primary care nurses and health visitors to develop as advanced practitioners and nurse consultants will be provided. The challenge for the nurses themselves must be for them to articulate their skills, to advance their practice (underpinned by evidence-based enquiry skills) and to market their contribution effectively to both their clients/patients and to commissioners of health/social care services.

Conclusion

This chapter has proposed that the 'reformed' health service requires a community healthcare workforce that is both fit for practice and fit for purpose, equipped with competencies that will enable practitioners to function across a range of priority, inter-professional care pathways both within hospital and within primary care settings (including a range of emergent community services). In designing the new workforce, we should be cognisant of the demand placed by service commissioners and providers to ensure flexibility within the workforce to accommodate to emergent needs in the population.

The chapter has recognised that the demand for healthcare, influenced by changes in disease pattern and treatment response, will evolve based primarily on the principles of co-design and the co-delivery of healthcare in partnership with users, carers and clinicians. The NHS 'choice' and personalisation agenda with emphasis being placed on 'care closer to home' has been a key driver for the Government's vision of primary care services, which has been characterised with concepts relating to new sources of patient engagement, personalised care packages and flexible access arrangements to a multiplicity of care providers.

The importance of providing a competent workforce that is prepared fully to confront challenges relating to inequalities in health and social care treatment responses will present key challenges to the profession as will the need to enhance clinical competence and leadership capability. The acquisition of clinical judgment skills in decision making and care planning has also been identified as key drivers for change in care practice.

The key policy directives that have shaped our reformed health service in recent years have been derived from the Health and Social Care Act 2012, which sets out the vision for healthcare reform for the next decade and beyond. The key principles that are enshrined with the Act have been analysed and embedded throughout the text.

More specifically, the Prime Minister's (DH 2010b) review of the future contribution that nurses can make to the reformed health service has been used to inform relevant chapters in this new edition. Nurses and health visitors continue to be central to government plans as identified in the Commission's Report. For example, nurses and health visitors play key roles in establishing new models of primary care and social enterprise and are integral to developing care pathways as part of the multidisciplinary team.

In summary, the health service has engaged in a period of self-reflection and re-examination of personal and public values, thus reinforcing the need for clients to assume personal responsibility for their own social and healthcare needs. The reduction in dependency upon inpatient care in our hospitals has assisted in the transfer of care 'closer to home' and to our naturally occurring neighbourhood support systems. Care in the community and investment in public health/primary care strategies will become an increasing feature of our healthcare philosophy and, in partnership with a rationalised (and smaller) acute sector, will provide the context for our healthcare system for the foreseeable future.

The significant role that our local health and social care services play further reinforces the Government's commitment to primary care and the transformation of services. Lord Darzi in his vision for primary and community care, for example, advised that:

> Community services are in a central position to deliver the Next Stage Review of the NHS, and of critical importance in delivering our vision for the future of primary and community care...Increased influence for community staff in service transformation, through a commitment to multi-professional engagement in practice based commissioning and the piloting of more integrated clinical collaborations (DH 2008c, p. 1).

If this vision is to be achieved, then the importance of leadership for primary care nursing must be acknowledged and responsive systems put in place to facilitate the emergence of innovative practice in local practice settings. Nurses and health visitors must also continue to advocate for their clients, families and communities and engage in raising health-related issues for inclusion in local and government policy agendas. Above all, they must demonstrate confidence and competence to assess risks and to practise safely in accordance with their professional code of practice (NMC 2008). Our primary care practitioners need to be prepared to respond to an increasingly well-informed public that is keen to have a bigger say in their care and treatment. The overall thrust of this new edition has been to re-focus and reform our understanding of primary and community care practice within the context of a rapidly evolving health service.

References

Buchan, J. (2008) *Nursing Futures, Future Nurses*, Queen Margaret College, Edinburgh.

Cipd. (January 2010) *Building productive public sector work places – delivering more with less – the people management challenge.* Cipd, London.

Department of Health (DH) (2008a) *High quality care for all: NHS Next Stage Review (Final Report – Lord Ara Darzi)*, Cm 7432. DH, London.

DH (2008b) *Delivering Care Closer to Home – Meeting the Challenge.* DH, London.

DH (2008c) *NHS Next Stage Review: Our vision for primary and community care: what it means for nurses, midwives, health visitors and AHPs.* The Stationary Office, London, Gateway Reference 10096.

DH (2010a) *Equity and excellence: liberating the NHS.* White Paper, Cm 7881. The Stationary Office, London, Gateway Reference 14385.

DH (2010b) *Front line care – report by the Prime Minister's Commission of Nursing and Midwifery in England.* Prime Minister's Commission of Nursing and Midwifery in England, London.

DH (2011) *The NHS in England: the operating framework for 2012/213*, DH, London.

DH (2012) *NHS future forum – summary report*, Second Phase, Professor Steve Field, Chair, London.

Ham, C. (2011) *A Chance to go Back to Basics on Health and Social Care Reform?* The King's Fund, London.

Mathers, C. & Loncar, D. (2006) Projections of global mortality and burden of disease from 2002 to 2030. PLoS Medicine, **3** (11), 2011–2030.

Nancarrow, S.A., Moran, A., Enderby, P., *et al.* (2006). *The Impact of Workforce Flexibility on the Costs and Outcomes of Older Peoples' Services: A Policy and Literature Review*, p. 120. University of Sheffield, Sheffield.

NHS London (2007) *Healthcare for London: a framework for action*, NHS London, London.

NHS London (2010) *Workforce for London progress report*, NHS London, London.

Nursing and Midwifery Council (NMC) (2008) *The Code – Standards of Conduct, Performance, and Ethics for Nurses and Midwives*, NMC, London.

Office for National Statistics (2011) *National population projections 2010-based statistical bulletin, 26 October 2011*. Office for National Statistics, London.

Parliament (2012a) Health and Social Care Act, c. 7, London.

Parliament (2012b) *Caring for our future: reforming care and support*, Cm 8378. HM Government, London.

Royal College of Nursing (2011) *Transforming Community Nursing*. Royal College of Nursing, London.

Wanless, D. (2004) *Securing good health for the whole population: final report: February, 2004*. HM Treasury, London, Gateway Reference 2004.

2

Community Development and Building Capacity

Kate Potter[1] and Jane Wills[2]

[1]Faculty of Society and Health, Buckinghamshire New University,
High Wycombe, UK
[2]Faculty Health and Social Care, London South Bank University, London, UK

Introduction

Primary care organisations and community care agencies have been placed at the centre of health service development in the major changes that have taken place in the organisation of health services in recent years. In addition to their role in the treatment of ill health and the commissioning of secondary care services, they are also expected to take the lead in improving the health of their local populations. For the community nurse, supporting a community and enabling community action entail an ability to understand and address the social context in which people live and the political, social and economic factors that influence behaviour, together with the ability to identify and address community priorities through community engagement. Moves to greater public involvement and patient-centredness pose a challenge to the culture of health care professionals that fosters a belief in professional expertise and does not value lay understandings and priorities. Understanding relationships with the community and such issues of power and politics is a key competence for community nurses (NMC 2004).

This chapter commences with a short outline of the policy context for community development and approaches to health improvement and then explores some of the associated terms of 'empowerment' and 'community development' and the related concepts of social capital, capacity building and social inclusion. The second half of

Community and Public Health Nursing, Fifth Edition. Edited by David Sines,
Sharon Aldridge-Bent, Agnes Fanning, Penny Farrelly, Kate Potter and Jane Wright.
© 2013 John Wiley & Sons, Ltd. Published 2013 by John Wiley & Sons, Ltd.

the chapter moves on to discuss some of the challenges and opportunities commonly associated with community development approaches including appropriate and compatible methods of evaluation. The implications of these approaches for the community nurse conclude the chapter.

The current context for community development practice

This section outlines the underlying themes of national policies and strategies and how they relate to communities and community development.

Recent years have seen a retreat from traditional welfare support to a focus on greater choice, more devolved services and individual rights as patients are seen as consumers of services. These values have given rise to specific strategies and policy initiatives, including

- Devolved services allowing local flexibility and freedom, with additional 'earned autonomy' for best performing services
- Quality assurance and service accountability through clear standards and performance criteria
- Patient-centred services that reflect the changing needs and aspirations of better-informed and more assertive patients/public
- Partnership working to erode professional barriers and enable the delivery of seamless services
- A positive focus on disadvantaged or excluded groups
- A community focus to build capacity and encourage communities to be active providers as well as users of services

Government policy has emphasised the importance of participation by users and the public in the modernisation agenda for health and social care for over a decade. A Joint Strategic Needs Assessment conducted by every area provides the evidence base for commissioning to meet local health and well-being needs, and its process is a means of engaging communities (DH 2007). The 'Health and Social Care Act 2012' (Great Britain Parliament 2012) was proposed on the basis of putting the patient first. The Act sets up a new national body, HealthWatch England, as a statutory committee of the Care Quality Commission to represent the views of users of health and social care services, other members of the public and Local HealthWatch organisations.

Alongside the focus on involvement and participation by patients and the public, there has been a renewed focus on 'the community' as the site where needs are both defined and met. The Public Health White Paper 'Choosing Health' refers to how 'the environment we live in, our social networks, our sense of security, socio-economic circumstances, families and resources in our local neighbourhood can affect individual health' (DH 2004, p. 77). Policy initiatives have attempted to address many of the characteristics of community. There has been a raft of regeneration initiatives intended to transform the country's most deprived and excluded areas and initiatives targeting local areas of need such as Sure Start centres. There is a recognition that some population groups such as migrants or older people are marginalised, harder to reach or excluded from mainstream services. For example, in the United Kingdom, the concept of social inclusion/exclusion has gained currency as a way of focusing on populations that do not make use of opportunities to participate in society. Under the coalition government created in 2010, the concept of community acquired a different meaning. Political efforts attempted to build the 'Big Society' in which power will be transferred from the state to people, individuals, neighbourhoods or communities using laypeople in the delivery of care – both as volunteers and in non-professional paid roles (Cabinet Office 2010).

The Marmot review 'Fair Society, Healthy Lives' (DH 2010) is a wide-ranging analysis of inequalities in health and society and the wider factors that affect people at different stages. The Health and Social Care Act 2012 (Great Britain Parliament 2012) introduces a new duty for local areas to reduce health inequalities in relation to access and outcomes. The Public Health White Paper 'Healthy Lives, Healthy People' (DH 2010) also asserts the need to tackle health needs at different stages of life and key transitions, instead of tackling individual risk factors in isolation. It reflects the view of the Marmot review that early interventions and giving every child a start in life are central to health improvement.

Defining the terms

This section discusses the key terms and concepts used when exploring the potential for promoting health in a participatory way: community, community development and empowerment, social capital and social inclusion.

Defining community

The meaning of the word 'community' has also long been contested in sociological and policy terms. Jewkes and Murcott (1996) claim there are at least 55 different definitions in use. It is often conflated with neighbourhood, yet many different kinds of communities exist. Geographically defined communities are convenient for agencies that want to work within boundaries, but living in the same place does not necessarily guarantee a common view. More recently, the emphasis has been on communities of interest with shared needs such as 'teenage mothers' or 'people with learning disabilities'. Marginalised communities are those whose contributions are invisible. They may experience discrimination and may not make use of traditional or mainstream services. Examples of such groups are asylum seekers, Gipsies and Travellers and homeless people. Other communities are those defined by service use; by shared interests or occupation; or by characteristics such as culture, religion and sexual orientation. Understanding who comprises the community and in what ways they share needs or concerns is vital to practice. Laverack (2004) identifies four characteristics of community:

- Spatial dimension, that is, a place or location
- Interests, issues and identities that link otherwise heterogeneous groups
- Shared needs and concerns that can be achieved through collective action
- Social interactions and relationships that bind people together

The question of who to involve in a 'community' is similarly complicated. Early attempts to increase participation focused on a strategy of involving those who were most accessible, who tended to be local leaders. For example, attempts to reach ethnic minority groups frequently employ strategies of contacting faith leaders or using existing groups that meet at religious buildings. Identifying 'activists' and those used to participating in groups – those in tenant groups or parents' associations – may also be seen as ways of increasing involvement and getting a 'lay voice'. Where there is no clear constituency, these representatives tend to be drawn from voluntary sector agencies. 'These constraints result in the community representatives being drawn from one small part of the voluntary sector, the larger funded organisations' (Jewkes & Murcott 1998, p. 855).

The Health Visitor Implementation Plan 2011–2015 (DH 2010) describes different levels of service for communities from universal services for all families with children under five years old to 'universal partnership plus' for families with children with complex needs. Targeting services according to levels of need is based on several different rationales. An ethical rationale argues that targeting the most vulnerable and marginalised is needed to supplement a universal service if the needs of all population groups are to be met equally. An economic rationale argues that it is more cost-effective to provide resources to meet needs effectively rather than spend resources later to address the multiple social effects (e.g. acute and chronic ill health) resulting from a failure to meet needs. A scientific rationale rests on a notion of risk. Epidemiological evidence identifies population groups on the basis of their behavioural risk factors, environmental risk conditions, their health outcomes (i.e. ill health or premature death) or ease of access to care and services (Naidoo & Wills 2010).

Defining social capital

Understanding the networks that exist within a community provides opportunities to identify routes through which less visible members need to be engaged. Personal networks can both sustain communities and contribute to the effectiveness of community activity. It is not surprising then that there has been so much interest in the concept of social capital, the term used to describe networks and shared norms that facilitate coordination and cooperation for mutual benefit and create civic engagement. It is a relatively new concept that has aroused considerable debate about how it should be defined and measured. It originated with the work of Robert Putnam in Italy and the

USA (Putnam *et al.* 1993; Putnam 2000). Putnam found that the very poor living in urban areas in the USA who have a few relatively intense family or neighbourhood ties are trapped in their poverty, whereas those with a wider network of weaker contacts do better.

A body of evidence exists to suggest that low social capital and social exclusion arising from poverty or discrimination are linked to poor health. Wilkinson (1996, 2005, 2000) has argued that the level of inequality in a society is crucial in determining a range of factors, from the overall life expectancy of a population through to levels of violence and teenage birth rates. Low social status, poor friendship networks and difficult early childhood experience contribute to psychosocial insecurity, anxiety and people's sense of whether they are valued and appreciated. These are major sources of stress and may contribute to pathways which link a variety of social problems to relative deprivation and adverse health outcomes. It has also been demonstrated that where the levels of social capital are high, associated health benefits are evident. For example, reductions in infant mortality and increases in life expectancy (Putnam *et al.* 1993); lower levels of deaths from stroke, accidents and suicide and improved survival from heart disease (Kawachi & Kennedy 1997); and lower levels of common mental disorders (De Silva *et al.* 2005) have all been linked to social capital. Greater social capital may also affect health directly through the diffusion of knowledge and healthy norms. Cohesive neighbourhoods are also more able to ensure the availability of services through lobbying or development of other services and provide more opportunities for self-esteem and mutual respect. Children growing up in areas with high social capital learn through witness and experience about civic responsibility amongst people with no personal ties. The concept of social capital is helpful in considerations of how to work with communities as it provides a framework to examine the processes through which formal and informal social connections and networks can protect people against the worst effects of deprivation and health inequality.

Defining empowerment

The key process involved in community development is individual and community empowerment. 'Empowerment' is a notoriously slippery concept that is widely used but differently understood. In a broad sense, it means 'individuals acting collectively to gain greater influence and control over the determinants of health and the quality of life in their community, and is an important goal in community action for health' (Nutbeam 1998, p. 354). The process will aim to strengthen the range and quality of organisational capacity and capability in communities both at the level of networks and local activities but also increase participation and influence so that communities can begin to identify needs and lobby for change.

If individuals are to become empowered, they need first of all to recognise their own powerlessness. Paulo Freire, a Brazilian educationalist, worked on literacy programmes with 'poor peasants' in Peru and Brazil and saw education as the political and social means of changing power relationships (Freire 1972). He described a process of 'conscientisation', a change in awareness and knowledge concerning a person's own position in the world in relation to others. The rise in consciousness of their situation enables individuals to identify their own needs, rather than having them prescribed by others. The central tenets of empowerment are described as the exercise of power, information sharing and involvement in decision-making.

Defining capacity building

The related concept of 'community capacity' refers to the set of assets or strengths possessed by a community. 'Capacity building' is a systematic approach to build the confidence and ability of individuals, community and voluntary groups/organisations to influence decision-making and service delivery. This could include enabling communities to provide and manage services and programmes to meet community needs. So it may be used in a functional way to equip people for particular jobs through skills training or vocational learning and accreditation, or it may involve personal or organisational development. The term 'releasing capacity' or 'asset-based' community development (http://www.abcdinstitute.org) is often preferred to 'capacity building' to reflect the view that local people are not 'empty vessels' and may already have valuable experience, knowledge and skills that need identifying and enabling. Community capacity building involves three main types of activity:

- *Developing skills* – learning and training opportunities for individuals and groups and sharing through networks and mutual support to develop skills, knowledge and confidence
- *Developing structures* – developing the organisational structures and strengths of community groups, communities of interest and networks
- *Developing support* – developing the availability of practical support to enable the development of skills and structures

Defining community development

There is no one widely accepted definition of community development. The Community Development Exchange (www. cdx.org.uk) describes it as a way of working with communities whose key purpose is to build communities based on justice, equality and mutual respect. It starts from the principle that there are assets within any community that can be channelled into collective action to achieve the communities' desired goals. It may be radical and progressive challenging professional monopolies of power and information and attempt to tackle disadvantage and inequalities, or it may be interpreted simply as a way of working in communities in which programmes or services reach out to or are located in communities. These projects may be designed and delivered according to the needs of communities but tend to be set within government or health professionals' agendas (Gilchrist & Taylor 2011). Community development, on the other hand, prioritises issues identified by the community themselves and seeks improvements in quality of life – material, environmental or social – that may

Table 2.1 Characteristics of community-based versus community development models (after Labonte 1998)

Community based	Community development
Problem, targets and action defined by sponsoring body	Problem, targets and action defined by community
Community seen as medium, venue or setting for intervention	Community itself the target of intervention in respect to capacity building and empowerment
Notion of 'community' relatively unproblematic	Community recognised as complex, changing and subject to power imbalances and conflict
Target largely individuals within either geographic area or specific subgroup in geographic area defined by sponsoring body	Target may be community structures or services and policies that impact on the health of the community
Activities largely health oriented	Activities may be quite broad based, targeting wider factors with an impact on health, but with indirect health outcomes (empowerment, social capital)

indirectly lead to better health. Table 2.1 illustrates some of the differences between community-based work and community development work.

Defining community engagement

Community engagement refers to the process of getting communities involved in decisions that affect them. This includes the planning, development and management of services, as well as activities which aim to improve health or reduce health inequalities (NICE 2009). The ways in which communities are involved in decision-making and the design and delivery of programmes and services have been the subject of much debate. Several writers have developed typologies of participation (Arnstein 1969; Brager & Specht 1973; Wilcox 1994) that describe levels or stages of participation. These models make a hierarchical distinction between approaches to involvement according to the amount of power sharing involved and the degree of influence over decisions, attempting to distinguish between consultation, participation and empowerment. People can be involved in the services that affect or may affect them at a variety of levels and in a number of ways, ranging from very little to complex relationships:

- *Information* – ensuring that relevant information about service planning reaches the public, for example, surveys, leaflets and focus groups
- *Consultation* – asking people's views and advice about plans, policies and services, for example, public meetings and consultation documents
- *Participation* – identifying a problem and asking the public to make a series of decisions within defined limits, for example, the site of a health care facility
- *Partnership* – working together to set objectives, make plans and decide funding priorities, for example, patients and carers in service planning groups
- *Delegated control* – giving authority and money to a community to plan services, choose providers and run the services

BOX 2.1   Degrees of participation

1. Youth-initiated, shared decisions with adults: When projects or programmes are initiated by the youth and decision-making is shared amongst youth and adults. These projects empower the youth, at the same time enabling them to access and learn from the life experience and expertise of adults.
2. Youth-initiated and directed: When young people initiate and direct a project or programme. Adults are involved only in a supportive role.
3. Adult-initiated, shared decisions with the youth: When projects or programmes are initiated by adults but the decision-making is shared with the young people.
4. Consulted and informed: When young people give advice on projects or programmes designed and run by adults. The youth are informed about how their input will be used and the outcomes of the decisions made by adults.
5. Assigned but informed: Where young people are assigned a specific role and informed about how and why they are being involved.
6. Tokenism: Where young people appear to be given a voice, but in fact have little or no choice about what they do or how they participate.
7. Decoration: Where young people are used to help or 'bolster' a cause in a relatively indirect way, although adults do not pretend that the cause is inspired by the youth.
8. Manipulation: Where adults use young people to support causes and pretend that the causes are inspired by the youth.

Box 2.1 illustrates the Ladder of Participation applied to youth participation in a model developed by Hart (1992). It highlights the debate about levels of participation and their benefit for the individuals concerned and for decision-making. Somewhat controversially Hart suggests that shared decision-making by children with adults is the most desirable.

The role of community health professionals

This section discusses

- Why community nurses should be engaging in community development work
- How it relates to their scope of practice
- The competences and aptitudes required to carry out this kind of work

Community health professionals, with their considerable knowledge and unique roles within the local communities they serve, have long been identified as being in an ideal position to be at the forefront of initiatives to tackle healthy lifestyles and inequalities

(CPHVA 1999; DH 2001; DH 2011a). They possess an abundance of knowledge about the health and social needs of their communities and about how those needs can be met. Their everyday experience of home visiting and their long-term knowledge of individuals, families and networks built up over time are valuable resources. As a result, they are well placed to identify community leaders and build alliances with local groups. Community health practitioners also have a role to play in the recruitment and support of lay health workers from the local community who are key players in community health development programmes.

Working within a community development framework can provide community nurses with a number of opportunities and challenges. Some of these opportunities are about building partnerships and more responsive services. Some of the challenges relate to issues of professional autonomy, bureaucratic accountability and fear of loss of professional power. A fundamental shift is required to enable practitioners to change their focus of practice in order to address not only the individual and the family but also the wider community. Community development necessitates a change in 'mindset' from a task- to a community-orientated form of practice recognising the individual as part of a collective group with specific needs. As one participant in the South West 'Connecting Communities C2' project put it:

> Obviously we need programs and projects and targets and sustainability and knowledge management, but we don't want to lose sight that we are trying to work with people to get people to do something and that is our focus...so it's about building relationships with people and the organisations they are in, it is building networks with people and through people in organisations.

Practitioners wishing to be more proactive in their communities require skills, training and support to do so. The practice of community development and capacity building is not only a set of skills about working with people but also a set of principles and way of working based on respect, facilitating participation and working and learning together. In order for this to occur, community development must become an integral part of the fundamental role of the community practitioner. One of the key areas in the National Occupational Standards for the Practice of Public Health is 'Work in partnership with communities to assess their health and well-being needs (https://tools.skillsforhealth.org.uk/competence/show/html/id/2422/)', and the associated standards are listed in Box 2.2. The Federation for Community Development Learning has also developed a set of National Occupational Standards for Community Development Work designed for community development workers and activists, for those adopting a community development approach within their work and for those commissioning or managing community development work. The new Health Visitor Implementation Plan (DH 2011a) will also require health visitors to increase community participation in projects to increase health and well-being, and school nurses are also expected to have a public health leadership role within their communities (DH 2011b). Community nurses and specifically health visitors and school nurses

BOX 2.2   National Occupational Standards for Public Health: PHP22 Work in partnership with communities to assess health and well-being and related needs

1. Interact with communities in ways which
   a. Demonstrate that they are equal partners in improving health and well-being
   b. Encourage effective relationships and participation
   c. Respect people's roles and responsibilities
   d. Facilitates their involvement
   e. Enable them to think through and share their feelings about their health and well-being
   f. Facilitate opportunities for identifying health and well-being and related needs
2. Develop people's confidence in you so that they are able to think and say what they want to knowing that you will listen to them.
3. Select and use methods and approaches for assessing health and well-being that
   a. Encourage people's active participation
   b. Facilitate a broad range of views
   c. Are sensitive to the culture of the community and the broader context in which it is set
   d. Ethically manage conflicting values
   e. Promote people's diversity and rights
   f. Engage their interest in improving health and well-being
   g. Are recognised as evidence-based good practice
   h. Are capable of gaining sufficient, valid and reliable information about the concerns and priorities of communities
   i. Are the most likely to develop a sufficient appreciation of the context of people's lives and of the opportunities, constraints and threats which affect them
   j. Make effective use of inter-agency and partnership arrangements
   k. Are sustainable and make effective use of resources

therefore need to develop their knowledge and skills to interact effectively at community level.

By 2015, it is hoped that all specialist community public health nurses will have accessed either by distance learning or within their training a module encompassing:

- Human ecology/population health and epidemiology
- Social capital/social marketing/social networks
- Building networks and understanding communities

- Building community capacity
- Influencing and developing policies and strategies for health and well-being
- Public health and inequalities (DH 2011c)

The aim of this education is to allow experienced practitioners to expand their knowledge and develop their confidence in the area of community development. Newly qualified health visitors and school nurses will be prepared to work in a practice area delivering the new service models (DH 2011a,b). The case study in the succeeding text is an example of how practitioners have worked with clients and other agencies to jointly plan a project with the aim of improving health outcomes for children and families within the communities in which they work.

There are numerous examples of community development activities facilitated by health care professionals from the radical transformation achieved by health visitors in the 1990s on estates in Redruth and Falmouth in Cornwall to the work by a family worker with Edenbrook Parents Group http://www.dsdni.gov.uk/vcni-community-capacity-building.pdf) to develop a capacity plan and activities including a drug awareness programme for parents; a programme for adults including parents as co-educators (basic English and Math), IT (use of email and web), sewing skills, healthy cooking and keep-fit; and a health awareness programme. What all such examples show is that community work takes time and change happens slowly but confidence can be built with the right encouragement and people can then develop their own action plans. For health care professionals, recognising that they do not have superior knowledge or power can be a challenge but also rewarding as people have tremendous capacity to learn and develop if given safe and comfortable space to do it for themselves.

The latest policy initiatives which are encouraging community practitioners to play a strong leadership role in community development and building community capacity allow them to fully demonstrate the four principles of public health nursing, searching for health needs, stimulation of awareness of health needs, influencing policies affecting health and the facilitation of health-enhancing activities (NMC 2004). A community development approach may necessitate new skills and new ways of thinking as illustrated in Case Study 2.1, and it can also pose organisational challenges. Although community development and building capacity has long been recognised within the remit of professional practice and community involvement and civic engagement are an integral part of the policy framework, local agendas within the NHS have not always been compatible with the philosophy and aims of community development. Long-term involvement with communities is essential for strategies to develop and to be effective. However, this conflicts with the dominant emphasis upon performance management, targets and the desire for immediate results. Crucially, this approach and the issues identified by communities may conflict with operational caseload demands or the traditional remit of the service. As public health nurses move into the newly formed public health teams within local government (DH 2010), there are likely to be increased opportunities for greater engagement with the communities in which they work.

Case study 2.1 of a project to improve levels of exercise in pre-school and primary school children

A student health visitor and school nurse were both placed in the same area for their practice placement. As part of the assessment for their public health module, they were required to identify a significant health need within their area and develop a project which would help address the need.

Identified health need

The practitioners had a considerable amount of knowledge gained from working in the area, and information from the health profile of the borough published on the Association of Public Health Observatories website (http://www.apho.org.uk) confirmed that

- Deprivation was higher than average and that around 19 300 children lived in poverty.
- Around 23.7% of Year 6 children were classified as obese (higher than the national average).
- Estimated levels of adult physical activity were also worse than the national average.

Health promotion advice on the importance of regular exercise and healthy eating was given to parents at the Children's Centre and the local school. Parents raised the problem of the children having a safe and attractive play area.

The school nurse and health visitor worked with a family centre worker to gather information on what would be acceptable in the area using a survey and focus groups. At one of these focus groups, a number of the local mothers identified that there was a suitable area behind the local community centre which had been left derelict since the centre had been built.

Aim of the project

- To create a safe play area for children up to seven in the area.

Methodology

A working party was formed. Members included local parents, a health visitor, a school nurse, the Children's Centre manager and a community development officer from the local authority.

Local opinion was canvassed by distributing questionnaires to parents via the school and in local GP surgeries and the Children's Centre. There was overwhelming support for the project, and a number of parents offered to take an active part in the project.

continued

Case study 2.1 *(Continued)*

The local council who owned the property agreed to the development and provided a small grant to pay for the clearing of rubbish and re-landscaping of the area. Funding for play equipment was obtained via sponsorship from local businesses and various community fundraising activities.

Outcome and benefits for the community

- A well-maintained and safe play area for young children
- Socialisation of parents within the play area led to less isolation
- Participation in the project gave many parents the sense of belonging to the community

What this project demonstrated is the importance of identifying the needs that the community themselves prioritise and recognising that poverty and social deprivation may influence many aspects of life. The practitioners involved in this project had to learn to work across many sectors and boundaries (partnership working); how to network, negotiate and influence to gain funding; how to work with people with differing capabilities; how to get community ownership and develop local leaders to create sustainability; and how to gain visibility for the project so the community felt there was a 'quick win'.

Conclusion

Community development covers a spectrum of approaches to interacting with local communities and community involvement from working with established health programmes such as smoking cessation groups based in a community to facilitating community needs outside of mainstream services. In this chapter, we have seen examples of practice where communities decide for themselves what the problem is to other examples where the practitioner is imply providing the opportunity or framework for community input to services.

Primary care organisations clearly recognise the importance of public involvement but historically have focused on individuals as patients and understand involvement from this perspective of consulting with patients as users of services. As well as being an unfamiliar field, community development may also be viewed as a threat to professional expertise and autonomy. The shift required is significant to move to a position where members of the public are valued as equal experts and public involvement is regarded as other than a 'time-consuming indulgence'. Reliance solely on the medical model of health and professional expertise ignores many fundamental socio-economic determinants of health and fosters an unhealthy dependency and passivity amongst patients and the public. An understanding of the benefits of community engagement and skills in supporting community development are vital aspects of the role of the community health practitioner today.

References

Arnstein, S. (1969) A ladder of citizen participation. *Journal of American Institute of Planners,* **35** (4), 216–224.

Brager, G. & Specht, H. (1973) *Community Organizing,* Columbia University Press, New York.

Cabinet Office (2010). *Building the Big Society* (Briefing Note) (online). Available from http://www.cabinetoffice.gov.uk/news/building-big-society. Accessed on 20 November 2012.

Community Practitioners and Health Visitors Association (CPHVA) (1999) *Joined up Working: Community Development in Primary Care,* CPHVA, London.

Department of Health (DH) (2001) *Health Visitor Practice Development Resource Pack,* DH, London.

DH (2004) *Choosing Health: Making Healthy Choices Easier.* DH, London.

DH (2007) *Guidance on Joint Strategic Needs Assessment.* DH, London.

DH (2010) *Healthy Lives, Healthy People: Our Strategy for Public Health in England.* DH, London.

DH (2011a) *Health Visitor Implementation Plan 2011–2015: Call to Action.* DH, London.

DH (2011b) *Getting it Right for Children, Young People and Families – Maximising the Contribution of the School Nursing Team: Vision and Call to Action.* DH, London.

DH (2011c) *Educating Health Visitors for a Transformed Service.* DH, London.

De Silva, M., MecKenzie, K., Harpham, T. & Huttly, S. (2005) Social capital and mental illness: a systematic review. *Journal of Epidemiology and Community Health,* **59**, 619–627.

Freire, P. (1972) *Pedagogy of the Oppressed,* Penguin, Harmondsworth.

Gilchrist, A. & Taylor, M. (2011) *A Short Guide to Community Development,* Policy Press, Bristol.

Great Britain Parliament (2012) *Health and Social Care Act.* HMSO, London.

Hart, R. (1992) Children's Participation: From Tokenism to Citizenship, UNICEF, New York.

Jewkes, R. & Murcott, A. (1996) Meanings of community. *Social Science and Medicine,* **43** (4), 555–563.

Jewkes, R. & Murcott, A. (1998) Community representatives: representing the 'community'. *Social Science and Medicine,* **46** (7), 843–858.

Kawachi, I. & Kennedy, B. (1997) Socio-economic determinants of health: Health and Social Cohesion: why care about income inequality? *British Medical Journal,* **314**, 1037.

Labonte, R. (1998) *A Community Development Approach to Health Promotion: A Background Paper on Practice, Tensions, Strategic Models and Accountability Requirements for Health Authority Work on the Broad Determinants of Health.* Health Education Board of Scotland, Research Unit on Health and Behaviour Change, University of Edinburgh, Edinburgh.

Laverack, G. (2004) *Health Promotion Practice: Power and Empowerment,* Sage, London.

Marmot, M., Allen, J., Goldblatt, P., et al. (2010) *Fair Society, Healthy Lives. Strategic Review of Health Inequalities in England post-2010.* DH, London.

Naidoo, J. & Wills, J. (2010) *Public Health and Health Promotion: Developing Practice,* Balliere Tindall, London.

NICE (2009) *Public Health Guidance PH9 An Assessment of Community Engagement and Community Development Approaches including the Collaborative Methodology and Community Champions,* NICE, London.

Nursing and Midwifery Council (NMC) (2004) *Standards of Proficiency for Specialist Community Public Health Nursing.* NMC, London.

Nutbeam, D. (1998) Health promotion glossary. Health Promotion International, **13** (4), 349–364.

Putnam, R. (2000) *Bowling Alone: The Collapse and Revival of American Community,* Simon Schuster, New York.

Putnam, R., Leonardi, R. & Nanetti, R.N. (1993) *Making Democracy Work: Civic Traditions in Modern Italy*, Princeton University Press, Princeton, NJ.

Wilcox, D. (1994) *A Guide to Effective Participation*, Pavilion, Brighton.

Wilkinson, R. (1996) *Unhealthy Societies*, Routledge, London.

Wilkinson, R. (2000) *Mind the Gap: Hierarchies, Health and Human Evolution*, Weidenfeld, London.

Wilkinson, R. (2005) *The Impact of Inequality. How To Make Sick Societies Healthier*, Routledge, London.

3

Multi-Sector Working and Self-
Community Health Care

Jenni Burton

Faculty of Society and Health, Buckinghamshire New Ui.. .isity,
High Wycombe, UK

Introduction

This chapter explores contemporary community health care in the United Kingdom,
with a particular emphasis on the growing importance of multi-agency partnership
working and the impact that collaborative initiatives are starting to have on the individual, the local community and the broader shape of community health care delivery.
With strong roots emerging from Canada and North America, multi-sector working
can be defined as the coordination of valuable resources to maximise scope for improving the health, safety and well-being of citizens. Tamarack's Communities Collaborating
Institute (CCI) refers to multi-sector working as

> Together we create increased credibility, capacity and capital for the world.

Community collaboration is an evolving feature of global, national and local
government-driven initiatives and provides an impetus for innovative ways to solve
community problems and promote systems changes. An Executive Summary Report
'Multi-Sector Community Collaboration – Assessing the Changing Environment'
(Changing Environment Team 2003) from the USA refers to multi-sector working as

Community and Public Health Nursing, Fifth Edition. Edited by David Sines,
Sharon Aldridge-Bent, Agnes Fanning, Penny Farrelly, Kate Potter and Jane Wright.
© 2013 John Wiley & Sons, Ltd. Published 2013 by John Wiley & Sons, Ltd.

...boration is a partnership formed by representatives of at least two sectors ...vate and public organisations and community members) to solve problems ...on the whole community (Deith, Changing Environment Team 2003, p. 1).

...chapter will address the following aspects of community health care across multi-...ncy partnerships with an emphasis on how this operates in the United Kingdom:

- To explain what multi-agency, multi-sector working means in practice and the impact for health care initiatives in the United Kingdom.
- To explore some of the key drivers for multi-sector working and why this is such an important way forward in community health improvement initiatives.
- To analyse some of the underpinning influences of multi-agency partnership working from individual, historical, cultural and political perspectives.
- To refer to the direct link between community health planning and an increased focus on self-management of health and increased collaboration with service users and their family relatives.
- To focus on three real contemporary health concerns in the United Kingdom and provide case examples of local partnership working which harnesses expertise and local knowledge to improve local community health care.

The identified aspects of community health care joint sector working will refer to specific examples of health concern in the United Kingdom and provide contrasting examples of how a collaborative, community response can deliver meaningful and effective ways to tackle pressing health concerns. The three rising health concerns identified are dementia, obesity and childhood asthma. According to Mathers and Loncar (2006), there will be ten primary areas of health concern leading to death which will affect large numbers of the population by 2030. Three of these ten leading health challenges are dementias, upper respiratory tract disease and heart disease linked to obesity. The exemplars selected within the chapter will be explored within the context of the vastly changing national health movements and government-driven changes to the way that local health plans and services are delivered. Some of the key drivers for multi-agency working will also be explored.

Context for multi-sector working in the United Kingdom

Over the past few years there have been an increasing number of initiatives in the United Kingdom where different agencies and community groups have responded collectively to health issues triggered by economic, environmental and demographic challenges in this country. An important development has been the creation of new partnerships such as between the NHS, universities, industry and the private and independent sector. Higher education has a part to play in developing collaborative courses to ensure that effective public health delivery involves different disciplines and agencies and also has a strong commitment to public participation. An example of this is the Swansea University MSc 'Public Health and Partnerships in Care' course. This course has a holistic framework covering health, social care and the importance of sustaining employability for healthcare workers by complying to the 'UK Public Health Career Framework' competencies (Swansea University 2012).

Bucks New University is also working with a range of statutory and third-sector organisations to lay foundations for a new 'Health and Care Alliance'. The Alliance aims to support multi-agencies to develop career progression for workers, drive up quality standards and support the development of new roles and new ways of working within community health and social care services (Bucksinghamshire New University 2012a).

The transformation of the health care system over very recent years is set to accelerate even faster with wide-scale changes to professional roles, the restructuring of health services, transition of some public healthcare services to local authorities and economic cutbacks. Changes to health care support worker roles, for example, have meant an increase in the numbers of staff moving from traditional primary health care services to secondary, preventative roles within the community. These new, emergent roles are numerous and include mentoring, support brokerage, home-based intermediate care and advanced health care support workers in community nursing settings. These role transformations are impacting on practice, training and personal development needs for a changing workforce. Initiatives such as shared (inter-agency) training, conferences and budget pooling are some of the vital measures being taken to respond to structural changes in community health care delivery. These changes have a direct effect on individual workers.

An increasingly prominent feature of the NHS infrastructure is the increase in the tendering and procurement of health care services by private and independent companies (all of whom have been awarded 'Qualified Provider' status) which has shifted the traditional domain of public health delivery and is set to accelerate as this century progresses. A controversial example of privatisation and the diminishing power of the NHS can be illustrated by the tendering process in Devon County Council and Devon NHS where two private, profit-making companies have been shortlisted to provide front-line health care services for children. Serco and Virgin Care have been shortlisted to take on the running of complex and high-profile areas of health care for children to include child protection, mental health care, health visiting and palliative nursing for children at the end of life.. The President of the Royal College of General Practitioners (RCGP), Clare Gerada, expressed concern about the increasing privatisation of the national health care system:

> Contracts will be commercial in confidence. GP'S will end up rubber stamping them; any company for profit will put shareholders before patients. We will find the NHS as we know it fragmented. (Lawrence 2012, *The Guardian*, 15 March 2012)

This is perhaps an extreme example of how private enterprise alone can provide an increase in the consumerist ethos of mixed market economy and that, in order to temper this, it is vital to involve the local community and citizens in the health-enabling emphasis promoted by the government.

An important aspect of community collaboration is the empowering impact this can have on individual service users who should hold central stage position within the ethos of partnership working. The transformation of adult social care and the personalisation of social care (DH 2008, *Transforming Social Care*) and increasingly also health care delivery in England provide a philosophical context to the focus on individual self-management and control. The emphasis on self-management is echoed by the NHS Chief Executive Report 'Innovation, Health and Wealth' 2011 (DH 2011a), which is committed to increasing the pace and scale of technologies to assist patients and their families which are targeted in high-need areas. As a direct result of the Chief Executive's Report (2011), the NHS Institute (2012) 'High Impact Innovations' Reports began to be published throughout 2012. Some of the targeted areas include the provision of support for carers of people with dementia, increased use of technology to access health care services, increased national programme of assistive technologies, reducing waiting time for children assessed as needing wheelchairs and better website information to promote the dissemination of new innovations and advise the public of how to provide feedback on them.

Progress in spearheading multiple-agency collaboration can be exemplified by Bucks New University's 'Centre of Excellence in Tele-Health and Assisted Living' (Buckinghamshire New University 2012b). The centre is the result of a fusion of financial investment and innovation initiated by Buckinghamshire County Council, Stoke Mandeville NHS Trust, Aylesbury Vale District Council, Buckinghamshire Business First and Buckinghamshire New University. This multi-agency venture aims to deliver holistic and creative responses to assist people with longer term disabilities to accommodate to modern daily living and to provide the impetus to enable and empower people to remain in their own homes and receive preventative health care support as a preferred alternative to receiving more invasive hospital treatment.

The focus on self-management of health and the importance of community cohesion is further strengthened by the coalition government's emphasis on society's role and responsibilities to tackling local issues and merging resources across health and social care for mutual benefit. Critiques of the principles of transformation, local control and the removal of the national welfare state argue that this can be disempowering and can, in effect, create a neoliberalist society, thereby reducing eligibility to health and social care and a resultant reduction in public spending. A strong opponent of the shrinking of the welfare state is writer Ian Ferguson. Ferguson argues that public policy is shaping the lives of individuals but that this can reduce their status as customers without the real purchasing power to make realistic choices about their health and social care needs. Ferguson is concerned that the safeguards built into the post-war health reforms in Britain may be reduced with the reduction of public services, thereby placing increased risks upon the individual and their families (Ferguson 2009).

Certainly it could be argued that the fast pace of change to the context of health delivery and the emphasis on a holistic and integrated approach to community health care in the United Kingdom has had the effect of reducing or eliminating boundaries across health, social care and communities. The following section will explore some of the drivers for multi-sector working and identify some of the tensions and opportunities created by partnership working and community health care delivery.

Key drivers for multi-agency working

Reflecting on the historical background of multi-sectoral working, there has been a rich and resourceful journey over the years to develop community health care and move away from traditional forms of healthcare delivery, where this is relevant and beneficial for the person and their family relatives. The shape of primary health care has continued to develop and extend as the importance of their status as first-line health services has been strengthened. The promotion of health care in communities is therefore not a new concept; the World Health Organisation (WHO 1987) stated that the main social target of governments and WHO should be the attainment:

> by all the people of the world by the year 2000 of a level of health that will permit them to lead a socially and economically productive life (WHO 1987, p. 11).

The importance of the international health scenario has become increasingly essential in the pledge to achieve 'health for all' with the emphasis on rising costs of health care and a need to move away from the hospital-orientated focus of health improvement. In its place has been a move towards a more personalised and fluid recognition of primary, secondary and preventative health care measures.

A central impetus for this change has been the recognition that people understand their own health issues and need to take control of their treatment and management plan. An example of this is the positive work carried out within local health promotion services to work with people to change their own behaviour and take responsibility for their own health and well-being. This may be illustrated by 'stop smoking' initiatives which were launched in England in 2009 and were based in primary care locations such as GP surgeries and involved practice nurses as primary change agents. In one of the pilot projects based in Rotherham, Yorkshire, referrals for support to stop smoking increased by 49% as a result of this initiative. A report (Staines 2009) links the success rate to an increased awareness of the health issues related to smoking. This success has been achieved by a joined-up approach to prevention of smoking and secondary respiratory disease through direct work with individuals and broader cultural, political and structural changes such as public media campaigns, imposed restrictions on smoking in public places and limits on tobacco advertising.

Major changes to NHS and Commissioning have moved along the continuum of breaking down the barriers between health and social care. There has undoubtedly been a strong political steer to these changes. The NHS and Community Care Act (DH 1990), for example, outlined a reformed strategic framework for the provision of all health care in England and defined the key role of primary care trusts (PCTs). The Government White Paper 'Our Health, Our Care, Our Say: A New Direction for

Community Services' (DH 2006) also declared a major commitment to consult and collaborate with patients and listen to their views. The then Health Minister Lord Darzi's new vision for the NHS (DH 2008) took this vision further by seeking to promote self-management, increased partnership working, enhanced quality standards and the breaking down of organisational barriers.

These changes heralded a major policy shift that was enshrined within the *Health and Social Care Act*, 2012, which abolished PCTs and announced the creation of Health and Wellbeing Boards to be located within local authorities (Act of Parliament, The *Health and Social Care Act*, 2012):

> A more integrated health and social care remit and scope for more joined up approaches to sharing resources and acting on patient choice and autonomy. (Health and Social Care Amendments Bill, DH 2012a)

At the heart of the new policy changes has been the creation of the NHS Commissioning Board and the inauguration of local Clinical Commissioning Groups (the latter replacing PCTs). Clinical Commissioning Groups will work closely with their local authority partners to coordinate and monitor funding and resource allocation across localities in response to local population need. There is an accompanying need to sharpen the focus on local community cohesion and the intrinsic role of society to take on the ownership of community health issues. The emphasis on greater patient involvement, tackling health inequalities and an increased emphasis on education and training can be summarised in a government slogan 'No decision about me, without me' (Health and Social Care Amendment Bill 1,2,12).

The central initiative of the new *Health and Social Care Act* is the governmental drive to reduce bureaucracy of the NHS and strip back managerial levels, therefore saving money to be reinvested in the delivery of front-line health care . The new Act also provides a legal foothold to shift the responsibility of the financial management of the nation's public health to local authorities. The progression towards a more flexible and personalised response to the health and welfare of individuals and their communities is therefore regarded to be a vital component of multi-sectoral change, thus maximising resources across the health and social care spectrum:

> From a cultural perspective changes to systems, roles, responsibilities and everyday life are inevitable (Burton *et al.* 2012, p. 96).

The changes that are being applied to the commissioning of social care and increasingly also to health care are a significant factor in the promotion of personalisation and personal health budgeting for service users. Such cultural shifts have also promoted an increase in the personal ownership of our own health:

> This government trusts people to take charge of their lives and we will push power downwards and outwards to the lowest possible level, including individuals, neighbourhoods,

professions and communities as well as local councils and other local institutions (Communities and Local Governments, Burton *et al.* 2012, p. 106).

The integration of health and social care may be a step forward in recognising that the individual, the family and the community need to be fully involved in their own health and well-being and acknowledge that resources can be utilised more effectively when pooled together. Evidence of partnership working, for example, is bountiful within school settings where parents and children themselves are increasingly seen as co-producers in the quest to promote and improve the health of children and young people across localities. The role of the school nurse, for example, has recently been reintroduced as a high-profile advocate for children's health and well-being. The school nurse role introduced in the 1930s was a significant albeit forbidding figure with the responsibility for checking height, weight, hearing and sight and, of course, checking heads for lice! The term the 'nit nurse' was commonly used and portrayed a formidable perspective of a highly respected and integral part of the school system. The coalition government is now increasing the number and role of the school nurse as part of the new Health and Wellbeing Boards located within local authorities.

The Department of Health published their vision and model for school nursing in March 2012: 'Getting it right for children, young people and families' (DH 2012b). The implementation of the strategy that is enshrined within this vision is dependent upon collaboration between the Department of Health, Department for Education, key partner public and private organisations, professionals and children and young people themselves. The vision profiles the school nurse remit as central to a universal partnership that includes the child, the family, teachers and other professionals. A direct quote from a school nurse taken from *The Guardian Professional* (16 May 2012) encapsulates the essence of the role:

> I like being able to be an advocate for the school child. In some ways we are the voice for that child to make sure that they have the best health care possible and the optimum health (Ross 2012, p. 2.)

Examples of multi-sector working and self-management initiatives

The next section provides an exploration of several different and contrasting case studies that reflect some of the contemporary health concerns confronted within the United Kingdom. These are real examples of how local communities are working together to tackle emerging and increasing health issues commonly experienced within society by pooling local knowledge and resources and embracing role changes and the focus on managing health locally. These examples also recognise the strength of personal choice and control and, in line with this, the need for the adoption of a macro, structural approach to tackle escalating and shared health concerns. It is this dual-focused approach that forms the core of multiple co-working.

Dementia

750 000 people in the United Kingdom have dementia; this number is expected to double in 30 years (DH 2011b). The National Dementia Strategy 'Living Well With Dementia' (2011b) sets out a national vision to improve national awareness of dementia, early diagnosis and treatments. An increasing and concerning trend in the United Kingdom is for people to develop dementia at an earlier age. The Alzheimer's Society has identified that recorded numbers of people under 65 years old with dementia are more than 17 000 in the United Kingdom. These numbers may in reality be three times higher due to difficulties in early diagnosis and eligibility for help, support and treatment for younger patients and their carers.

The Care Services Improvement Partnership (CSIP 2007) has devised a practical toolkit to offer advice and examples of positive practice which involve people who have dementia in the planning, delivery and evaluation of their services, including health-based, social care or domiciliary support. The ethos of the CSIP promotes the view that people with dementia can express a view and with the right support can identify their personal preferences and needs whilst ensuring dignity, respect and the well-being of the individual. *Dementia 2012: A National Challenge* was spearheaded by the Alzheimer's Society, published in March 2012. This important research study identified five top solutions to tackle dementia, following consultation with people who have dementia and their family carers:

• Better understanding of dementia and less social stigma
• More public awareness of the condition
• More local activities and opportunities to socialise
• More community spirit
• More tolerance and patience

Arising from the top solutions were a range of key recommendations – one being a more collective education and training approach across health and social care agencies involving all key stakeholders. Across the country initiatives have already been happening over the last few years in support of the roll-out of this strategy. The following multi-agency approach to the National Dementia Strategy in Gloucestershire is summarised later as one example.

The Dementia Training and Education Strategy for Gloucestershire utilised evidence and expertise from a number of local organisations including the Older People's Mental Health training group and the Partnerships for Older People's Project (POPP) to develop a county-wide strategy for dementia training and education in March 2008. A 3-year implementation plan and dedicated resources have created a multi-agency pathway with clear core competencies and 'Kitemarked' training which includes a new dementia 'passport'. The training emphasis is on person-centred dementia care.

Priority groups were identified to engage in training programmes within care homes, domiciliary care services, and management teams and also included carers and primary care services.

The results have proven to be positive with increased cross sector working, high uptake of training and delivered across the identified target groups. One spin-off has been a reduction in referrals to the NHS and an improvement in the quality of person-centred dementia care provided across sector service agencies. Also evident has been an increase in flexible use of resources, increased knowledge of different professional roles and organisational cultures and a more responsive way of channelling resources to meet the needs of local community.

The National Dementia Strategy (February 2011b) has spearheaded many local partnership forums across the United Kingdom. Luton Borough Council, for example, has initiated a partnership model of joint commissioning (the Joint Commissioning Strategy, *People with Dementia* Working in Partnership 2010/2015). The partnership involves NHS Luton, Luton and Dunstable Hospital, Luton Borough Council, Age Concern and other local organisations. A particularly strong focus is placed on preventative intervention and the vital role of self-help in recognising that the personal ownership of health and well-being is crucial to reducing the risk of developing dementia. The strategy stresses the importance of at least 15 minutes of vigorous exercise a day, a healthy balanced diet and stimulation of the mind and body by engaging in activities of interest as part of daily life. The strategy also promotes the linking together of existing local dementia campaigns, mapping and auditing current services and providing a clear and transparent basic care pathway for people to follow and to signpost and navigate them to the help needed.

Obesity

The lifestyle choices and increasingly sedentary lives of people in the United Kingdom have triggered a real concern about the increased weight of children and adults. Combined factors such as diet choices, increasingly office-based occupations and an increase in the interest in sedentary computer-based leisure pursuits for children and adults have all compounded to raise alarm about the health of communities across the United Kingdom. The Foresight Report 'Tacking Obesities: Future Choices' (The Foresight Report 2007) predicts that if current trends continue by 2050, 60% of men and 50% of women and 26% of children and young people in the United Kingdom will be obese. In addition, cases of type 2 diabetes will rise by 70%, cases of strokes will rise by 30%, and cases of coronary heart disease will rise by 20%. The Foresight Report is the largest ever UK study into obesity backed by the Government and complied by 250 experts. The report stressed that obesity must no longer be targeted as an individual problem but it must be recognised that much broader societal and environmental factors are at play.

Obesity is recognised as one of the major public health issues in the developed world. The Medical Research Council funded research into obesity at Imperial College, London, in 2007 which identified that in England alone obesity is the cause of 9000 premature deaths each year and that obesity can reduce life expectancy by 9 years (Medical Research Council 2007, p. 1).

The rising concern about childhood obesity has also initiated a wide-scale enquiry and a National Audit Report *Tackling Child Obesity: First Steps* (National Audit Report 2003). Three national departments – the Department of Health, Department for Education and Department for Culture, Media and Sport – have joined forces with local partnership forums comprising public and private organisations to take a broad view about the behaviours that are intrinsic to obesity in young children under 11 years of age. A broad-based approach has been taken to make sweeping local community changes such as improving the health quality of school meals and the provision of better open, green spaces for leisure and play within localities.

In Manchester a multi-agency approach to tackling obesity was established by the Manchester Alliance for Community Care: 'Tackling Obesity and Promoting a Healthy Weight, A Briefing' (Manchester Alliance for Community Care 2010). The resultant programme is geared towards community practitioners and managers within the voluntary and community health sectors. A 'Health and Well-Being Network ' was also proposed. The programme aims to tackle issues around obesity and overweight with the focus on a positive environment and culture and a multi-agency approach. The key objectives for the network are

- To make obesity a priority for all
- To promote healthy behaviours
- To tackle the obesogenic environment
- To invest in prevention
- To invest in treatment

The research briefing also linked together community projects, such as the 'Food Futures' project started in 2007 (Food Futures Strategy for Manchester 2007) and the 'Sport and Physical Activity Alliance' set up in 2008 (Manchester's Sport and Physical Activity Alliance: 'A Vision for Sport and Physical Activity' 2008). It was discovered that community development projects such as these can be more proactive and 'tuned in' to what motivates local people and identify which initiatives could best encourage people to make important health changes in their own lives. Ideas such as healthy eating lunch clubs, cooking classes, play schemes for children, more active modes of local transport, gardening projects, promotion of breast-feeding for babies, peer support weight management groups and community cafes are all examples of resultant action emanating from this initiative.

Stakeholders across a range of local organisations meet bimonthly to share information and ensure a 'joined-up approach' to create pathways and identify benefits to link up with Manchester's Healthy Weight Strategy.

Asthma

The NHS has increasingly promoted an early intervention approach to respiratory disease. In the United Kingdom over one million children have asthma, which is the most common respiratory disease in children. 5.4 million people in total in the United Kingdom have asthma and receive treatment. Surprisingly the United Kingdom has the highest rate of asthma symptoms in children worldwide (Asthma UK 2012). This costs the NHS around £1 billion a year.

The coalition government has initiated partnership consultation across PCT's NHS, allied health providers and voluntary organisations to agree clear outcomes to promote good respiratory health and reduce health inequalities. Published in July 2011, the Department of Health 'An Outcomes Strategy for Chronic Obstructive Pulmonary Disease (COPD) and Asthma' sought to respond to the high mortality rates in the United Kingdom for COPD and asthma (DH 2012c). Premature mortality for asthma in 2008 was 1.5 times higher than the European average. The outcomes strategy recognised that improving respiratory health is both a health and social care concern which also needs to take account of environmental factors which can exacerbate asthma and other breathing conditions. There was also realisation that wide-scale health issues such as asthma must be tackled by crossing boundaries and pooling resources. The central vision for the strategy has five shared objectives:

* Respiratory health and good lung health
* Early and accurate diagnosis
* Active partnership between professions
* Chronic disease management
* Tailored evidence-based treatment for each individual

In 2012 Asthma UK delivered the 'Triple A' Avoid Asthma Attacks campaign (The Triple A 'Avoid Asthma Attacks' Campaign). This is a UK-wide initiative to reduce hospital admissions, focused on particularly identified 'asthma hot spots' in the United Kingdom such as Ealing in West London. Prior to the project starting, hospital admissions for children in Ealing were the highest in London. The 'Triple A' project organises NHS nursing specialists to work closely with teachers in primary schools, the children themselves and their families across local communities to reduce the impact of the consequences of asthma on the lives of children. Since 2009, 2500 schools and 'Early Years' staff have received training on asthma awareness, and close working with GP practices has helped to identify children who have been admitted previously to hospital due to asthma attacks. This in turn has reduced the number of hospital admissions as increased preventative work with schools, education staff, GP practices and families has reaped positive results. One NHS Ealing asthma nurse specialist was tasked with the role of working across local communities to reduce the impact of asthma on children's lives and advised that

> By helping parents and school staff understand how serious asthma is we not only want to reduce hospital admissions but ultimately hope to prevent children dying from asthma. (Asthma UK 30 April 12)

The pooling of pressure across different organisations can also strengthen the impact for changing legislation where children's health and welfare may be at risk. This is illustrated by one campaign that allowed schools to keep emergency asthma kits on-site. Asthma UK has also called for a change in legislation to overturn the ruling that blue reliever inhalers are 'prescription only' medicines making it illegal for schools to keep a spare inhaler on their premises. The campaign has been supported by the RCGP, the Primary Care Respiratory Society and charities including 'Education for Health' and the George Collen Memorial Fund (Asthma UK, 2012).

Concluding reflections

An important synergy between the Manchester community approach to obesity, the co-produced dementia training alliance in Gloucestershire and the grass-roots approach to reducing asthma in children in Ealing is the emphasis placed upon healthy communities and away from individual blame or medical ownership of the issues. The focus on local people being fully involved, taking control and working out their own solutions by being more informed about their health appears to be the driving force and impetus for the multi-sector alliances.

Another reflection arising from the case exemplars is the move away from purist biological, medicalised treatment regimes alone when responding to community health issues and a more holistic recognition that society has created unhealthy ways of living which can be combated with a combined effort and the sharing of local resources and reference to both medical and social models of health and social care (Riddell & Watson 2003).

A selection of examples of multi-sector working have been explored to highlight the proactive and practical ways that social, cultural and environmental influences can be approached to promote shared responsibility of health and well-being for society. The combined impact of an ageing population, climate change, fiscal crisis and escalating health concerns such as diet, dementia and respiratory disease has created an increasing and urgent need to pool resources, remodel services and address pressing issues in a joined-up, holistic way. There appears to be a layering of interdependency when exploring individual, local, national and global health concerns which requires a very macro and organic perspective. It also seems apparent that more vulnerable sectors of a society may be disproportionately affected by poor health. A combination of unacceptable housing conditions, poverty, a poor diet and restricted education, employment and leisure opportunities can also accumulate to create intersectional risk and result in more chance of health problems linked to environmental issues (Greenfields *et al.* 2012).

Research into the need to develop sustainable systems of health and social care recognises that certain sectors of the population are more susceptible to threats such as climate change, significant cuts in public spending and an increased demand for care and support for certain groups, for example, older people. Research into the importance of sustainable development (Evans *et al.* 2012) makes a clear link with health and social care services and the need to promote health, well-being and equality when considering the natural environment and how to maximise sustainable growth:

> Sustainable development is about social justice and well being for all, about living environments in which everyone can flourish and be safe. A sustainable development approach to health and social care means the vulnerable in our society will be better placed to withstand the social, economic and climate pressures we are all facing (Evans *et al.* 2012, p. 748).

As with all structural innovation which impacts on the lives of people and their communities, the influence of multi-sector working on the delivery of primary health services has received mixed research outcomes. Partnership working has been a central plank of 'New Labour's' policies since 1997 (Perkins *et al.* 2010). The importance of a modernised health and social policy to improve health and reduce health inequalities has been widely researched. Perkins's research looked at the impact of partnership working to improve local health planning and in fact arrived at some mixed findings. In essence, the summary findings led to an overemphasis on gaining 'quick wins' by focusing on younger people rather than those members of the community with more deep-rooted health concerns. A lack of physical and financial resources was often the reason for reduced success in partnership working, and a limited focus on action-orientated outcomes diluted the impact of some of the partnership work carried out.

A learning point from the research was the vital need to share and disseminate information across different organisations. Often it was the practical hurdles such as different information and databases across separate agencies which hampered progress. Another substantial area of learning gained was the complexity of health improvement needs across localities and involving diverse organisations, particularly where other departments such as education, housing and employment needed to be involved. By identifying and agreeing the common barriers that impeded progress, new strategies were identified to build on and create a raised awareness of the complexity of tackling health care inequalities.

Economic globalisation, demographic shifts and technological developments have also impacted on health and social care delivery, both nationally and internationally (Reisch & Jayshree 2012). This has heightened the politicisation of health and social care professions and the strong emphasis on anti-discriminatory practice, a focus on equitable service delivery and value of the individual within increasingly diverse religious and cultural dynamics within societies. Strength-based models of self-management, resilience and empowerment (Ligon 2002) fit well with the model of an organic multi-agency approach to community health care. Individuals are seen as central to the bigger picture and able to shape their lives as major stakeholders in their own health and welfare. Ligon captured this well in stating that

> A strength perspective acknowledges that the client possesses knowledge, abilities, resilience, coping and problem solving skills that are there to be employed. ...the professional worker's role is to facilitate the process, to serve as a bridge to the client's own resources, to move ahead and seek solutions (2002, p. 99).

In conclusion, the chapter has journeyed through the key drivers pushing the multi-sectoral agenda for community health care forward. The overriding feature has been the politicisation of health delivery transformation and the personal investment of the individual as an integral component of the community collaboration process. Real examples of multi-agency working have clarified experiences in action across the United Kingdom and have reinforced the message that resources can be most effectively deployed when shared and openly disseminated for the common good of all. The challenge to find new and effective ways of coordinating health and other primary care services will undoubtedly continue. The complex interweaving of factors influencing the health of the individual and their communities will require increasing emphasis given to collaborative partnership working at political, cultural and local levels.

References

Alzheimer's Society (2012) *Dementia 2012: A National Challenge* (Online). Available from http://www.alzheimer's.org.uk/dementia2012. Accessed on 5 September 2012.

Asthma UK (30 April 2012) *Avoid Asthma Attacks Campaign; The Triple A Campaign* (Online). Available from http://www.asthma.org.uk/campaigns/thetriple-a-avoid-asthma-attacks-campaign. Accessed on 15 October 2012.

Buckinghamshire New University (2012a) *Care and Health Alliance* (Online). Available from http://bucks.ac.uk.research/research institutes/care health alliance. Accessed on 25 September 2012.

Buckinghamshire New University (2012b) *Centre of Excellence in Tele-Care and Assisted Living (CETAL)* (Online). Available from http://bucks.ac.research/research_institutes/cetal. Accessed on 28 September 2012.

Burton, J., Toscano, T. & Zonouzi, M. (2012) *Personalisation for Social Workers; Opportunities and Challenges for Frontline Practice*, McGraw Hill, Oxford University Press, Maidenhead, UK.

Care Services Improvement Partnership (CSIP) (2007) *Strengthening the Involvement of People with Dementia; A Resource for Implementation*. CSIP, York.

Changing Environment Team (2003) *Executive Summary; Multi Sector Community Collaborations – Assessing the Changing Environment* (Online). Available from http://www.uwex.edu/ces/pdande/evaluation. Accessed on 10 September 2012.

Lord Darzi, K.B.E. (2008) *High quality care for all: NHS next stage review (final report)*. Stationary Office, London. Gateway ref. 10106, page 92.

Department of Health (DH) (1990) *The NHS and Community Care Act*, HMSO, London.

DH (2008) *Transforming Social Care*. LAC (DH). DH, London.

DH (2006) *Our Health, Our Care, Our Say: A New Direction for Community Service*, DH, London.

DH (2011a) Chief Executive Report, *Innovation, Health and Wealth*, Electronic Publication ref. 16978. Crown copyright, London.

DH (2011b) *Living Well with Dementia; A National Dementia Strategy*. DH, London.

DH (2012a) *Amendments to the Health and Social Care Bill*. DH, London.

DH (2012b) *Getting it Right for Children, Young People and Families*. DH, London.

DH (2012c) *An Outcomes Strategy for Chronic Obstructive Pulmonary Disease (COPD)*. DH, London.

Evans, S, Hills, S. & Orme, J. (2012) Doing more for less? Developing sustainable systems of social care in the context of climate change and public spending cuts. *The British Journal of Social Work*, **4** (2), 744–764.

Ferguson, I. (2009) *Reclaiming Social Work: Challenging Neo-Liberalism and Promoting Social Justice*. Sage, London.

Food Futures Partnership (2007) *Food Futures – a Food Strategy for Manchester – 2007*. Manchester Joint Health Unit, Manchester.

Greenfields, M., Dalrymple, R. & Fanning, A. (2012) *Working with Adults at Risk from Harm*. Maidenhead, UK, McGraw Hill, Oxford University Press.

Joint Commissioning Strategy (2010) *People with Dementia Strategy, Luton 2010–2015*. Luton Borough Council (Online). Available from http://www.luton.gov/uk/..../LutonDocuments/..../People%20with%20dementia%draft%20strategydoc. Accessed 10 September 2012.

Lawrence, F. (2012) *NHS Reforms: The School Nurse's View. The Guardian Newspaper* (Online). Available from http://www.guardian.co.uk/society/2012. Accessed on 14 August 2012.

Ligon, J. (2002) Fundamentals of brief treatment In: *Crisis Intervention Handbook: Assessment, Treatment and Time-Limited Cognitive Treatment* (eds. Roberts & Greene). pp. 96–100. Oxford University Press, New York.

Mahmud, T. (2012) *Better Patient Feedback, Better Healthcare*. M+K Publishing, Maidstone.

Manchester Alliance for Community Care (2010) *Tackling Obesity and Promoting a Healthy Weight, A Briefing*. MACC, Manchester (Online). Available from http://www.macc.org.uk. Accessed on 3 September 2012.

Manchester Sport and Physical Activity Alliance (2008) A Vision for Sport and Physical Activity – 'Getting Manchester Moving' – 2008–2013, Manchester Sport and Physical Activity Alliance, Manchester

Mathers, C. & Loncar, D. (2006) Projections of global mortality and burden of disease from 2002–2030. *PLoS Medicine*, **3**, 2011–2030.

Medical Research Council (2007) *Achievements and Impact Report; Obesity* (online). Available from http://www.mrcac/ukAchievementsimpact/obesity/indexhtmcached-similar. Accessed on 3 October 2012.

National Audit Report (2003) *Tackling Child Obesity: First Steps*. HC (2005–2006) 801.

National Health Information Systems (2011) *The Role of Effective Multi-Sector Collaborations*. Asia Pacific Leadership Forum on Health Information Systems. Department of Health, London.

National Health Service Institute (2012) *High impact innovations*. Published Reports; High Impact Innovations Website; Author Holmes, L., 10 July (Online). Available from http://www.innovation.nhs.uk. Accessed on 6 November 2012.

Parliament (27 March 2012) *The Health and Social Care Act*. Ch 7, London.

Perkins, N., Smith, K., Hunter, D., Bambra, C. & Joyce, K. (2010) *What Counts in What Works? New Labour and Partnerships in Public Health*. The Policy Press, .

Reisch, M. & Jayshree, S. (2012) The new politics of social work practice; understanding context to promote change. *British Journal of Social Work*, **42** (6), 1132–1150.

Riddell, S. & Watson, N. (2003) *Disability, Culture and Identity*, Pearson Prentice Hall, London.

Ross, H. (2012) *How to Get Ahead in School Nursing. The Guardian Professional* (Online). Available from http://www.guardian.co.uk/healthcare2012. Accessed on 15 October 2012.

Staines, R. (2009) *New Stop Smoking Initiative to be Launched in England.* Nursing Times.net. (Online). Available from http://www.nursingtimes.net/stop.smoking-initiative… .5002288articlecachedsimilar. Accessed on 20 September 2012.

Swansea University (2012) MSc *Public Health and Partnerships in Care* Course (Online). Available from http://www.swan.ac.uk/humanandhealthsciences/mscpgdpg/publichealth-site….partnershipsincare. Accessed on 23 August 2012.

The Foresight Report (2007) *Tackling Obesities: Future Choices Project.* webarchive.national-archives.gov.uk/+/www/obesityCDH_079713cached.similar. Accessed on 21 October 2012.

Willis, A. & Coupland,T. (2009) *The Dementia Training and Education Strategy for Gloucestershire: A Multi Agency Approach for Gloucestershire that Supports the National Dementia Stategy.* Dementia Training and Education Strategy Group for Gloucestershire, Gloucester.

World Health Organization (WHO) (1987) *Health for All Declaration of WHO Conference on Primary Health Care*, Alma Ata, Geneva.

4

Moving Care Closer to Home

Susan Procter

Faculty of Society and Health, Buckinghamshire New University, Uxbridge, UK

Hospital provision: A brief history of the last 50 years

Historically health care has been synonymous with hospital care, and for many people today it still is as evidenced by the public protests which occur every time the closure of a hospital service is considered. There has, however, been a substantial reduction in the number of hospital beds over the last 50 years. It is very difficult to get exact figures because of changing structures in the NHS; however, all evidence points to a reduction in hospital beds of about 80% since the 1960s. Armstrong (1998) identified that the number of hospital beds in Great Britain peaked in the 1960s when there were 488,013 beds in the NHS. The number gradually declined until by 1990 there were only about 255,054 hospital beds remaining in the NHS. In February 2013 the Department of Health (2013) published the average number of daily and occupied beds in England in all NHS organisations between October 2012 and December 2012 as 136,076. In mental health Leff (2001) identifies that of the 130 psychiatric hospitals functioning in England and Wales in 1975, only 14 remained open in 2001 with fewer than 200 patients in each. The Care Quality Commission (CQC) identified a reduction of 4,000 hospital beds between June 2010 and March 2012 (CQC 2012).

In order to understand the reasons driving this reduction in hospital beds, it is important first to understand the factors that gave rise to the growth in hospital provision initially. Armstrong (1998) attributed growth in hospital provision during the early twentieth century to a benign faith in the care provided by hospitals and in particular

Community and Public Health Nursing, Fifth Edition. Edited by David Sines,
Sharon Aldridge-Bent, Agnes Fanning, Penny Farrelly, Kate Potter and Jane Wright.
© 2013 John Wiley & Sons, Ltd. Published 2013 by John Wiley & Sons, Ltd.

in the merits of extended bed rest as an appropriate response to most medical conditions. Hospitals removed potentially dangerous or infectious individuals from society providing safe spaces where they could be cared for. This created a sense of public safety whilst maintaining compassion and care for these individuals. Hospitals and the people they cared for became a thoroughly worthy cause.

According to Armstrong (1998), the reasons for the decline in hospital provision during the second half of the twentieth century were twofold. The first reason was a growing awareness that hospitals did not provide a safe environment in which to recover from illness. Throughout the 1960s and 1970s, there was increasing evidence of the problems of cross infection in hospitals, noise levels, sleep deprivation and isolation from families which led to a recognition that hospital admission was not always in the best interests of the patient and could in fact cause considerable harm to patients. Secondly the dangers associated with bed rest started to be evidenced from about the 1950s onwards. Corcoran (1991) identified over 50 years of scientific evidence demonstrating the specific damage done to each of the body systems by prolonged bed rest and inactivity. He identified that both ageing and inactivity lead to strikingly similar kinds of physical and psychological deterioration.

The reduction in hospital beds has been accompanied by a reconfiguration of hospital services. Imison (2011) has estimated an 85% reduction in the number of acute hospitals from a baseline of 1962 and suggests that the number of sites at which elements of highly specialist care are delivered has reduced even further. According to Imison (2011) in England, general acute care is now delivered in just over 200 hospitals, and at the same time the average size of hospitals has grown from 68 beds, as indicated by the Ministry of Health 1962, to just over 400 beds, the average acute trust (which may have multiple hospital sites) has just over 580 beds.

Centralisation of hospital services has been supported by major developments in medicine and surgery which require both clinical and technical staff and equipment to become more specialised and therefore more centralised (Imison 2011). Maximising the use of complex technology and maintaining the skills and competencies of highly specialised staff require a volume or patient throughput that optimises productivity, and this requires centralisation of specialist teams and equipment onto fewer, larger sites. There is growing evidence of the benefits of centralisation of hospital services through specialisation. NHS London has estimated that the reconfiguration of stroke services across London into specialist centralised stroke units will save 400 lives a year. As Imison (2011) points out, this strategy is based on evidence which shows that there was more than a fourfold difference between the lowest and highest performing hospitals when measuring the number of patients who died within 30 days of having a stroke. However, for many conditions specialisation makes only a marginal improvement in outcomes, and other factors such as nurse staffing levels or 24/7 consultant cover are more important in determining outcomes than specialisation (Imison 2011). Imison (2011) also points to the reduced reliance on bed rest as a driving factor in the reduction in hospital beds.

The reduction in hospital beds has been accompanied by an increase in the use of ambulatory care. The term ambulatory care covers a wide range of interventions where patients are treated and discharged on the same day. Ambulatory care is increasing with advances in medical technology and includes surgical and medical procedures, diagnostic procedures, dental procedures and a variety of other clinical interventions delivered in a health care setting during a normal working day. As a result, hospital activity, now measured in finished consultant episodes rather than bed days, has continued to increase driven by progressive increases in day cases and a progressive reduction in the time patients need to spend in hospital for their treatment. There were 17.5 million finished consultant episodes in 2011/2012, an increase of 1.1% on the previous year (Health and Social Care Information Centre 2012).

The early 1990s saw the development of a cluster of predominantly long-term conditions which came to be defined as ambulatory care sensitive (ACS) conditions; these are clinical conditions for which the risk of hospital admission can be reduced by timely and effective ambulatory care, usually provided by primary, community or outpatient services (Bardsley *et al.* 2013). The aim here is to provide early intervention to prevent the patients' condition from deteriorating to the point where emergency admission to hospital becomes necessary. More recently attention has shifted to ambulatory emergency care (AEC). Here an acute event has developed but can be managed with appropriate emergency input without requiring an overnight stay in hospital (NHS Institute for Innovation and Improvement 2010).

Despite increasing evidence of the effectiveness of early intervention in ACS conditions and AEC, provision nationally is patchy and there is very little evidence that the potential gains from particularly managing ACS conditions have been realised (Bardsley *et al.* 2013).

Wistow (2000) points out that the closure of hospital beds was largely accounted for by the care in the community policy which aimed to replace long-stay elderly, mental health and learning disability hospitals with community provision (Leff 2001). The impact of these policies on community provision is evident in CQC (2012) data which shows that at 31 March 2012 there were 13,134 residential care homes with 247,824 beds registered in England and 4,672 nursing homes with 215,463 beds. The increases in residential and nursing home care have been accompanied by increases in self-care. The CQC Report (2012) registration figures show that as at 31 March 2012, there were 6,830 agencies providing domiciliary care (also known as home care) across England. This is an increase of 16% since the July 2011 figure reported in the previous year's State of Care report and continues the long-term trend towards people continuing to live in their own homes and communities with appropriate support.

Despite the growth in residential and nursing home care, it is currently estimated that 65% of people admitted to hospital are over the age of 65 and that this group accounts for 70% of bed days occupied (Cornwell *et al.* 2012). It is estimated that 25% of hospital beds are occupied by people with dementia (Lakey 2009). Frail elderly and people with dementia increase length of stay, readmission and inter-ward transfers (Cornwell *et al.* 2012).

Imison *et al.* (2012) identified significant variation in the use of hospital beds by people over 65 admitted as an emergency. They found that this resulted in almost equal part from variation in rate of admission and variation in length of stay. Rate of admission was the dominant driver for hospitals with the highest and lowest rates of bed use. Imison *et al.* (2012) also found that if all primary care trusts (PCTs) achieved the rate of admission and average length of stay of the lowest 25th percentile, 7,000 fewer hospital beds would be needed across England. Interestingly they found that areas with higher proportions of older people have proportionately lower bed use. They speculate that where there is a large elderly population, providers have worked together to address the needs of this population as it will have been identified as a priority in their strategic plans. In areas where the proportion of elderly people is lower, other population needs may take priority.

Hurst and Williams (2012) in a review of hospital productivity found that spending in the NHS has grown by an average of 7% per year since 2000. This growth is now over and the NHS is facing a freeze on growth. At the same time it is facing increasing demands brought about by advances in medical technology, increasing consumer expectations and demographic trends. To address this, there is an increased emphasis on efficiency particularly in the hospital sector. New techniques for measuring efficiency are being introduced including frontier methods. Frontier methods are based on benchmarking. In essence the best achieving hospitals, on a given indicator, are identified, and the distance that other hospitals lie from the frontier is measured in percentage terms. In practice the frontier measurement should include quality and outcomes or effectiveness as well as activity. In reality because quality and effectiveness are very difficult to measure, frontier measures tend to just measure activity; consequently quality and outcomes are subsumed under activity as productivity. This approach to measurement drives increases in hospital throughput but does not necessarily give rise to real improvements in health outcomes within the whole system of health care. Appendix C of the report by Hurst and Williams (2012) gives a synopsis of the difficulties of measuring efficiency in hospital care.

Trends in productivity have been available for hospital and community health services in the United Kingdom since 1974. These trends demonstrate improvements in productivity (measured primarily as activity) following the introduction of general management in the mid-1980s and again following the introduction of the internal market in the 1990s (Hurst & Williams 2012). Productivity fell in the NHS by 16.7% during the period of rapid expansion in NHS funding between 2001 and 2008 (Hurst & Williams 2012). However, this does not include quality-adjusted productivity. There is also evidence of considerable variation in productivity between the best and the worst performing hospitals, and it is these variations that are being examined to identify productivity improvements within the NHS to maintain costs whilst meeting increasing demand.

International comparisons on hospital productivity also indicate room for considerable improvement in the NHS. The Organisation for Economic Co-operation and Development (OECD) international comparisons of hospital length of stay (which exclude day cases) suggest that average hospital length of stay in the United Kingdom, at 7.7 days in 2009, remained above the OECD average at 7.2 days. The USA reported 4.9 days, Sweden reported 5.7 days and Denmark 4.8 days (OECD 2011). The average length of stay in hospital identified in Denmark has been linked to the quantity and quality of its long-term care services which include a significant number of specialists working in the community outside hospitals (Hurst 2002). Comparisons such as these alert the Department of Health to the scope for further reductions in NHS spending on hospital provision.

Hurst and Williams (2012) highlight the findings of McKinsey & Company, who prepared a report for the Department of Health detailing potential efficiency savings in the NHS. Using predominantly benchmarking techniques, McKinsey suggests that savings of between £13 and £20 billion were potentially available in the NHS as a whole over the following 3–5 years. About 45% could come from improvements in technical efficiency, that is, the introduction and diffusion of new technologies; about 35% from improvements in allocative efficiency, that is, the reallocation of resources to more cost-effective services; and about 20% from a shift of hospital care to the community.

The concerns about a focus on activity and improving productivity without measuring quality were addressed by the Department of Health via the introduction of QIPP – Quality, Innovation, Productivity and Prevention. This was a large-scale transformational programme for the NHS, designed to involve all NHS staff, clinicians, patients and the voluntary sector. The intention was to improve the quality of care the NHS delivers whilst making up to £20billion of efficiency savings by 2014–2015, to be reinvested in front-line care. From 1 April 2013 this programme will transfer to the NHS Commissioning Board. More recently the Department of Health has introduced Commissioning for Quality and Innovation (CQUIN) targets. This will transfer to the NHS Commissioning Board for review for the 2014/2015 planning round. Under CQUIN one fifth of the value (0.5% of overall contract value) is to be linked to the achievement of national CQUIN goals, where these apply. In other words contract funding will be withheld from those NHS providers who fail to meet their CQUIN targets. Central to CQUIN is the safety thermometer. The NHS Safety Thermometer has been designed to be used by front-line health care professionals to measure a snapshot of harm once a month from pressure ulcers, falls, urinary infection in patients with catheters and treatment for venous thromboembolism (VTE). Additionally the NHS is introducing the friends and family test that sets response targets on feedback from patients and staff. Commissioners will be empowered to incentivise high-performing trusts, in response to meeting or exceeding targets on the friends and family test on improvement against the NHS Safety Thermometer (excluding VTE), particularly pressure sores; improving dementia care, including sustained improvement in finding people with dementia, Assessing and Investigating their symptoms and Referring for support (FAIR); and VTE – 95% of patients being risk assessed and achievement of a locally agreed goal for the number of VTE admissions that are reviewed through root cause analysis (NHS Commissioning Board 2012).

These targets go some way towards measuring the quality of care delivered and to promoting harm-free care to counter the tendency to increase hospital activity without any information of the impact of productivity improvements on quality of care. They still, however, only focus on harm-free care; they do not measure improvements in health outcomes at an individual or population level which may be crucial to managing overall demand for NHS services and containing costs whilst realising higher levels of individual and population health (Wanless 2002).

Given these changes over the last 50 years, it is timely to consider the role of nursing within a reconfiguration of hospital care. Like health care and the NHS, nursing is primarily associated with hospital care. This is evidenced in the assumptions that underpin nurse training where hospital placements still dominate the curriculum in the majority, although not all, of nurse training courses and to access community nurse training will result in a second registration. Training as a hospital nurse is still required before you can train as a community nurse. Many courses leading to community nursing registration require applicants to have had experience of working as a registered nurse in hospital as an entry requirement for community nursing programmes. Given the changing scale and design of hospital services and the evolution of care closer to home as the primary platform for the delivery of care services as against treatment services, the feasibility of hospitals as a platform for nurse training and for entry to community nursing programmes is coming under considerable strain. In order to distinguish between activity, harm-free care, patient outcomes and improvements in patient and population health, it is useful first to review some of the interpretations and definitions surrounding the terms 'health' and 'care' and the actual and potential contribution nurses in general and community nursing in particular make towards health outcomes.

Health care: What does it mean?

In the United Kingdom health care like hospitals is synonymous with the NHS. Yet only a cursory review of definitions of health and definitions of care will indicate that most health is created by organisations and institutions including industry, employers and families outside of the NHS, whilst most care is delivered predominately in family and friendship units.

In reviewing what is meant by the term health, it is possible to classify definitions according to two main categories (Procter 2000): (1) selective definitions that define health as the absence of diagnosable disease and/or disability and (2) universal definitions that recognise health as a product of social determinants such as income, housing and education and the impact these factors make on lifestyle opportunities and choices in relation to factors such as diet, exercise and stress (Blane *et al.* 1996; Laverack 2004; The Marmot Review 2010).

Selective definitions of health

Selective definitions of health tend to be derived from biomedical frameworks in which health and illness split the population into two camps, those who are not currently exhibiting manifestations of illness or disease processes and are, therefore, by definition healthy and those who are exhibiting symptoms of illness and disease processes and who consequently come forward or are brought forward for treatment in order to restore health or ameliorate symptoms. Hospitals whose function is still to investigate and provide treatment for disease processes whether as inpatients or as ambulatory care clearly promulgate this definition of health. Selective definitions therefore define health as the absence of disease (Tones & Green 2004; Naidoo & Wills 2009). Selective definitions of health can include health as functional capacity to fulfil one's role (Arnold & Breen 1998). This closely resembles Talcott Parsons' description of the 'sick role' (Parsons 1979). According to Parsons, the onset of a disease or disability reduces a person's functional capacity and consequently gives rise to the need for them to adopt the 'sick role'. By adopting this role the individual can be excused from partici-pating in their normal social duties. Their absence from their social roles is tolerated so long as the individual is seen to be striving towards regaining health, and this includes obtaining medical treatments and following medical advice. This introduces a moral imperative on those who succumb to disease to seek the appropriate interven-tions provided by the NHS.

However, there is evidence that selective definitions of health as the absence of dis-ease make only a marginal contribution to improving health outcomes (McKeown 1979; Tarlov 1996) and that real impact on improving health outcomes can only be achieved through working with universal definitions of health that address the social, economic and environmental inequalities (The Marmot Review 2010) which delay the onset of disease and reduce the progression of the disease and therefore lengthen life expectancy.

Universal definitions of health

Universal definitions of health are definitions that apply to the whole population regardless of individual differences. They tend to recognise health as a relative rather than absolute state in which each individual strives constantly to maintain their health rather than merely being healthy. Health is therefore a lifelong pursuit and one that people with serious diagnostic conditions, such as ischaemic heart disease or those who are terminally ill, can still strive to achieve.

Universal definitions of health include health as growth. Arnold and Breen (1998) have described how within the health as growth perspective individuals are seen as hav-ing a capacity for growth that can be nurtured and supported throughout the person's lifespan. Growth is viewed as a progressive lifelong activity, a 'striving towards' rather than a realisation of an end point. Health as growth encompasses Maslow's notion of self-actualisation (Maslow 1987). Here a person feels themselves to be an autonomous, free-thinking individual who is able to realise their own goals whilst maintaining a constructive relationship with their natural, cultural and familial environment. Maslow recognises that the achievement of higher levels of enlightenment are based on the pro-vision of basic human necessities such as food, shelter, warmth, security and education clearly indicating that in achieving health these basic needs must be met.

Closely allied to definitions of health as growth are the concepts of health as independence, the exercise of autonomy (Doyal & Gough 1991), empowerment (Tones & Green 2004) and self-determination (Seedhouse 1986). This collection of theories of health derives from humanistic traditions which recognise that humanity is distinguished by respect for individual self-determination and the exercise of free will (Doyal & Gough 1991). Using this collection of theories, health is a personal goal that people choose and can be different for different people; no one standard definition can be derived or applied. Multiple interpretations and choices need to be accommodated. In using concepts such as autonomy, self-determination and independence to define health, it may be necessary to distinguish between objective and subjective definitions of autonomy. People who possess the power to exercise considerable autonomy in a social structure may not necessarily possess the personal characteristics associated with a moral use of autonomy. Humanistic definitions of health, as autonomy exercised within a moral framework, imply that behaviours by individuals and groups who abuse objective power or who exercise autonomy in a way that damages others within social systems could be classified as manifestations of ill health. Sex offenders frequently fall into this category, but in theory it could be extended to include bullying and even the perpetuation of national or institutional discrimination and oppression.

The concept of well-being as a definition of health became prominent following its incorporation into the 1946 definition of health produced by the World Health Organization which stated

> Health is a state of complete physical, mental and social well-being and not merely the absence of disease and infirmity. (WHO 1946)

This definition locates well-being as a universal construct that applies to all individuals regardless of their underlying physiological or psychological state. However, health as well-being may not equate easily with other definitions of health given earlier. A temporary sense of well-being may be achieved through the use of drugs or alcohol or through other behaviours such as domination or control, which using alternative definitions of health (described earlier) may be deemed unhealthy. Any attempt to develop well-being as a definition of health needs to relate personal experiences of well-being to healthy forms of individual and collective behaviour.

Finally Seedhouse (1986) has described health as the realisation of potential. This definition, in many ways, integrates both selective and universal definitions of health. According to Seedhouse (1986), health is stratified by genetic endowment, but should not be stratified by environmental or social conditions. Work for health is about striving to reduce the obstacles that prevent a person from realising their full physical and psychological potential. The more physical and psychological problems they have, the more input they are going to need to overcome the obstacles to realising their potential. Interventions are selectively applied to individuals according to an identification of the particular configuration of obstacles preventing them from realising their full potential. However, whilst work at an individual level is of necessity selective and in many cases individualised, in working to create situations in which individuals can realise their full potential, Seedhouse (1986) suggests, work for health must address and overcome the obstacles to health embedded in social and political structures, including oppression and domination. Health as the realisation of potential, therefore, also includes a whole systems approach in working to overcome the structural obstacles embedded in social systems that prevent people from realising their full potential regardless of their individual physical and psychological state.

The preceding discussion of definitions of health indicates that although health care is synonymous with the NHS and the NHS is synonymous with hospital care, hospitals have only a very minor role to play in creating health. Most health is created in domains far removed from hospital services, in community, work, travel, family, education and leisure environments. As both the Marmot Review (2010) and Wanless (2002) point out, as a nation we can only avoid rationing NHS services and make real efficiency savings in health care by addressing the determinants of overall population health using the principles underpinning universal definitions of health.

However, in reality the NHS in general and hospitals in particular tend to adopt the selective definition of health as the absence of disease and in the face of disease the promotion of functional capacity and adjustment to circumstances. This definition of health is powerful in determining who can access resources as it provides a clear set of parameters for identifying the population in need of NHS interventions and for defining the boundaries of NHS provision. It also forms the basis of a legitimate contract between the patient and the health-care practitioner. The patient has a moral obligation to adopt the sick role and in so doing enters into a contract with the NHS to adhere to the advice and treatments provided. Increasingly this access is being mediated by the evidence base. Access to treatments can only be legitimised and paid for by the state if there is an expert consensus that the evidence for the effectiveness of the intervention produces improvements in health outcomes for the individuals treated. Just looking after people because they are frail or dependent is at best a temporary function of the NHS until more suitable caring provision can be found elsewhere, normally with the family but failing that through social services or the charitable or third sector organisations. Caring as a public service has therefore transferred to the community.

Caring and nursing: Where are we now?

The publication of the Francis Report (2013) has highlighted some serious issues in relation to the provision of hospital care. Care as a concept and as a practice is elusive and difficult to define. Much of this difficulty derives from its universal appeal as a defining feature of humanity. Brykczynska (1997) in a review of the literature on caring suggests that at a philosophical level caring is frequently characterised as a moral obligation and a human imperative. It is also depicted as an ethical way of being, which results from moral development. Here people understand the value of caring and use the principles of caring to guide their behaviour (Watson 1985). For Benner and Wrubel (1989), caring is fundamentally about values. It is about the things (people, projects, events) that really matter to us. Caring is simultaneously about 'being connected' – 'fusing thought, feeling and action – knowing and being and differentiating' (Benner & Wrubel 1989, p. 1). Through caring we know what we value and what we wish to be connected with or to and are able to identify those things that are less important to us. Here again caring has a universal quality to it, enabling us to chart a course through life by attending to the things we value most.

Bulmer (1987) in his discussion of caring distinguishes between 'care as labour' and 'care as communal action'. For Bulmer family care and informal local care are sacrosanct, whilst the role of health and social care organisations is supportive and redistributive as indicated in the more public area of 'care as communal action'. The intimate aspects of 'care as labour' or tending provided by families, or substituted by nurses, nursery nurses, child minders, nannies and residential care workers if finances and economic and social policy permits, and the emotional labour (Smith 1992) of individual psychological and social support associated with care as labour remain private and obscure. Lawler (1991) in an anthropological study of hospital nursing in Australia highlights how the intimate work undertaken by nurses providing physical care for patients breaks social taboos rendering such work secret. It is generally avoided as an unsocial topic by those not directly engaged in it and is, therefore, difficult to publicise or scrutinise.

More recently Fine (2007) has identified how care has gone public. Significant changes in the status of women and opportunities for personal and economic development mean that care is no longer confined to the home and assigned to women to provide. A care industry is developing which is professionalising care within market-based provision as the increases in residential, nursing home and domestic service provision described earlier illustrate. However, in going public the tensions that exist between the privatised and intimate work associated with care as labour performed by family members and the public accountabilities associated with care as communal action have not been addressed. Going public has simply made these tensions more visible and the public services more accountable as exemplified in the Francis Report (2013).

As the findings of the Francis Report (2013) indicate, by far the biggest concerns were located in the provision of personal care, the intimate care associated with nursing. It is here that many of the most difficult ethical and moral dilemmas of service provision are located. They are difficult because rather than there being a continuum from formal to informal (family) care within which the intimate care associated with nursing could be located, a number of writers have suggested that the two forms of care (formal and informal) are fundamentally incompatible. Bulmer (1987) relates this to the distinction made by Max Weber between bureaucratic modes of action which are governed by a rational–legal authority (characterised by policies, guidelines, procedures and audits) and affective modes of action, which are governed by traditional or cultural authority and motivated by values, feelings and emotions which are difficult to codify and measure and incorporate in written procedures and processes. Fine (2007) has proposed a social division of care to represent the distinctions between paid and unpaid care but has also identified the emergence of shared care as a new form of practice and the need to research the practice of caring whether it is unpaid or paid to provide evidence of how the different domains of caring can be integrated.

Nursing at the interface between paid and unpaid care

One of the most obvious parallels between hospital nursing and family care is that both provide 24-hour care in the form of actually ensuring continuity of care for the person(s) being cared for. Family care is characterised as being unpaid and based in the home where it becomes a 24-hour 'on-call' responsibility (James 1995). Hospital nursing is characterised by access to nursing care, although not the same nurse carer, throughout the 24-hour period. Like hospital nursing a carer's life is, therefore, circumscribed by the alternative arrangements they can make for caring. A failure in these arrangements, for whatever reason, pulls the carer or nurse back into their caring role.

Whilst hospital nursing is characterised by 24-hour provision, community nursing has struggled to replicate this aspect of care outside of hospital settings. However, if care is to move closer to home, then this is perhaps one of the key structural changes in community care that needs to be addressed. If hospital admissions are to be reduced and increasingly elderly patients are maintained in their home environment and not subjected to the physical and mental health risks of hospital admission, then understanding the provision of 24-hour care in the community becomes critical. However, rather than thinking about 24-hour care as being a 24-hour provision, one possible alternative is to think about the nature of nursing work as 'the management of the 24 hour life space of the patient' (Procter 2000).

This description suggests that in managing the 24 hour provision of care in the community, nurses are not expected to be present for 24 hours but nurses do need to understand the needs of the patient over the 24-hour period. Nurses need to consider how patients manage their medications, diet, exercise or any other aspect of their illness or treatments over the 24-hour life space of their daily life. For frail or vulnerable patients, they need to consider whether they will be able to access sufficient food and fluids, access their medications, access the toilet and get sufficient rest and possibly even sufficient social interaction over a 24-hour period. The concept of the 24-hour life space also applies to the wider community in relation to public health issues of access to healthy food, fresh air and exercise. This approach to community nursing resonates with universal definitions of health described earlier.

Focusing on the 24-hour life space of the patient places nursing in a very special relationship with the patient. It means that nursing operates at the interface between creating dependency and promoting independence, between partnerships with patients based on professional expertise and definitions of need and partnerships based on patient expertise and definitions of need and between a 'nanny state' of interference and a 'self-reliant' state which can give rise to neglect. Nursing operates initially and primarily within a legislative context where free access to medical treatments and technology is enshrined within government policy legislation, but no similar free access to personal care is guaranteed or expected. At a fundamental level nursing, therefore, derives legitimacy to practise from the needs for personal care which arise out of medically directed interventions (Kuhse 1997). Through this legitimacy, however, nursing is able to develop a body of theoretical and practical knowledge and expertise about 'care as labour' that has relevance to situations beyond the narrow confines of medical interventions and may be relevant in informing wider social policy concerns about the distribution of care within the community addressed by policies defined by Bulmer (1989) as 'care as communal action' which arise at the interface between the provision of paid and unpaid care.

Facilitating self-care over the 24-hour life space of the patient requires nurses to enter into an ongoing caring relationship with the patient. Tarlow (1996) in a qualitative study of the components of a caring relationship identified time, being there and talking of any kind as essential requirements for caring to begin and to be sustained. Sensitivity, acting in the best interests of the other, caring as feeling, caring as doing and reciprocity all featured as essential components in maintaining ongoing caring relationships. Reciprocity between the carer and the person being cared for was found to be critical to the quality of the caring relationship as it developed. The person being cared for must respond in a way that perpetuates the caring process. If the person being cared for fails to respond, the carer can become demoralised. Reciprocity between nurses and patients has been identified in a number of studies where patients often work hard to shape relationships with nurses and to give something back to nurses in exchange for the care received (Bridges *et al.* 2009). Maben *et al.* (2012) using observation and interviews on a range of elderly care wards demonstrate how this circular relationship created 'good patients' who worked with the nurses to help the nurse help them and less favoured patients whose care frequently lacked compassion. In their work Maben *et al.* (2012) replicated earlier findings where patients were keen to comply with nurse expectations of their behaviour as they were fearful of a worsening of care experience if they were seen as a nuisance or a problem by nursing staff.

Caring therefore embodies an ongoing process of supportive, affective and instrumental interchanges embedded in reciprocal relationships. These aspects of care are difficult to bureaucratise and rationalise as they are based on the quality of the interpersonal relationship that develops between the carer and the person being cared for, and it is this that creates both the challenge and satisfaction to be derived from undertaking care work.

The preceding discussion on the theory and practice of caring highlights its links to universal definitions of health which promote growth, independence and autonomy. At a theoretical level it suggests that the achievement of a caring relationship is integral to providing patients with the support required to enable effective self-care and reduce dependency on NHS services, in particular hospital services. Further research is required to identify the processes by which nurses and other health care professionals are able to achieve these relationships and the potential of these relationships to improve self-efficacy and universal health outcomes. In working with patients, nurses and other health care professionals need to be able to distinguish the type of relationship required to meet the immediate and longer-term health care needs of the patient and to identify whether the local service configuration, multi-disciplinary team and resources available are conducive to the development of a longer-term caring relationship.

Public health and care closer to home

Gray (2013) has identified what he describes as five giant problems confronting health care in the United Kingdom and every other country. These are

1. Failure to prevent preventable disease
2. Harm to patients, not only from errors but also from overuse of services
3. Inequity
4. Waste of resources
5. Unwarranted variation in access, quality, cost and outcome

In addressing these five giants, Gray (2013) advocates a systems approach to service planning which starts with an epidemiological analysis of the prevalence of the illness, disease or frailty and plans service provision on an analysis of the needs of the population for health care. This is radically different from the way in which most community nursing roles have developed or are planned. As Hurst (2006) points out, the size and mix of the community nurse workforce are largely historical and rarely based on any explicit analysis of population need. In a study designed to provide managers with a staffing profile for the 304 English PCTs, Hurst (2006) found that the number of community practitioners per head of population fluctuated widely not only between but also within organisations and there was very little evidence of systematic workforce planning based on an analysis of need. Hurst (2006) points to the need to develop more robust community workforce planning models which take account of the multi-disciplinary team and relate directly to population demand. Lack of a planned approach to community services was also found in a study of the nursing contribution to chronic disease management (Procter *et al.* 2012). Here a number of innovative nurse-led services both in hospital and in community settings were explored. In each case the initiation and continuation of the nurse-led service were highly dependent on support and championing by local GPs or medical consultants. The findings indicated a bottom-up approach to service development without the necessary integration with strategic planning required to sustain the service beyond the life of the champions.

Given this situation it is difficult to see how the five giants identified by Gray (2013) will be addressed. It is clear that current approaches to workforce and service planning in community care give rise to considerable variation in access to services leading to inequities, potential waste of resources and a failure to prevent preventable disease as evidenced by the variation in admission to hospital of elderly people found by Imison *et al.* (2012). There is clearly a need for a much more systematic understanding of the components of community care and the integration of the components to support moving care closer to home. Two approaches to integration of care to reduce hospital admissions are advocated: the first focuses on the improving disease management of specific conditions (Bodenheimer *et al.* 2002) and the second on integrating health and social care provision (Ham & Oldham 2009).

Bodenheimer *et al.* (2002) first proposed the chronic care model in order to improve disease management in primary care which the authors recognise constitutes a major rethinking of primary care services. The chronic care model takes place within three overlapping domains: (1) the entire community with its full range of resources and public and private approaches to health; (2) the health-care system including the payment and structures which can build in incentives which are conducive to improving disease management or act perversely to channel behaviours in ways that do not support this model of care, for example, paying hospitals for increasing activity; and (3) the organisation and structure of provider organisations. Within these three overlapping domains, Bodenheimer *et al.* (2002) identified six essential elements of the chronic care model:

1. Community policies and resources – This includes linkages with local resources and facilities such as exercise programmes, day care and self-help groups.
2. Health care organisation – This includes the infrastructure within which chronic care is delivered. It requires leaders of health care organisations to prioritise chronic care models and to build financial incentives to support the model into the funding streams and to remove perverse financial incentives.
3. Self-management support – This recognises that patients themselves provide most of the care for long-term conditions; the more well educated and motivated they are, the more the condition is likely to be controlled and demand for services reduced.
4. Delivery system design – The structure of medical practice needs to change. Physicians should focus on treating acute exacerbations and working with patients with complex needs or whose condition is unstable. Routine monitoring of care is delegated to nurses and other healthcare professionals so that division of labour is clear.
5. Decision support – The evidence base for most chronic conditions identifies clear clinical standards for optimal care management often detailed in national service frameworks in the United Kingdom. These guidelines should be integrated into the daily delivery of care.
6. Clinical information systems – Computerised information systems serve three functions: (1) sending out reminders or alerts for routine monitoring to improve compliance with guidelines, (2) providing feedback on how well each patient's disease is being managed and (3) creating registers for managing individual care and providing information for population-based planning of resources including staffing resources.

The second approach focuses much more on the integration of health and social care services providing generic support within integrated teams of GPs, nurses, social workers, physiotherapists, occupational therapists, care coordinators and health care assistants. Integration of health and social care in the United Kingdom is fraught with organisational difficulties as health and social care have different funding sources, information sources, governance arrangements, eligibility criteria and employment terms and conditions, any or all of which can act as significant barriers to integration (Watson *et al.* 2003). In the United Kingdom Torbay is often held up as an example of where effective integration of health and social care has been achieved (Thistlethwaite 2011).

The following factors were all found to be critical to the success achieved by Torbay in integrating health and social care:

- have a clear vision based on making a positive difference for service users and be sure to keep this in sight at all times.
- Start from the bottom up by bringing together front-line teams and align these teams with general practices and their registered populations.
- Consider how simple and inexpensive innovations like the appointment of health and social care coordinators can make a major impact.
- Keep the faith in what you are doing even when all those around you may be losing their heads as a consequence of organisational and other changes that may hinder rather than help the cause of integration and service improvement.

Improvements to patient care were achieved by the zoning of patients into geographic population groupings and the integration of health and social care provision within each geographic zone which worked to meet the needs of all patients within the zone. Service provision was characterised by the principles and service delivery responses in Table 4.1.

The two models presented earlier provide exemplars for community development to reduce hospital admissions and move care closer to home. There are clear obstacles

Table 4.1   Service provision characterised by the following principles and service delivery responses

Improved overall access to services	Single point of access for patients to all service provision in each geographic zone
Shortened time from identification of need to delivery of community services	Informal and formal multi-disciplinary teamwork
Simplified decision-making processes	Unified single management system including financial delegation to local managers
Increased efficiency of processes of assessment	Informal and formal multi-disciplinary teamwork (e.g. single nursing and occupational therapy assessment)
Eliminate 'buck passing' – take responsibility for addressing patient problems even if they are not part of the professionals normal care domain	Staff in zones work together as a team to create a shared vision. Whole systems approach with hospitals, primary care, social care and mental health encouraged to work in partnership in zones

that have to be overcome for these models to be successfully implemented. However, it is clear that a good understanding of the issues will enable community nurses to take on leadership roles in bringing about the integration of community and primary care necessary for care to move closer to home.

Conclusion

This chapter has demonstrated the transformation in NHS provision over the last 50 years from a service dominated by the bricks and mortar of hospitals to one where the patients' ability to effectively promote their own health and manage any deterioration in health is the fulcrum of health care provision. Care has clearly come home. However, although the theories for care closer to home are well articulated and a variety of models for achieving care closer to home have been eloquently described, the evidence suggests that in reality patients still expect to be admitted to hospital if they experience a deterioration in their health and hospitals are struggling to manage the increasing demand produced by a rapidly ageing population. Increasing hospital beds would simply recreate the problems of harm to patients through inactivity and cross infection that gave rise to the closure of hospital beds in the first instance. The NHS is under severe strain and if unpalatable options like rationing of services are to be avoided, community care must step up and implement the models of care which have been demonstrated to reduce reliance on hospital services whilst simultaneously improving the quality of care received by patients.

References

Armstrong (1998) Decline of the hospital: reconstructing institutional dangers. *Sociology of Health & Illness*, 20 (4), 445–457.

Arnold, J. & Breen, L.J. (1998) Images of health. In: *Health Promotion Handbook* (S. Gorin & J. Arnold). St. Louis, Mosby.

Bardsley, M., Blunt, I., Davies, S. & Dixon, J. (2013) Is secondary preventative care improving? Observational study of ten year trends in emergency admissions for conditions amenable to ambulatory care. *BMJ Open*:e002007. doi:10.1136/bmjopen-2012-002007

Benner, P. & Wrubel, J. (1989) *The Primacy of Caring: Stress and Coping in Health and Illness*, Addison-Wesley, California.

Blane, D., Brunner, E. & Wilkinson, R. (eds) (1996). *Health and Social Organisation*. Routledge, London.

Bodenheimer, T., Wagner, E.H. & Grumbah, K. (2002) Improving primary care for patients with chronic illness. *The Journal of the American Medical Association*, 288 (14), 1775–1779.

Bridges, J., Flatley, M. & Meyer, J. (2009) Older people's and relatives' experiences in acute care settings: systematic review and synthesis of qualitative studies. *International Journal of Nursing Studies*, 47, 89–107.

Bulmer, M. (1987) *The Social Basis of Community Care*, Allen and Unwin, London.

Brykczynska, G. (1997). A brief overview of the epistemology of caring. In: *Caring the Compassion and Wisdom of Nursing* (G. Brykczynska), 1–9. Arnold, London.

Care Quality Commission (CQC) (2012) *The State of Health Care and Adult Social Care in England 2011/12*. The Stationary Office, London. Available from http://www.cqc.org.uk/sites/default/files/media/documents/cqc__soc_201112_final_tag.pdf. Accessed on 8 March 2013.

Corcoran, P.J. (1991) Use it or lose it – the hazards of bed rest and inactivity. *Western Journal of Medicine*, 154, 536–538.

Cornwell, J., Levenson, R., Sonola, L. & Poteliakhoff, E. (2012) *Continuity of Care for Older Hospital Patients: A Call for Action*, The Kings Fund, London.

Department of Health (DH) (2013) *Data, Statistics and Transparency, Bed Availability and Occupancy October to December 2012*. DH, London. Available from http://transparency.dh.gov.uk/?p=19745. Accessed on 8 March 2013.

Doyal, L. & Gough, I. (1991) *A Theory of Human Need*, Macmillan, Basingstoke.

Francis, R. (2013) *Independent Inquiry into Care Provided by Mid Staffordshire NHS Foundation Trust January 2005–2009, Vol 1*, The Mid Staffordshire NHS Foundation Trust Inquiry, Stationary Office, London.

Fine, M. (2007) The social division of care. *Australian Journal of Social Issues*, **42** (2), 137–149.

Gray, M. (2013) *Better Value Health Care*. Available from http://www.bvhc.co.uk/challenges/. Accessed on 12 March 2013.

Ham, C. & Oldham, J. (2009) Integrating health and social care in England: lessons from early adopters and implications for policy. *Journal of Integrated Care*, **17** (6), 3–9.

Health and Social Care Information Centre (2012) *Hospital episode statistics: admitted patient care 2011–12 Summary Report*. Crown Copyright. Department of Health, London.

Hurst, J. (2002) The Danish health care system from a British perspective. *Health Policy*, 59 (2), 133–143.

Hurst, K. (2006) Primary and community workforce planning and development. *Journal of Advanced Nursing*, 55 (6), 651–798.

Hurst, J. & Williams, S. (2012) *Can NHS hospital do more with less?* The Nuffield Trust, London.

Imison, C. (2011) *Briefing Paper – Reconfiguring Hospital Services*. The Kings Fund, London. Available from http://www.kingsfund.org.uk/sites/files/kf/briefing-on-reconfiguring-hospital-services-candace-imison-kings-fund-september-2011.pdf. Accessed on 8 March 2013.

Imison, C., Poteliakhoff, E. & Thompson, J. (2012) *Older People and Emergency Bed Use*. The Kings Fund, London. Available from http://www.kingsfund.org.uk/sites/files/kf/field/field_publication_file/older-people-and-emergency-bed-use-aug-2012.pdf. Accessed on 8 March 2013.

James, A. (1995) *Managing to Care: Public Service and the Market*, Longman, London.

Kuhse, H. (1997) *Caring: Nurses, Women and Ethics*, Blackwell, Oxford.

Lakey (2009). *Counting the costs*. Caring for people with dementia on hospital wards. Report, Alzheimer's Society, London.

Laverack, G. (2004) *Health Promotion Practice Power and Empowerment*, Sage, London.

Lawler, J. (1991) *Behind the Screens: Nursing, Somology and the Problem of the Body*, Churchill Livingstone, Edinburgh.

Leff, J. (2001) Why is care in the community perceived as a failure? [Editorial]. *British Journal of Psychiatry*, 179, 381–383.

Maben, J., Adams, M., Peccei, R., Murrells, T. & Robert, G. (2012) Poppets and parcels': the links between staff experience of work and acutely ill older peoples' experience of hospital care. *International Journal of Older Peoples Nursing*, 7, 83–94.

McKeown, T. (1979) *The Role of Medicine. Dream, Mirage or Nemesis?* Blackwell, Oxford.

Maslow, A.H. (1987) *Motivation and Personality*, Harper Collins, New York.

Naidoo, J. & Wills, J. (2009) *Foundations for Health Promotion*, 3rd edn. Elsevier, London.

NHS Commissioning Board (2012) *Commissioning for Quality and Innovation (CQUIN) 2013/14 Guidance*. Crown Copyright, Department of Health, London.

NHS Institute for Innovation and Improvement (2010) *Delivering Quality and Value Directory of Ambulatory Emergency Care for Adults*. Department of Health, London.

OECD (2011) *Health at a Glance: OECD Indicators*. OECD publication, Paris.

Parsons, T. (1979) Definitions of health and illness in the light of American values and social structure. In: *Patients, Physicians and Illness*, (ed E.G. Jaco), pp. 120–144. Free Press, New York.

Procter, S. (2000) *Caring for Health*, Macmillan, London.

Procter, S., Wilson, P., Brooks, F. & Kendall, S. (2012) Success and failure in integrated models of nursing for long term conditions: multiple case studies of whole systems. *International Journal of Nursing Research*. Available from http://dx.doi.org/10.1016/j.ijnurstu.2012.10.007. Accessed on 25 May 2013.

Seedhouse, D. (1986) *Health: The Foundations for Achievement*, John Wiley, Chichester.

Smith, P. (1992) *The Emotional Labour of Nursing*, Macmillan, Basingstoke.

Tarlov, A.R. (1996) Social determinants of health: the sociobiological translation. In: *Health and Social Organisation towards a Health Policy for the 21ˢᵗ Century* (eds D. Blane, E. Brunner & R. Wilkinson). Routledge, London.

Tarlow, B. (1996) Caring: a negotiated process that varies. In: *Caregiving Readings in Knowledge, Practice, Ethics and Politics* (eds S. Gordon, P. Benner & N. Noddings). University of Pennsylvania Press, Philadelphia.

The Marmot Review (2010) Fair Society Healthy Lives. Strategic Review of Health Inequalities in England post-2010. Institute of Health Equity, University College London, London.

Thistlethwaite, P. (2011) *Integrating Health and Social Care in Torbay*, The Kings Fund, London.

Tones, K. & Green, J. (2004) *Health Promotion Planning and Strategies*, Sage Publications, London.

Wanless, D. (2002) *Securing Our Future Health – Taking a Long Term View*. HM Treasury, London.

Watson, J. (1985) *Nursing: Human Science and Human Care*. Appleton-Century-Crofts, Norwalk, Conn.

Watson, B., Myelotte, A. & Procter, S. (2003) Health and social care collaboration: the case of a community outreach service for patients with COPD. *Nursing Times*, 99, 17.

WHO (1946) *Preamble to the Constitution of the World Health Organization as adopted by the International Health Conference*, New York, June 19–22.

Wistow, G. (2000) Home care and the reshaping of hospitals in England: an overview of problems and possibilities. *Journal of Management in Medicine*, 14 (1), 7–24.

5

Evidence-Based Practice and Translational Research Applied to Primary Health Care

Penny Farrelly

Faculty of Society and Health, Buckinghamshire New University,
High Wycombe, UK

Introduction

This chapter aims to assist the reader to understand a range of research methods used when exploring community and public health practice. The chapter can also be read as a 'stand-alone' text that provides the community health care practitioner with the necessary information required to consider how research methodologies, methods and findings are applied in every day practice.

The chapter considers

- Issues relating to evidence-based nursing
- The design of research studies with selected research examples that demonstrate the application of the research process and use of research in community nursing practice
- Research methods
- General research issues
- Ethical issues

Evidence-based practice

Evidence-based practice (EBP) has many definitions. The most widely cited definition of EBP is adapted from Sockett *et al.*'s definition of evidence-based medicine (EBM). This states that EBM is

> the conscientious, explicit and judicious use of current best evidence in making decisions about the care of individual patients. The practice of evidence-based medicine means integrating individual clinical expertise with the best available external clinical evidence from systematic research (Sockett *et al.* 1996, p. 71).

This definition highlights the need to draw on both the professional's clinical experiential knowledge and the best external evidence. Neither is enough on its own. As Sockett and his colleagues point out, clinical practices become out of date if new evidence is not drawn upon. However, the clinician must be aware of what evidence is appropriate to integrate into their practice. This can prove to be a difficult and time-consuming task, but it is an essential skill in implementing EBP.

In the current age of quality assurance and clinical governance, health care staff must strive to provide the best quality of care they can. This recognises Sockett's argument that EBP is 'conscientious', meaning that it requires thought and a questioning attitude to be applied to patient care.

There are many reasons why nurses should engage in EBP. These include

- The increasing complexity of health care decisions and clinical decision making.
- Ensuring that care is provided safely and effectively.
- The Department of Health's directive that services and treatments should be based on the best evidence of what does and does not work (DH 1997).
- The need to provide the most effective care in the most productive manner.
- Compliance with the Codes of Professional Conduct.
- The nurse's ability to make informed judgments is of importance to patients and assists nurses' in being valued members of multidisciplinary teams.
- Nurses do not have the time to read extensively. The pragmatic process of appraising and using the literature benefits patients whilst also expanding the nurses' knowledge base.

The problem lies in attempting to define 'evidence'. In the past nursing as a profession has been guilty of relying on trial and error and custom and practice, building up a body of knowledge from what does and does not appear to work. Clearly this is unacceptable for patients who expect more from today's nurses who are required to make informed clinical decisions based on recent evidence of clinical effectiveness. Nurses generally have little time to engage in extensive reading of multiple research articles so it is advisable to access a systematic review which summarises the results from a large number of high-quality research studies. These can be found on a wide range of topics relevant to nursing in the online Cochrane Library. If, however, this fails to answer the specific question that needs answering, then a full literature search of articles published in scientific journals should be conducted. A number of bibliographic databases are available to assist practitioners to search the literature. The most commonly known are

- CINAHL (nursing-related journals)
- MEDLINE

The main barrier to evidence-based nursing care is the lack of ability to critically evaluate research on the part of the nurses. Practice settings may also be resistant to change which may limit the ability of the nurse to provide evidence-based care. However, there will always be a desire to improve the care of our patients. The spiralling cost of health care and the need for more accuracy in clinical decision making proves the need for evidence-based health care and for engagement with the research process.

Designing the study

When designing a research study, it is important to ensure that the research design responds appropriately to the type of research question being considered and the type of evidence required to inform the study. Examples of research designs frequently used in primary health care research include experimental research and clinical trials, descriptive and explanatory surveys, case studies and participatory approaches. Many of these designs are concerned with evaluation, which is a key interest for primary care research. As Gray (2009) observes, the methodology chosen

> will be influenced by the theoretical perspectives adopted by the researcher, and, in turn, by the researcher's epistemological stance (p. 19).

A range of different research methods and analysis tools will be applied, depending upon the research question to be answered.

Translational research

Overview

Translational research is becoming a popular system, particularly in the USA, of moving scientific discoveries from the scientist at 'the bench to the bedside'. This method allows for the faster development of innovation so that research becomes disseminated rapidly for use by multi-disciplinary teams with the aim of improving the effectiveness of clinical interventions and patient experience.

Turning clinical research discoveries into marketable products is a difficult and often lengthy process, so ways of improving the efficiency of early adoption and implementation are important. For example, an inventor may need to do further work on the proof of concept of a technology to link skills in the physical sciences to those in biology and medicine. They may also need to bring together the right combination of business expertise to develop the product and position it within the market – anticipating ahead what the market will be looking for and deciding how the innovation will be introduced alongside other competitors. Translational research helps to overcome such obstacles, bridging the gap between basic research and a marketable product. Funding schemes such as those provided by 'Technology Transfer' at the Wellcome Trust therefore aim to advance the development of an innovation to the point where it becomes attractive for others – such as venture capital firms, industry or public–private partnerships – encouraging the take-up of the challenge of producing a product that is suitable for the market. This will mean that new innovations will become available to the general public in a much more speedy and efficient manner.

Experiments, randomised controlled trials and quasi-experiments

The experimental approach, referred to as the 'randomised controlled trial' (RCT), has been widely applied to the study of interventions on human subjects, and as Parahoo (2006) notes: 'Nursing like all other health professions, needs to justify it's practice on sound evidence', and a double-blind RCT is seen as a gold standard in the hierarchy of evidence.

In order to decide on the specific design for the trial, researchers need to be clear from the outset of their aims and should be sure that the method they choose to research their subject is 'fit for purpose' (Newell & Burnard 2011). Study design incorporates every stage of the study including decisions about sampling, size, the techniques by which the subjects will be allocated to a treatment (or non-treatment group), how the intervention will be introduced, the statistical applications required and the methods by which the study outcome will be evaluated.

The phenomena under study are broken down or reduced to smaller components known as 'variables'. Smoking, for example, may be broken down into variables which are chosen because they are assumed to have explanatory value that will contribute to theory testing, prediction and new knowledge. Subjects recruited to take part in studies need to be representative of the population from which they are drawn and bear sufficient similarity to the type of individuals likely to benefit from the intervention. Clear inclusion criteria therefore should be identified for this purpose. It is important that variables related to class, age, gender and ethnicity are taken into consideration.

For example, it has been shown that studies have been undertaken with a bias towards white middle-class males with a risk that the needs of women, ethnic minority groups and older people will be overlooked. The famous Framingham Heart Study undertaken in the USA, for example, provided detailed knowledge of the risk factors associated with cardiovascular disease in white middle-class men but did not take sufficient account of the specific risks for women and people of different ethnic backgrounds (www.framingham.com; www.nhlbi.nih.gov/about/framingham/riskabs.htm).

A study of people with strokes who had not been admitted to hospital used an RCT to assess the impact of offering them a package of occupational therapy for up to 5 months, compared with a control group who received 'routine practice' (Walker *et al.* 1999). The results were very encouraging in that the measures used to assess activities of daily living and 'carer strain' suggested that the intervention produced more favourable results compared with the people in the control group. The main differences between an experimental and a quasi-experimental design are that both approaches involve an intervention; however, a quasi-experimental study does not include randomisation in its sampling frame and such studies are referred to as controlled trials without randomisation and quasi-experiments also do not have control groups in their design.

A 'placebo' group may also be added to the experimental and control groups. In such instances the placebo group receives a modified version of the treatment or intervention. The reason to introduce a placebo group into the study design is twofold. First, it helps to discount bias on the part of researcher or patient in their judgment (whether favourable or otherwise) towards the experimental intervention. Second, it provides a control for the frequency of spontaneous changes that may occur in the patient, independent of the intervention under study. Placebos are very often used in experimental studies for testing the effectiveness of drugs or other interventions.

Health impact assessments

Health impact assessment (HIA) is an evaluation strategy designed to measure the effects of public policies on individual and community health. HIA is recommended in *Saving Lives: Our Healthier Nation* (DH 1999) and is of two types: prospective (the impact of a new policy on health is evaluated ahead of its introduction to maximise the potential benefits) and retrospective (the impact of a policy is monitored following its introduction). HIA can also be used to inform better decisions for future policy and practice at a local, national and international level (World Health Organization 2012).

Because HIA is such an important part of government commitment to implementing an effective public health agenda, primary care practitioners need to be aware of the methodologies currently being developed. These methodologies can be applied to a variety of projects, policies and programmes and are represented diagrammatically in Box 5.1 (DH 1999):

A dedicated website (www.hiagateway.org.uk) has been dedicated to the dissemination and implementation of HIA. The website contains case studies written by practitioners and policymakers with personal experience of using this evaluative methodology. The case studies included in the site present examples of how using HIA has provided opportunities to increase community participation as well as a mechanism to evaluate

BOX 5.1   Evaluative tools

The choice of evaluative technique in any appraisal of policy will depend partly on the question to be addressed and partly on availability of data. These approaches to evaluation are summarised here:

- *Cost-effectiveness analysis (CEA)* – If alternative (non-health care) policies yield the same type of effect, but at different volumes, then CEA is the appropriate evaluative technique, and the output of the analysis will be expressed in terms of cost-effectiveness (CEA) ratios, that is, 'cost per unit of effect'.
- *Cost utility analysis (CUA)* – This is a special case of cost-effectiveness analysis where the effects are measured in some generic way such as quality adjusted life years (QALYS).
- *Cost benefit analysis (CBA)* – This type of analysis enables an assessment to be made of the worth of implementing a policy or not (rather than implementing policy A vs. policy B). CBA converts all costs and benefits to monetary terms: if the value of the costs exceeds the value of the benefits, then this suggests that it is not worthwhile to implement the policy.

the impact of a range of cross-sectoral initiatives including transport, air quality, nutrition and sports facilities (www.hiagateway.org.uk/contacts/personal_experiences). The case studies illustrate the broad remit of public health and the need for the community practitioners to be aware of local initiatives that may impact on and go beyond their own roles. This approach will form a key component of how Public Health England transacts its evaluative role in the future.

Surveys

Most people are familiar with surveys either as investigators or respondents. There are two types: the descriptive survey used to collect biographical, demographic and attitudinal information and the explanatory survey set up to find out 'why'. The Office for National Statistics regularly conducts a whole range of routine and special surveys. The national census is the prime example of a survey that describes the total population. More usually a representative sample has to be drawn. The 2011 Census revealed very useful information which could be invaluable for community health care practitioners, in terms of ideas for further research, such as

- On census night the population in England and Wales was 56.1 million, 53.0 million in England and 3.1 million in Wales. This was the largest the population had ever been.
- The population of England and Wales grew by 3.7 million in the 10 years since the last census, rising from 52.4 million in 2001, an increase of 7.1%. This was the

largest growth in the population in England and Wales in any 10-year period since census taking began, in 1801.

- The median age of the population in England and Wales was 39. For men, the median age was 38 and for women it was 40. In 1911, the median age was 25.
- The percentage of the population aged 65 and over was the highest seen in any census at 16.4%, that is, 1 in 6 people in the population was 65 and over.
- There were 430,000 residents aged 90 and over in 2011 compared with 340 000 in 2001 and 13 000 in 1911.
- In 2011, there were 3.5 million children under 5 in England and Wales, 406 000 more than in 2001.

Whilst the census represents the largest survey carried out in Great Britain, it is of equal importance for practitioners to realise that small-scale studies are valuable for giving insights on local situations while identifying areas for further enquiry.

Case studies

Case studies allow the researcher to gain in-depth perspectives on a situation or an incident (Bell 2005; Parahoo 2006). The case study can be combined with a range of qualitative methodologies. Ethnography, for example, involves participant observation and interviewing during extended periods of fieldwork.

Scholes *et al.* (2008) used a case study approach in their evaluation study whereby the focus of the case study was the organisation rather than the individual, thus allowing a picture of the cumulative experiences to be built up. Data were collected by participant observation and interviews with a range of stakeholders and analysed within the prism of the organisations involved.

Different methodologies and methods give you new insights

Knutsson *et al.* (2008) undertook a study which looked at children's experiences and needs when visiting relatives on an intensive care unit. The study found that the children did not appear to be frightened by the visit and instead 'it generated feelings of release and relief' (p. 155). This hermeneutic study allowed the author's insight into the thoughts and feelings of the child respondents, thus establishing what the children thought rather than what adults thought the children thought!

In relation to long-term conditions, epidemiological data will provide information about how many people have a particular condition, how old they are and where they live. Studies such as that by Clark *et al.* (2008) complement that data. Clark *et al.* looked at the complexities of informal care giving for people with chronic heart failure using semi-structured interviews with informal careers. Clark *et al.* concluded that the management of heart failure was a shared and ongoing responsibility between the patient and the carer and although the carer had limited clinical knowledge, their expertise was in the effect of the condition on the patient.

Participatory approaches for community research

A number of research approaches are available to primary health care researchers that involve local participants and contribute to empowering and improving their lives and communities. Community participation is also a key health promotion concept (Strachin *et al.* 2007; Pearson 2008). Readers will be familiar with action research, a popular methodology with health care researchers (Bell 2005; Parahoo 2006). Action research is usually associated with participatory and collective forms of research although at its most extreme it can be set up as an experiment in which an 'intervention' is tested and its outcomes monitored (Coghlan & Brannick 2005).

The central tenet of action research is the cyclical process of intervention, evaluation and feedback with researchers and participants working closely together. Action and other participatory forms of research balance generalisable knowledge and benefit to the community by collaborating as experts and as equals in the research process (Macaulay *et al.* 1999).

The public health agenda described earlier with its emphasis on partnership working and the major NHS reorganisations that are currently underway, particularly within Clinical Commissioning Groups and community provider services, suggests the appropriateness to the community practitioner of understanding the principles of action research to gain insights into the process of developing complex relationships and managing change.

Participatory appraisal

Participatory appraisal (PA), a community research approach, encapsulates the current government commitment to eliminate social exclusion and reduce poverty. It involves multi-agency and partnership working to assess needs and involves local communities in order to effect and evaluate change. It also demonstrates the range of methods available to primary health care practitioners.

Pain and Francis (2003) describe PA as 'participatory approaches (methodologies and epistemologies that aim to effect change for and with research participants)'. Investigators involved in participatory methods are concerned with issues of empowerment and the relationship between research and action. The aim of PA is to enable those from marginalised groups to make their needs known while at the same time encourage debate within communities and agencies involved in developmental work with them.

Feurstein's model of participatory evaluation has been adapted by Smithies and Adams (1993) to systematise an approach that is subject to competing agendas and unpredictable outcomes while maintaining a commitment to community development. The model is presented as a cyclical process and emphasises the importance of capacity building to equip local people to develop local initiatives. The model offers a framework that evaluates and builds on any initiatives forthcoming from the PA.

Data collection methods

Methods are the techniques of doing research: asking questions, observing people and groups, analysing case records and sifting through historical documents and local newspapers (Pope & Mays 2000; Bell 2005; Parahoo 2006).

A variety of research methods can be used within a study, irrespective of the underlying paradigm and approach. The use of a multi-method research approach is described as 'triangulation' by which more than one method is used and/or groups of people are studied within the same project (Foss & Ellefsen 2002). This has the advantage of validating the findings as data are from different sources, different paradigms and different subjects, thus affording a more comprehensive understanding of the phenomenon being studied.

Data management, analysis and interpretation

How data are analysed in a study will depend on the research questions being asked and the methodologies and methods being used. Data analysis is often the most time-consuming part of the research. For example, if it takes 2 months to collect data, it is likely to take 4 months to analyse and interpret them. In order for researchers to retrieve their data easily and accurately for analysis and interpretation, it is important that during data collection, they develop systems to ensure this. In quantitative studies, it is likely that the data are coded, collected and recorded on standardised forms, for example, self-administered questionnaires and structured interview schedules.

In qualitative studies, the researcher develops ways of recording fieldwork notes during participant observation, such as by keeping index cards to record observations as events take place, for example, mealtimes in a day nursery. Interviews are (with the participants' permission) most often tape-recorded and then transcribed to facilitate analysis of the interview contents.

In large-sample surveys, data are likely to be stored in a computer. This will potentially ease and speed up data analysis. If the sample is small, it may be quicker to analyse the data by hand. Data, it should be remembered, are only as good as the operator who enters them into the computer and the logic that inspires decisions about statistical tests. Preparing data for analysis may also be very time-consuming. Data analysis produces summary statistics (e.g. frequencies and average – mean, median and modes) and appropriate statistical significance tests (Greenhalgh 2006).

Statistical analysis can be undertaken using such programs as Statistical Package for the Social Sciences (SPSS) or Minitab and textual analysis, for example, the 'Nudist' and 'Ethnograph' programs, which are constantly being revised. Statistical tests are based on probability theory, and a statistician is usually consulted to advise on the appropriate test given the sample size, type of data and questions being asked. In short, the data are manipulated statistically in order to ensure the results have not occurred by chance. The importance of logic in interpreting results cannot be underestimated.

A 'significant' result does not mean that 'cause' and 'effect' are automatically established. First, the researcher must ensure that a number of conditions are met if causality between variables is to be demonstrated. Sometimes an accidental link may bind independent and dependent variables together in a 'spurious' relationship, confounding results or muddling the picture (Greenhalgh 2006).

The hallmark of the qualitative research process is that coding and analysis take place alongside data collection. The researcher then decides what future data should be collected and from where and whom they should be obtained. During the process, in-depth descriptions, interpretations and theoretical perspectives are generated. Phenomena are then described through narratives and accounts as a way of understanding, explaining and making inferences. Latent and content analysis can be used to analyse transcripts and develop themes and categories (Field & Morse 1998; Holloway & Wheeler 2002).

Melia (1982) in her now classic study used grounded theory, now further developed by Strauss and Corbin (1994), and in-depth interviews to study student nurse socialisation. Analysis yielded six conceptual categories, which were then used as a framework for presenting substantive issues raised by the students. The categories were 'learning and working', 'getting the work done', 'learning the rules', 'nursing in the dark', 'just passing through', 'doing nursing' and 'being professional'. From 'nursing in the dark', for example, she derived further categories, which she labelled 'coping with the dark', 'fobbing off the patient' and 'awareness contexts'.

In PA, analysis is collaborative and collective and, as described in the example in the succeeding text, permits a variety of needs and concerns to be expressed. Processed data are referred to as 'findings' or 'results'. Methods of data analysis vary according to the underlying research approach. Qualitative research is presented through words and narratives and quantitative research through numbers and statistical manipulations and also in tables and graphs (Holloway & Wheeler 2002; Greenhalgh 2006).

A multi-method evaluation of a clinical educational innovation

A multi-method evaluation was undertaken by Scholes *et al.* (2008) to evaluate the impact on practice of an education innovation, the development of physical assessment skills modules for nurses. The approach was a 360-degree evaluation and as many stakeholders as possible were involved in the evaluation. Interviews, both face to face and telephone, were undertaken with the alumnae of the course, the general practitioners or other medical staff they worked with and, where appropriate, patients and carers. The nurses' managers were also interviewed in order to determine if their expectations of the nurses post-course had been met. Observations of the interactions between the nurses and the patients they were examining were also undertaken. The sample was purposive and recruitment relied on local contacts. The multi-method approach allowed the researchers to build up a picture of the impact of the nurses' development physical assessment skills on a range of stakeholders. Comparisons were made between the findings and the literature.

Different perspectives were elicited by the different methods. Interviews allowed the researchers and participants to explore issues related to the topic in more depth; the telephone interviews were more focused and used a more predetermined format. However, the telephone interviews, by saving on travel time, allowed the researchers to widen their sample using the semi-structured schedule that had been employed during face to face interviews.

Example of PA

Pain and Francis (2003) undertook a project with homeless young people, young people who had been excluded from school and people who were working with these young people. The aim of the project was to explore the experiences of the homeless and excluded young people in order to understand the experiences of victimisation and concerns about crime and disorder. The authors employed a range of data collection methods such as interviews and observations. However, they also used participatory diagramming whereby the young people used tools such as Post-its and coloured pens to identify, discuss and prioritise issues. Where solutions were identified, the participants were encouraged to act on them if they wanted to. The data from the project were verified with the participants.

General research issues

Validity, reliability and generalisability

Regardless of methodological considerations, all researchers must consider issues of validity and reliability. In quantitative research, reliability refers to the extent to which methods and settings are consistent over time, across groups and between researchers. Validity refers to the accuracy and truth of the data being produced in terms of the concepts being investigated, the people and objects being studied and the methods of data collection and analysis being used.

For qualitative researchers the social context in which data are collected is important to consider. During field observations, for example, as researchers become increasingly familiar with the research setting, they are able to check the accuracy and recurrence of data in a number of different situations and from a variety of participant perspectives.

Validity and reliability are important concepts in large-scale studies, such as clinical trials and surveys, if the studies are to be generalisable. This is a particular concern in undertaking systematic reviews to ensure the robustness of the findings.

Meta-analysis takes account of these issues by reviewing the populations, methodologies and findings of a number of studies on a given topic. Statistical analysis is then applied to assess the significance of the combined results. Results from qualitative research are not normally generalisable to the wider population due to the small sample sizes and contextualised nature of the findings.

However, such findings have theoretical generalisability in terms of their ability to relate the results to raise awareness about experiences of others and the implications for practice. One of the authors of the previous edition of this chapter conducted a phenomenological study (Vydelingum 2000), and despite the small purposive sample, the findings of this study have nonetheless given important insights into the experiences of South Asian patients in hospital. The isolation and loneliness encountered by patients due to communication difficulties should make nurses more aware of such experiences and hopefully discuss these issues with relatives. Nurses would be able to pay more attention to the information given to South Asian patients and relatives about their conditions and aftercare and ensure that supportive domiciliary services are mobilised.

In qualitative research, concepts of validity and reliability are not easily transferable. There is a lot of debate and controversy about the best ways to evaluate qualitative research (Sandelowski 1993; Koch 1994). However, Guba and Lincoln (1989) proposed four main methods for establishing rigour in qualitative studies – dependability, credibility, transferability and confirmability:

- *Dependability (reliability)* – Findings of the study need to be consistent and correct to be dependable, so that anyone reading the study will be able to evaluate the sufficiency of the analysis and results from the research process.
- *Credibility (internal validity)* – The extent to which readers and participants can recognise the meaning that they give to the situations or contexts or the 'truth value' of the results.
- *Transferability (generalisability)* – How the results in one context could be 'transferred' to comparable situations or participants. In some cases, due to the small-scale samples utilised, theoretical transferability could be achieved.
- *Confirmability (objectivity)* – This method requires an audit or decision trail for readers who can judge the study for the intellectual honesty, researchers' bias and openness to sensitivity to the methods.

Presentation and dissemination

Presentation and research dissemination are essential so that findings are made available to be used and applied by others. Researchers may change their style of presentation according to their audience. Indeed, the *Journal of Advanced Nursing* is highly respected by a nursing professional, but to the non-researcher, articles here may appear 'jargonistic', using language that is difficult to understand. However, in the *Nursing Times* the language is more accessible and easier to understand by the field-level practitioner. The convention in quantitative research is to maintain objectivity and authority by writing in the third person. Qualitative, and particularly feminist, researchers prefer to write in the first person. In this way, they write themselves into their research accounts and make their methods and findings more transparent to the reader.

The notion of networks is an important part of the modernised health service and has been set up for the purposes of practitioners sharing expertise and knowledge across NHS trusts. The public health networks have been set up primarily to allow public health specialists and practitioners across community services to share good practice, manage public health knowledge and very importantly act as a source of learning and professional development. These networks also offer contacts with universities to support research, education and development and joint cross boundary collaborations across the health service.

The internet or world wide web (www)

The internet is useful for gathering and sharing information on web pages, by email and in forum discussions and newsgroups. It also influences the way research is conducted and disseminated. Although there has been massive investment in information technology, some practitioners still do not have access to the internet, and inequalities still exist between different parts of the country and different professional groups. This situation is improving as the NHS commits itself to ensuring that its employees have access to e-mail and a vast range of electronically accessible databases. It is essential that access and training are provided to practitioners because of the many uses of information technology and the net. Because information develops at such a fast rate, information published in more traditional media, such as books and journals, are in danger of being out of date before they are published!

Professional, ethical and information sharing issues are associated with research on the net. At present, it is extremely difficult to regulate the internet or hold individuals or companies responsible for unethical research practices. Copyright on the net is ambiguous, meaning not only is most information free and transcends boundaries, but also individuals and companies are not accountable for bad press of individuals, libellous remarks or improper research and ethical practices. Web service providers say they are unable to regulate what goes on their notice boards or is discussed in forums.

The main message to be taken from this by potential researchers is to be extremely cautious about the information received and transmitted via the internet. Currently, large amounts of information are available and positive and negative uses of the internet must be considered.

Research proposals

Monkley-Poole (1997) suggests

> There can be many reasons for writing a proposal apart from "pure" research. For example, similar principles can be applied to writing proposals to obtain resources to introduce change into clinical practice or undertake an audit of services. Proposals can also be

submitted to request funding to support study leave or attendance at a conference. In the health service, the move to the market with its emphasis on evidence based health care suggests the need for practitioners to attract monies to fund research and to clearly identify and document research activities being undertaken in the clinical areas.

A proposal puts forward the argument for why a piece of research is worth doing, how it will add to the body of knowledge and the plans and procedures necessary to successfully complete it. The applicant also includes a short curriculum vitae to demonstrate that he/she has the necessary experience for the job. When writing any proposal, it is important to consider the membership of the panel or committee who will be taking decisions based on its content since each member will have different backgrounds and biases. It is important to be clear and explicit when putting together the proposal especially if the people making decisions about it are likely to be unfamiliar with its approach. Another source of guidance for preparing and submitting a research proposal is provided by Punch (2006).

Ethical issues

Irrespective of paradigm, approach or method, research proposals should always be scrutinised for their ethical implications and submitted to an ethics committee for approval prior to commencement of the study. It is perhaps worth noting that people involved in research are called different things depending on the research design, for example, they are called *subjects* in experimental studies, *respondents* in surveys and *participants* in qualitative research such as ethnography or phenomenology, and by virtue of what they are called can give you an indication of the type of activities involved. Research subjects should also be fully informed of the study's implications before giving their written consent and be able to withdraw without prejudice at any time. Participant observation should not be covert and researchers using this method should be clear about their role.

All research activity must comply with the Research Governance Framework for Health and Social Care (DH 2010), as in general terms, health authorities and Clinical Commissioning Groups owe a direct and non-delegable duty of care to NHS patients. The framework clarifies responsibilities and accountabilities that define the setting in which negligence might occur and refers to the responsibility of researchers' employers.

Research ethics is managed through an 'Integrated Research Application System' (IRAS) which integrates research approvals for all health and social care/community care in the United Kingdom. This is an online system that can be accessed through the following website: https://www.myresearchproject.org.uk/Signin.aspx

All applications for ethical approval are processed through a single online portal. The IRAS application form includes a number of filters which organise the content of the application form. Links to any 'Site-Specific Information' (SSI) forms that are required as part of the application process are included in the portal depending on the information entered by the applicant. Following completion of the form, the application may be submitted directly via the portal to the appropriate regulatory body. An online tutorial and helpline are available on the IRAS website.

IRAS

- Provides a single system for applying for the permissions and approvals for health and social care/community care research in the United Kingdom.
- Enables researchers and students to enter the information about their project once instead of duplicating information in separate application forms.
- Uses filters to ensure that the data collected and collated is appropriate to the type of study and consequently the permissions and approvals required.
- Assists researchers and students to meet regulatory and governance requirements.

IRAS captures the information needed for the relevant approvals from the following research review bodies:

- Administration of Radioactive Substances Advisory Committee (ARSAC)
- Gene Therapy Advisory Committee (GTAC)
- Medicines and Healthcare Products Regulatory Agency (MHRA)
- Ministry of Justice
- NHS/HSC R&D offices
- NRES/NHS/HSC Research Ethics Committees
- National Information Governance Board (NIGB)
- National Offender Management Service (NOMS)
- Social Care Research Ethics Committee

The NHS research passport

Permission to undertake research in organisations other than the one the applicant is employed in has led to the creation of a research passport. The use of the research passport is recommended good practice by the Department of Health for all NHS organisations and researchers wanting to undertake research in NHS settings. It is not therefore mandatory and NHS organisations do not have to use it. The research passport provides one set of personal information required by human resource departments before they can issue an honorary contract. This includes one Criminal Records Bureau (CRB) check that is designed to reduce duplication created by multiple honorary contracts required for research purposes between NHS employing organisations:

> 'The Research in the NHS – HR Good Practice Resource Pack' consists of a 'Research Passport' system for HEI researchers who need to undertake their research within NHS

organisations; and standardised procedures for issuing 'Honorary Research Contracts' (HRCs) or 'Letters of Access' (LoAs), in line with the nature of the researchers' activity, and the NHS and/or employer's responsibility for that activity. (NIHR 2012)

Ethics committees are also found in universities, and students carrying out research as part of an academic award are expected to apply to their respective university ethics committees. Professional bodies, such as the Royal College of Physicians and the Royal College of Nursing, produce guidelines to assist researchers in considering the ethical dimensions of their research proposals (RCN 2009). Similar guidelines are available from the British Psychological Society and the British Sociological Association for researchers. The Association for Research in the Voluntary and Community Sector (ARVAC) has a set of ethical guidelines sensitive to the complex needs of the sector and which focus on the research subjects' rights. Researchers are urged to take account of equal opportunities, in terms of race, gender, disability and sexual orientation and the principles, values, objectives and agendas of the participants. The development of 'mutually beneficial relationships' between researchers and researched, set within the wider 'social, political and economic setting', is seen as key (ARVAC 2000, www.arvac.org.uk).

Unexpected ethical consequences can result from 'neutral', seemingly theoretical science; for example, the application of theoretical physics to the development of the atom bomb did untold harm and formed no part of Einstein's original intentions. Similarly, Darwin's theory of evolution was used by many Victorian biologists to advance pejorative racial stereotypes. This was especially true in Australia during the nineteenth century. Social Darwinism, as it was known, put forward racist stereotypes of aboriginal inferiority that tried to establish European cultural dominance. This approach continues to this day.

Unlike obviously intrusive clinical trials and research practices such as giving placebos rather than treatment or testing drugs with unknown side effects, qualitative research not involving patients or clients is often seen as exempt from the need to be scrutinised by an ethics committee. However, ethical implications of covert research, that is, research undertaken without the subjects' knowledge, are apparent when findings are reported without subjects ever having known they were being observed.

Consider, too, the ethical implications of interviews about feelings and emotions and the need to consider the participant's view with respect to research on women involving cervical screening (Howson 1999) or young women's experiences of abortion (Harden & Ogden 1999). Such interviews need to be carefully managed so as not to distress the interviewee.

Ethics committees

Ethics committees are set up to regulate good ethical practice in the conduct of health care research. In the United Kingdom the National Research Ethics Service (NRES) collaborates with colleagues to maintain a UK-wide system of ethical review that protects the safety, dignity and well-being of research participants whilst facilitating and promoting ethical research within the NHS. Through the granting of ethical approval, ethics committees are ensuring that health care research adheres to the basic principles of the Helsinki Declaration and the EU Convention on Human Rights.

The Human Rights Act 1998, active since 2000, contains numerous articles that are relevant to health care research. Protection of right to life (Article 2), prohibition of torture or degrading treatment or punishment (Article 30), right to liberty and security (Article 5), right to respect for private and family life (Article 8) and freedom of thought, conscience and religion (Article 9) should be included for consideration in study proposals to protect the interests and well-being of research participants. Further information on the requirements for ethics committees is available on local NHS provider websites and the Department of Health website, including NRES (http://www.nres.npsa.nhs.uk/).

Ethics committees require researchers to prepare written proposals to demonstrate the proposed study's adherence to ethical principles, such as autonomy, consent, justice, beneficence and non-malevolence. Practically, this may involve the signing of a consent form, following a full explanation of events, before the research commences. Informed consent signifies that the potential participants have had the opportunity to get satisfactory information or explanation about the research and their roles and expectations clarified. It is also important for researchers to allow the participants sufficient time to consider the information before making a decision, and they should also be offered guarantees that a refusal to participate in the research will not jeopardise the care or service they receive. Any nurse is within her rights to ask to see the consent form before allowing researchers' access to patients.

Research relating to people with mental health problems, with a learning disability or with children is problematic. This is because these groups are vulnerable to improper research practices. There is the issue of whether children, the people with learning disabilities and mental health service users may make informed decisions and give their full consent (or whether someone can consent on their behalf). Informed consent is particularly important if one considers the capacities of these groups as they are spelled out in law.

Conclusion

Research is the combination of systematic inquiry and a personal journey. The personal interests and style of each researcher and practitioner influence the questions asked and the approaches taken.

It is hoped that this chapter will generate ideas for the reader about the approaches and findings used for the study of community nursing and public health care and their application to practice. In particular, it identifies the knowledge base for primary health care and the topics and methodologies of relevance to the field. Reflective practice and research mindedness are described as part of the primary care practitioner's toolkit for recognising and drawing on experience which in turn contributes to the evidence base which informs research and practice. The world wide web plays an important part in making a wide range of materials electronically accessible as part of the policy, practice and research base. Issues such as ethics, proposal writing and funding are also raised to further assist primary care practitioners to apply and use research.

Research, in its various guises, is no longer an optional extra in the modern health service. Indeed, the current NHS agenda actively supports the development of a critical research culture. This chapter is designed to assist primary care and public health practitioners to shape a role for themselves within that culture in order to meet their own professional and personal needs and those of patients and clients.

Acknowledgments

The author wishes to acknowledge reliance on work included in Chapter 6 of the fourth edition of this text written by Vasso Vydelingum, Pam Smith and Pat Colliety who were the original authors of the previous version of this chapter.

Further reading

Audit Commission Reports – http://www.audit-commission.gov.uk
Cochrane database – www.cochrane.org
Department of Health – www.gov.uk
Eppi-Centre – http://eppi.ioe.ac.uk
Health Impact Assessment – http://www.hiagateway.org.uk
National Institute of Clinical Excellence (NICE) – http://www.nice.org.uk
The National Electronic Library for Health (NeLH) – www.library.nhs.uk
National Institute for Health Research – http://www.nihr.ac.uk/
The 2011 Census – www.statistics.gov.uk/census2011
The Public Health Electronic Library (PHel) – http://www.evidence.nhs.uk
York Centre for Systematic Reviews and Dissemination – http://www.york.ac.uk/inst/crd/

Journals

Links Page – http://www.sciencekomm.at/journals/medicine/nurse.html
Nursing Standard – http://www.nursing-standard.co.uk
The *Journal of Advanced Nursing* – http://www.blackwell-synergy.com/issuelist.asp?journal/jan
The *Nursing Times* – http://www.nursingtimes.net/
The *Sociology of Health and Illness* – http://www.blackwellpublishers.co.uk/journals/SHIL/

Ethics

National Research Ethics Service – http://www.nres.npsa.nhs.uk/
The Human Rights Act 1998 – http://www.gov.uk/acts/1998/htm

Funding

Directory of Grant Making Trusts – http://www.trustfunding.org.uk
Florence Nightingale Foundation – http://www.florence-nightingale-foundation.org.uk
Foundation of Nursing Studies – http://www.fons.org
National Institute of Health Research – http://www.nihr.ac.uk
The Association of Medical Research Charities – http://www.amrc.org.uk
The NHS Service Delivery and Organisation (SDO) Research and Development programme – http://www.sdo.lshtm.ac.uk

Statutory body

Nursing and Midwifery Council – http://www.nmc-uk.org

References

ARVAC Bulletin (2000) *Ethical guidelines*. Association for research in the Voluntary and Community Sector, Norwich.

Bell, J. (2005) *Doing your Research Project: A Guide for First Time Researchers in Education and Social Science*, 3rd edn. Open University Press, Buckingham.

Clark, A., Reid, M., Morrison, C., Capewell, S., Murdoch, L. & McMurray, J. (2008) The complex nature of informal care in home-based heart failure management. *Journal of Advanced Nursing*, 61 (4), 373–383.

Coghlan, D. & Brannick, T. (2005) *Doing Action Research in Your Own Organization*, (2nd edn). Sage, Thousand Oaks, CA.

Department of Health (DH) (1997) *The New NHS: Modern, Dependable*, Stationery Office, London.

DH (1999) *Saving Lives: Our Healthier Nation*, DH, London.

DH (2004) *NHS Improvement Plan: Putting people at the Heart of the Public Services*, DH, London.

DH (2010) *Research Governance Framework for Health and Social Care*, DH, London.

Field, P.A. & Morse, J.M. (1998) *Nursing Research: The Application of Qualitative Approaches*. Chapman and Hill, London.

Foss, C. & Ellefsen, B. (2002) Methodological issues in nursing research. *Journal of Advanced Nursing*, 40 (2), 242–248.

Gray, D. (2009) *Doing Research in the Real World*, Sage, London.

Greenhalgh, T. (2006) *How to Read a Paper: The Basics of Evidence-Based Medicine*, 3rd edn. BMJ Books/Blackwell, Oxford, Malden, MA.

Guba, E.G. & Lincoln, Y.S. (1989) *Fourth Generation Evaluation*. Sage, Newbury Park, CA.

Harden, A. & Ogden, J. (1999) Young women's experiences of arranging and having abortions. *Sociology of Health and Illness*, 21 (4), 426–444.

Holloway, I. & Wheeler, S. (2002) *Qualitative Research in Nursing*, 2nd edn. Blackwell Publishing, Oxford.

Howson, A. (1999) Cervical screening, compliance and moral obligation. *Sociology of Health and Illness*, 21 (4), 401–425.

Koch, T. (1994) Establishing rigour in qualitative research: the decision trail. *Journal of Advanced Nursing*, 19, 976–986.

Knutsson, S., Samuelsson, I.P., Hellstrom, A. & Bergborn, I. (2008) Children's experiences of visiting a seriously ill/injured relative on an adult intensive care unit. *Journal of Advanced Nursing*, 61 (2), 154–162.

Macaulay, A., Commanda, L., Freeman, W., et al. (1999) Participatory research maximises community and lay involvement. *British Medical Journal*, 319, 774–778.

Melia, K. (1982) 'Tell it as it is': qualitative methodology and nursing research: understanding the student nurse's world. *Journal of Advanced Nursing*, 7, 327–335.

Monkley-Poole, (1997) Research proposal writing and funding. In: *Research Mindedness for Practice* (ed. P. Smith). Churchill Livingstone, Edinburgh.

National Institute for Health Research (NIHR) (2012) Research in the NHS – HR Good Practice Resource Pack: HR Good Practice: Information for researchers, R&D and HR staff in Higher Education Institutions and the NHS. Available from http://www.nihr.ac.uk/systems/Pages/systems_research_passports.aspx. Accessed on 20 November 2012.

Pain, R. & Francis, P. (2003) Reflections on participatory research. *Area*, 35 (1), 46–54.

Parahoo, K. (2006) *Nursing Research: Principles, Process and Issues*, (2nd edn). Palgrave Macmillan, Basingstoke.

Parliament (2011) The National Census. Available from www.statistics.gov.uk/census2011. Accessed on 19 November 2012.

Pearson, P. (2008) Public health and health promotion. In: *Community Public Health in Policy and Practice*, (ed S. Cowley), 2nd edn, pp. 46–60. Balliere Tindall Elsevier, Edinburgh.

Pope, C. & Mays, N. (eds.) (2000) *Qualitative Research in Health Care*. BMJ Books, London.

Punch, K. (2006) *Developing Effective Research Proposals*, 2nd edn. Sage, London.

Royal College of Nursing (RCN) (2009) *RCN Guidance for Nurses*. RCN, London.

Sandelowski, M. (1993) Rigor or rigor mortis: the problem of rigor in qualitative research. *Advances in Nursing Sciences*, 16 (2), 1–8.

Scholes, J., Chellel, A., Scott-Smith, W., Volante, M., Coulter, M. & Colliety, P. (2008) *An Evaluation of an Educational Intervention (Physical Assessment Module) for the Non-Medical Workforce to Efficiently Provide Unscheduled Services Across the Primary and Secondary Sector in One SHA*. University of Brighton/University of Surrey, Guildford.

Smithies, J. & Adams, L. (1993) Walking the tightrope: issues in evaluation and community participation for health for all. In: *Healthy Cities: Research and Practice* (eds J. Davis & M. Kelly). Routledge, London.

Strachin, G., Wright, G. & Hancock, E. (2007) An evaluation of a community health intervention programme aimed at improving health and wellbeing. *Health Education Journal*, 66 (3), 277–285.

Strauss, A. & Corbin, J. (1994) Grounded theory methodology: an overview. In: *Handbook of Qualitative Research*. (eds N.K. Denzin & Y.S. Lincoln), pp. 273–285. Sage, Thousand Oaks, CA.

Sockett, D.L., Rosenberg, W.M.C., Gray, J.A.M., & Richardson, W.S. (1996). Evidence based medicine: what it is and what it isn't. *British Medical Journal*, 312 (January), 71–72.

Vydelingum, V. (2000) South Asian patients' lived experience of acute care in an English hospital: a phenomenological study. *Journal of Advanced Nursing*, 32 (1), 100–107.

Walker, M.F., Gladman, J.R.F., Lincoln, N.B., Siemonsma, P. & Whiteley, T. (1999) Occupational therapy for stroke patients not admitted to hospital: a randomised controlled trial. *The Lancet*, 354, 278–280.

World Health Organization (WHO) (2012) *Measuring Health Gains from Sustainable Development*. WHO, Geneva.

6

Integrating the Children's Public Health Workforce

Jane Wright and Kate Potter

Faculty of Society and Health, Buckinghamshire New University, High Wycombe, UK

The true measure of a nation's standing is how well it attends to its children – their health and safety, their material security, their education and socialisation and their sense of being loved, valued and included in the families and societies into which they are born (UNICEF 2007, p. 1).

Introduction

Transforming the lives of children and young people within modern society can only be achieved by a coordinated and comprehensive inter-professional approach that is provided across all sectors. This has been well documented over time, and this chapter will outline some of the fundamental principles about working together and the policies affecting children, young people and their families. Specifically, it will identify those professionals involved in an integrated children's workforce, explore the concept of the team around the child, identify the skills and knowledge needed to work within this sector and highlight the factors that affect young people's lives in the modern world. Although the focus of attention is community nursing in this book, the broad skills and knowledge needed to work with children and young people are common across all areas of practice. Therefore, these broad key skills will be explored as well as the more specific role of community public health nurses working with children, young people and their families.

Community and Public Health Nursing, Fifth Edition. Edited by David Sines,
Sharon Aldridge-Bent, Agnes Fanning, Penny Farrelly, Kate Potter and Jane Wright.
© 2013 John Wiley & Sons, Ltd. Published 2013 by John Wiley & Sons, Ltd.

The establishment of childhood and adolescence as distinct developmental stages with their own set of particular needs which are different from adults is a relatively new phenomenon. There is evidence to suggest that prior to the nineteenth century, childhood and the exploitation of children were not recognised in the public mind (Heywood 2001). Children were seen as young adults who were capable of work, could be sent to prison or even hanged if they broke the law (Heywood 2001). They were also viewed as the property of their parents (Hislop 2010). The 1861 census showed that one third of all children between the ages of 5 and 9 years and half of all 10- to 14-year-olds worked (Kirby 2003). The abuse of children then was not only from individuals, parents or communities but effectively by 'the state' as well.

Although the Victorian Era is most known for social reforms, interest in child welfare was evident much earlier. Thomas Coram was an early pioneer of child welfare in the eighteenth century, and he campaigned for 17 years to set up the Foundling Hospital in London. Foundlings were defined as abandoned babies with unknown mothers, and at the time, up to a thousand babies were abandoned in London per year. They were often left by the side of the road in the hope that someone would care for them but most died. Many were thought to have been babies of domestic servants who were unable to keep their babies and stay in work. Heartbreakingly, mothers often left tokens, such as buttons or even a nut, to identify their children in the hope they could return for them in the future (Coram 2012). More recent history has placed children and young people more firmly at the heart of health and social care policy with an acknowledgement that they need to be protected from harm, and there are many reasons for this. They have been recognised as a priority investment for the future economic stability of modern society, and their vulnerability has been more fully acknowledged in policy documents over the last 20 years, particularly since *The Children Act* in 1989 (HM Government 1989).

Developing a future healthy workforce begins with supporting families at a very early stage and ensuring that children and young people have equal opportunities for education and healthcare and access to work opportunities. Healthy children are likely to become healthy adults and this applies to both physical and emotional health and well-being. This can only be achieved with a concerted public health effort across all sectors.

Health indicators

A key factor in determining the health of children and young people is their economic status. Definitions of poverty change over time and, in particular, in response to economic crises where there are likely to be more people living below the defined poverty line. The Fiscal Studies Institute reported on living standards, poverty and inequality in the United Kingdom in June 2012 (Cribb *et al.* 2012). Year on year, the government has produced data about the distribution of wealth in the United Kingdom, and the recession in 2012 created a dramatic fall in the average income of people and a level of inequality which was last seen in the mid-1990s (Cribb *et al.* 2012). To assess the level of poverty, it is important to consider different indicators including living standards, income inequality and income poverty.

Living standards are measured by taking an average (mean) of household net incomes or the median (the midpoint of the distribution of those households). Since 2004, there had been a steady, gradual increase in the standards of living in the United Kingdom. However, during 2010–2011, the mean income fell by 5.7% and the median income by 3.1%. Just considering the average income in real terms, this represents a fall from £542 to £511 per week. For the lowest paid workers in this country, and in particular for those with children, this is a significant fall in household income.

As well as measuring the standard of living in this way, income inequality also needs to be measured. Cribb *et al.* (2012) argue that defining inequality is difficult as there are many interpretations, and they recommend that a range of indicators are utilised. Income inequality is commonly measured by the Gini coefficient which ranges from 0 to 1: the higher the score, the higher the level of inequality. During the 1960s and 1970s, the Gini scale was around 0.26 and it rose steeply during the 1980s and 1990s to 0.34. Between 2009 and 2010, it had risen again to 0.36. This prompted an independent report by government Adviser Frank Field on child poverty: *The Foundation Years: Preventing Poor Children Becoming Poor Adults* (Field 2010). Since then, the Gini scale has fallen to 0.34, and although still an unacceptable gap, it demonstrates that there is some progress and 300000 children have been removed from poverty since 2010 according to this definition (Cribb *et al.* 2012).

Income poverty is defined as 'the proportion of individuals with household incomes less than 60% of the contemporary mean' (Cribb *et al.* 2012, p. 10); this is known as the poverty line. This clearly measures whether those with the lowest incomes are keeping up in relative terms with higher income families. This is known as relative poverty, that is, relative to the rest of the population. A measurement of absolute poverty may be more accurate as it is less dependent on a comparison to others but more on how an acceptable standard of living is defined. You could argue that this is also difficult to define, particularly if you compared the United Kingdom with countries in the developing world where there is a very different standard of living.

Access to work is an important aspect of economic stability and the opportunities for young people vary considerably across the country. In 2011 there was the highest recorded level of unemployment amongst 16–24-year-olds; however, according to the Youth Unemployment Statistics, the level is slowly falling (Hough 2012). The rates remain high and this has an effect on the economic stability of the country, potentially creates unrest and affects the health and well-being of young people. It also has the potential to impact on the 'social order' of local communities. The summer riots of 2011 may be an example of this unrest and disaffection with our society, or it may simply be opportunists taking advantage of a situation. This 'fear' of anti-social behaviour in England led politicians to place increased emphasis on building communities and encouraging investment in social capital in government policy in an attempt to encourage communities to work together to improve the lives of local neighbourhoods and populations.

However, within this agenda of building community capacity, one could argue that there has also been a demonisation of young people and families and the blaming of parents for the behaviour of their children. 'Troubled' or 'dysfunctional' families were targeted for Family Intervention Projects by the Labour Government in their strategy for tackling anti-social behaviour during the late 1990s and early 2000s. In 2012, a report, 'Listening to Troubled Families', was published which explored the lives of 16 families from these intervention projects across the country (Department for Communities and Local Government 2012). This initial report introduced a project which has been funded by the government to further identify 'troubled families' and explore ways in which services and professionals can provide the support they need and, in particular, in order to tackle the cycles of deprivation, violence, mental health problems and substance misuse that may form a pattern across many families who are most at risk. Cross-sector working is the most effective way forward but there are still gaps in communication and cooperation across agencies.

In a world where the extremes of life can be witnessed firsthand in an ever-expanding global media and social network, the expectations for young people have changed, particularly in the United Kingdom. They witness the consequences of wealth portrayed by celebrities and reality TV shows such as the X Factor and want those lifestyles for themselves. Advertising by celebrities also fuels the craving for particular brands, and the concept of mass media consumerism was explored by a UNICEF report in 2011 which interviewed 250 children and young people in the United Kingdom, Sweden and Spain. This report followed on from a UNICEF investigation on child well-being in 21 affluent countries in 2007 which placed the United Kingdom in the bottom third of the table in five out of six measured domains. The 2007 study measured material well-being, health and safety, educational well-being, family and peer relationships, behaviours and risks and subjective well-being (UNICEF 2007). This is explored later in this chapter.

The 2011 UNICEF study talked to 250 children aged 8–14 across the three countries and found overwhelmingly that their well-being centres on time spent within a happy, stable family, having good friends and plenty of things to do, especially outdoors. The study also filmed the everyday lives of 24 families across the three countries. Crucially, there were clear differences between the United Kingdom and both Spain and Sweden. In the United Kingdom, parents struggled to give their children the time that they wanted to maintain their emotional well-being, whereas in the other countries, family life was woven into the 'fabric of everyday life' (UNICEF 2011, p. 1). A BBC documentary in 2011 on the British Family also plotted the history of the family in Britain and considered the dramatic changes in how parents view their children, the time that is spent with children, the emphasis on family life and what pressures there are for parents in today's society (BBC Two 2010).

Emotional health and well-being has become a public health focus rather than a concentration on physical health alone. All individuals will have their own view of what health means to them, and this will depend on their specific circumstances. For some, being healthy means never having a physical illness, not having to take any medications or being fully active. For others, being happy, having friends and family around them and being economically stable are important indicators of health.

The policy context

Every Child Matters (DH 2004) was introduced in 2004 by the Labour party. It sought to identify key outcomes for children and young people and was supported within the legal framework of *The Children Act 2004* (HM Government 2004a). The formalisation of an agenda which focused on children, young people and their families was driven by safeguarding tragedies such as the deaths of Maria Colwell in 1973, Jasmine Beckford in 1984 and Victoria Climbie in 2000. The common themes throughout these cases related to poor co-ordination of services and a failure to share information between agencies, but it took 30 years to establish a children's agenda. The Laming Report in 2003 highlighted that child protection cannot be separated from policies that are designed to improve children's lives as a whole (Laming 2003). He recommended that there should be both universal services for all children and young people and also specific, targeted services for those with additional needs. *Every Child Matters* (DH 2004) outlined health and social outcomes for children by emphasising the need to ensure that children and young people maximise their full potential given their individual circumstances. To achieve this, it is recognised that a multifaceted approach is essential with cooperation and effective communication across all professional agencies, families and the voluntary sector. Although the initial focus was on child protection, the agenda broadened out to consider more general outcomes for children and young people.

In addition to policy which focuses on health and social care, there is also a need to explore other policy which affects the lives of children such as education policy. Achieving positive outcomes for children requires a holistic approach which is informed from the ground as well as in the political arena. For example, there has been emphasis on early years education and a development of a common core of skills and knowledge that should be required of all those working in the children's sector. These core skills and knowledge include an emphasis on

- Effective communication with children, young people and their families
- An understanding of child development
- Supporting transitions
- Safeguarding and promoting children's welfare
- Multi-agency working
- Sharing information effectively

(HM Government 2004b)

A fully integrated workforce needs a common purpose, a philosophy which promotes safe and effective practice, and this can only be achieved by good communication

BOX 6.1   The health visitor implementation plan: the health visiting service: what it means for families

> - Your community has a range of services including some Sure Start services and the services families and the communities provide for themselves. Health visitors work to develop these and make sure you know about them.
> - Universal services from your health visitor and team provide the Healthy Child Programme to ensure a healthy start for your children and family (for example immunisations, health and development checks), support for parents and access to a range of community services/resources.
> - Universal Plus gives you a rapid response from your HV team when you need specific expert help, for example with postnatal depression, a sleepless baby, weaning or answering concerns about parenting.
> - Universal partnership plus provides ongoing support from your HV team plus a range of local services working together and with you, to deal with more complex issues over a period of time. These include services from Sure Start Children's Centres, other community services including charities and, where appropriate the Family Nurse Partnership.

across all sectors. A key to this is to consider the support that children and young people need throughout their life course, through the transitions that they make and recognition of the factors which will affect those transitions. The role of parents and how they are supported is also key to achieving positive outcomes for children and young people. In relation to community public health nursing, the 'Healthy Child Programme' (HCP) was introduced in 2009. Two documents were produced: 'The Healthy Child Programme: Pregnancy and the First Five Years of Life' (DH/DCSF 2009a) and 'The Healthy Child Programme 5–19' (DH/DCSF 2009b). The details of these recommended programmes are outlined later. These documents have set an agenda for achieving positive health outcomes but were recommendations rather than statutory requirements.

The Coalition Government in 2010 initiated a plan to improve the health of children by refocusing attention on the early years and increasing the health visitor workforce by 50% with the 'Health Visitor Implementation Plan: A Call to Action' (DH 2011a). Health visitors have always worked with a public health focus, and this document produced a model of care which highlighted the need for both universal and targeted services in a tiered system (see Box 6.1). The School Nurse Implementation Plan followed in 2012 (DH 2012a) but followed a similar pattern to the health visiting model (see Box 6.2). The NHS outcomes framework and the Child Public Health outcomes framework were published in 2012 and provide a complementary model for working in this arena (see Box 6.3).

BOX 6.2   The school nurse implementation plan

- Your Community has a range of health services (including GP and community services) for children and young people and their families. School nurses develop and provide these and make sure you know about them.
- Universal services from your school nurse team provide the Healthy Child Programme to ensure a healthy start for every child (e.g., immunisations, health checks). They support children and parents to ensure access to a range of community services.
- Universal plus delivers a swift response from your School Nurse Service when you need specific expert help (e.g., with sexual health, mental health concerns, long-term conditions and additional health needs
- Universal partnership plus delivers ongoing support by your SN team from a range of local services working together and With you, to deal with more complex issues over a period of time (e.g. with charities and your local authority).

The role of the specialist community public health nurse

The NMC (NMC 2004) defined the Standards of Proficiency for specialist community public health nurses (SCPHN); this was for health visitors, school nurses, occupational health nurses, health protection nurses and sexual health advisors. These standards are underpinned by the four principles of health visiting:

- Search for health needs
- Stimulation of awareness of health needs
- Influence on policy affecting health
- Facilitation of health enhancing activities
                    (Council for the Education and Training of Health Visitors 1977)

These four principles were revisited by Cowley and Frost (2006) and were still found to be pertinent to the role of both the health visitor and the school nurse. Table 6.1 shows how these principles remain key to the delivery of the HCP which has been adopted as the framework for services delivered by the children's workforce working either in health visitor or school nurse teams (see Table 6.1).

The HCP

The Coalition Government in 2011 made a commitment to the HCP. The HCP (DH/ DCSF 2009a, b) begins in pregnancy and progresses through to adult life. There are two

BOX 6.3   The NHS outcomes framework and the Child Public Health outcomes framework

---

A – NHS outcomes framework

Domain 1: Preventing people from dying prematurely

Improvement area
Reducing deaths in babies and young children

Indicators
Infant mortality
Neonatal mortality and stillbirths

Domain 2: Enhancing quality of life for people with long-term conditions

Improvement area
Reducing time spent in hospital by children and young people with long-term conditions

Indicator
Unplanned hospitalisation for asthma, diabetes and epilepsy in under 19s

Domain 3:   Helping people to recover from episodes of ill health or following injury

Improvement area
Preventing lower respiratory tract infections (LRTI) in children from becoming serious

Indicator
Emergency admissions for children with LRTI

Domain 4: Ensuring that people have a positive experience of care

Improvement area
Improving women's and their families' experience of maternity services

Indicator
Women's experience of maternity services

Improvement area
Improving the patient experience of children and young people in healthcare settings

Indicator
Improving children and young people's experience of healthcare

---

BOX 6.3 *(Continued)*

Domain 5: Treating and caring for people in a safe environment and protecting them from avoidable harm

Improvement area
Improving the safety of maternity services

Indicator
Admission of full-term babies to neonatal care

Improvement area
Delivering safe care to children in acute settings

Indicator
Incidence of harm to children due to 'failure to monitor'

B – Public health outcomes framework

Domain 1: Improving the wider determinants of health

- Children in poverty
- School readiness (placeholder)
- Pupil absence
- First time entrants to the youth justice system
- 16–18 year olds not in education, employment or training

Domain 2: Health improvement

- Low birth weight of term babies
- Breastfeeding
- Smoking status at time of delivery
- Under 18 conceptions
- Child development at 2–2.5 years (placeholder)
- Excess weight in 4–5 and 10–11 year olds
- Hospital admissions caused by unintentional and deliberate injuries in under 18s
- Emotional well-being of looked after children (placeholder)
- Smoking prevalence – 15 year olds (placeholder)

Domain 3: Health protection

- Chlamydia diagnoses (15–24 year olds)

Domain 4: Healthcare public health and preventing premature mortality

- Infant mortality
- Tooth decay in children aged 5

Table 6.1   The health visitor implementation plan

Domain	HV team activity	SN team activity
Search for health needs	The new birth visit including Family Need Assessment	Screening on school entry
	Recording breastfeeding statistics	School profiling
	Accessing local health need data from public health observatories	Immunisations
		Auditing drop in work
		Accessing local health need data from public health observatories
Stimulation of awareness of health needs	Weaning advice	Contributing to personal health and social education
	Breastfeeding support including clinics and drop-ins run in partnership with the midwifery service	Parenting groups
	Running parenting groups with Children Centre workforce	Working with teachers and parents
Influence on policies affecting health	Providing health data of local populations which will inform future policy	Providing health data of local populations which will inform future policy
	Membership of local policy forums	Membership of local policy forums
	Evaluating postnatal groups	Becoming practitioner members of working parties developing policy at the Department of Health
	Becoming practitioner members of working parties developing policy at the Department of Health	Working in partnership with other agencies with families where school children are subject to a child protection plan
Facilitation of health enhancing activities	Working in partnership with other agencies with families where children are subject to a child protection plan	Plan, implement and evaluate specific groups in an area (MEND)
	Plan, implement and evaluate specific groups in an area (e.g. Mini MEND)	

parts – 'Pregnancy and the First Five Years of Life', the framework for health visiting services, and 'From Five to Nineteen' – which together combine to support the effective provision of universal and progressive services. Universal services refer to what all children need (such as immunisations), and progressive services are those which target those with specific health needs. The HCP originated from the 'Every Child Matters' agenda introduced by the Labour Government in 2004 (DH/DfES 2004). Other drivers for the programme came from 'Health For All Children' (Hall & Elliman 2006) and the 'National Service Framework for children, families and maternity services' (DH 2004).

The key points of the HCP are

- Early intervention
- Safeguarding

- Parenting support
- Integrated services
- Preventative public health programmes
- Early identification of need and risk

The delivery of the programme has been the focus of the 'Health Visitor Implementation Plan' (DH 2011a) and the 'Vision and Model for School Nursing' (DH 2012). Both these documents refer to a strategy of delivering the HCP using four stages, 'Community', 'Universal', 'Universal Plus' and 'Universal Partnership – Plus' (see Box 6.1 and Box 6.2). Running alongside the four levels of service is safeguarding children. Munro (2011) identified that early intervention is a key component of reducing risk of harm to children and the children's workforce. Ensuring that all families are able to access the 'universal service' is key to identifying risk factors for children and young people.

Delivering the HCP

Health visitors and school nurses were seen by the Department of Health in 2009 as the lead professionals in the delivery of the HCP (DH/DCSF 2009a, b). This involves working in appropriately balanced skill mix teams where the knowledge and skills of the community staff nurse and nursery nurses are used effectively. The children's service should also be enhanced by working collaboratively with colleagues in Children Centres, schools, social care centres and the voluntary sector.

Pregnancy and the first 5 years of life

The recommended schedule: pregnancy (Universal Services)

1. Promotion of health and well-being. As well as routine antenatal care provided by a maternity healthcare professional, prospective parents should also be given information about local resources including Children Centres. Breastfeeding should be promoted at the earliest opportunity.
2. Preparation for parenthood. Antenatal classes should be designed to provide both information and social support, and there should be a focus on transition to parenthood. Services should be more responsive to the needs of fathers. Information should also be given on paternal rights and benefits.

This represents an important opportunity for health visiting teams to make contact with prospective parents and to introduce their service as well as identify clients who may need to access enhanced services.

The recommended schedule: pregnancy progressive services (Universal Plus and Universal Partnership Plus)

1. Extra support to be provided for parents who have had a history of mental health problems and are currently suffering from or have identified risk factors for developing problems in the ante- and postnatal period.
2. Specific services offered to mothers who smoke and those who are overweight and obese. Recognising the risk to their health and that of the baby.
3. Parents who are at higher risk (drug and alcohol misuse, severe mental illness, learning difficulties) should be provided with appropriate services by effective multi-agency working.

The recommended schedule: birth to 6 months (Universal)

Appropriate screening and health promotion are provided by midwifery and obstetric services until the new birth assessment at 10–14 days. Effective communication between midwifery and health visiting teams is essential to ensure the provision of the best care for infants and parents.

The focus of the universal service should be

1. *Infant feeding* – Emphasis is on sustaining breastfeeding and delaying the introduction of solids until 6 months.
2. *Promoting sensitive parenting* – Health visiting teams should be aware of the latest research into early brain development and the importance of calm loving care in achieving the best outcomes for the future.
3. *Maternal Mental Health* – There should be assessment of mother's mental health following guidelines from the Maternal Mental Health Pathway (DH 2012b). It is also important to consider the father's mental health and be aware of their risk of depression.
4. *Immunisation programmes* – Parents should be aware of the recommended immunisation programme for their baby (DH 2012c) and be given appropriate information to give informed consent.
5. *Promoting development* – Parents should be made aware of the importance of interactive activities on infant development and be encouraged to access groups in their local communities which will support them in gaining confidence in playing with their babies.

The recommended schedule: birth to 6 months (progressive services) (Universal Plus and Universal Partnership Plus)

1. Appropriate support and referral where infants have been diagnosed with health or development problems.
2. Extra support for babies who have feeding problems and help to sustain breastfeeding and delay weaning.

3. Helping families develop their positive and effective parenting skills using research based models (Solihull Approach, Family Partnership Model). Parenting interactions should be assessed and access to parenting programmes facilitated.
4. Listening visits for depressed mothers.
5. Couples who are finding new parenting is putting a strain on their relationship should be offered access to particular groups which address parental conflict.

Recommended schedule: 6 months to 1 year (Universal)

1. Health review at a year. This should assess the physical, emotional and social needs of the baby within the context of their own family. This contact should be an opportunity for parents to express concerns and discuss behaviour and any developmental issues. Growth should be monitored and again babies who are at risk of becoming overweight or obese should be identified. Health promotion should include addressing accident prevention, healthy eating and dental health. Opportunity should be taken to promote all aspects of the development of positive health, well-being and lifestyle.

Recommended schedule: 6 months to 1 year (progressive services) (Universal Plus and Universal Partnership Plus)

As for families with younger babies, extra support should be given where there are health or development problems, maternal depression, parents who smoke, feeding issues, parental conflict or poor parenting practices identified.

Recommended schedule: 1–5 years (Universal Services)

1. Continuation of the immunisation programme.
2. Two to two and a half year review. The focus of this review is the promotion of emotional development and communication skills. It is also the opportunity to support positive relationships. Health promotion should be aimed at obesity prevention and maintaining good dental health. Parents should be encouraged to enrol their children in early years education. Early years services are also tasked to carry out a review between 2 and 3 years on all children in their setting (DE 2012). It is hoped that this should lead to better integration of health and education reviews and a focus on preparing children for school (Tickell 2011).
3. Between 3 and 5 years the universal service should continue to support parenting and deliver the immunisation programme. The health visiting team should be working with early years services to provide appropriate health promotion.

Recommended schedule: 1–5 years (progressive services) (Universal Plus and Universal Partnership Plus)

1. The health visiting teams should continue to assess risk for children and their families and provide appropriate support from within their teams or refer to other agencies to meet identified needs.

2. Health visitors should ensure that their school nurse colleagues receive a detailed handover of records for all vulnerable children or families where extra concerns have been identified.

The recommended schedule: 5–11 years (Universal Services)

1. Information sharing between health visitor and school health and education on school entry. This will include information on developmental needs.
2. A health assessment including reviewing immunisation status and dental health and a height, weight, vision and hearing check. Height and weight are also reviewed as part of the National Child Measurement Programme (NCMP).
3. Support for emotional health and well-being for children and their families. School health teams can contribute to Social and Emotional Aspects of Learning (SEAL) in the school and also the Healthy Schools Initiatives. This may include contributing to the personal, social and health education programme in the school.
4. Support the Change4life campaign with regard to healthy eating and encourage this in the school setting (Change4life 2012).
5. Consider aspects of physical activity and advise schools and parents on the healthy weight of children and young people. School nurses may contribute to the Healthy Schools Initiatives.
6. Safeguarding and Child Protection as per *Working Together to Safeguard Children* (DCSF 2010).
7. Use of the Common Assessment Framework (CAF) is recommended within the HCP and development of the Team around the Child (TAC) for children identified with specific needs. School nurses are potential lead professionals for this work.
8. There should be clear referral routes for the school following any identified need through the school health team to more specialised services such as child and adolescent mental health services. The development of care pathways has been established in many areas.
9. Information and support should be available for parents through various means, including dissemination through the school health team, HCP websites, school websites or NHS choices.

The recommended schedule: 5–11 years (progressive services) (Universal Plus and Universal Partnership Plus)

1. Immunisations for children at risk. Check immunisation status and refer if necessary.
2. Supporting emotional health, psychological well-being and mental health. Targeted Mental Health in Schools (TaMHS) services can be accessed if available. Consideration of primary, targeted and specialist services (tiers 2, 3 and 4) for those children at risk of mental health problems. Again, clear referral routes and

responsibilities should be clarified by the school health team. Drop-in services for children and parents are established in some areas of the country.

3. Overweight and obese children. Advice, support, signposting and referral on to secondary services if necessary. There are projects being run by school nurses such as Mind Exercise, Nutrition, Do it (MEND) or the equivalent.
4. The child in need. Responsibility for the assessment of need in the CAF and TAC as the lead professional.
5. Health assessments for the looked-after child (LAC). Local authorities are required to ensure that a Strengths and Difficulties Questionnaire is completed for all their LAC. School nurses may be involved in health assessments with good opportunities to support LAC and promote health and help foster parents fill in these questionnaires.
6. Children with special educational needs. Health advice is required within the assessment of children with special educational needs. School nurses are available to schools to coordinate these health assessments.
7. Children with complex health needs should have a comprehensive care plan coordinated by the school health team. Care pathways can be developed to support children with particular needs. Policies should be in place to manage medicines in schools and school staff trained accordingly.
8. Support for young carers through the school health team.
9. Other support for parents and carers. The school nurse should be aware of specific projects that are set up to help families in need.
10. Support for parents with specific needs such as drugs and alcohol problems, mental health problems, learning difficulties or families where there is domestic violence.

Recommended schedule from 11 to 16 years (Universal Services)

1. A health review in year 7 (11–12 years). Some areas have developed a review process at the transition to secondary school which involves administering and reviewing questionnaires. The purpose of this review is to review immunisation status, to alert the school nurse to any health problems and also to highlight the role of the school nurse to young people entering secondary school.
2. Immunisation programmes (HPV and school leaver's booster immunisations).
3. Support for emotional health, psychological well-being and mental health. School nurses can contribute to PSHE programmes effectively to promote positive relationships and emotional well-being.
4. Promoting healthy weights as with the 5–11 schedules.
5. Sexual health and well-being. Local authorities and the NHS are expected to work together to provide accessible, confidential services for sexual health.
6. Ongoing support for children in need as with the 5–11 schedules. Includes safeguarding issues and consideration of additional needs.

Recommended schedule from 11 to 16 years: progressive services (Universal Plus and Universal Partnership Plus)

1. Emotional health, psychological well-being and mental health. Many secondary schools now have a drop-in service for young people to access one-to-one support and advice at tier one and tier two CAMHS.
2. Young people at risk from a range of problems such as drugs and alcohol, smoking or obesity should be supported within the school with school nurses acting as gate-keepers for referrals on to specialist services.
3. LAC. Adolescents need further support through this stage of development as there is evidence of poor outcomes and risk-taking behaviours.
4. Young people with special educational needs. The transition into adulthood and the workplace needs to be managed within a multidisciplinary team.
5. Young people with complex health needs also need transitional support as they move into adult services.
6. Young people in contact with the youth justice system. These young people may need additional support to reintegrate into the education system and consider their healthcare needs in the event of custody.

Recommended schedule: 16–19 years (Universal Services)

1. Immunisation status check.
2. Young people entering Further Education (FE). This group of young people is still in need of support for their own health and well-being. They may be at a vulnerable stage of development, and once they enter FE or Higher Education (HE), they may be susceptible to poor health and should be offered continuing support through the school health teams. This may be achieved through the Healthy FE programmes.
3. Emotional health and well-being. Young people and their families should have access to psychological well-being and mental health support.
4. Sexual health services.
5. Physical activity. There is a dropout rate from physical activity in the 16–19-year-olds. There is potential to work with young people through partnerships with sports coordinators and voluntary agencies to maintain participation in sporting activities.
6. Ongoing support. All opportunities for offering health information should be taken at this age; this will include forming partnerships with professionals such as youth workers and social care.
7. Ongoing safeguarding responsibilities. This age range is recognised as problematic in terms of safeguarding. Teams need to be aware of the ongoing risks in this age group and offer support and advice through accessible services.
8. Support for parents. Parenting teenagers can also be problematic and parents may be experiencing real difficulties with setting boundaries and communicating with their adolescents. School nurses are in a good position to give support and advice.

Recommended schedule: 16–19 years (progressive services) (Universal Plus and Universal Partnership Plus)

1. Immunisations for at-risk young people as with the other age groups.
2. Emotional health, psychological well-being and mental health. Referral to specialised services for young people at risk. Clear understanding of the role of school nurses and clearly identified referral routes. Clinical supervision should be considered here with specialist services.
3. Drug and alcohol misuse. Consideration of local specialist services as well as support and advice through drop-in centres. Also for consideration should be those leaving schools for FE and, later, HE.
4. Smoking cessation. Accessible support and referrals to NHS services if necessary.
5. Consideration of at-risk groups:
   a. Looked-after young people and the transition to FE and the work place.
   b. Young people with complex welfare needs. May be ongoing from earlier ages.
   c. Young people with special educational needs as with the 11–16 age range.
   d. Young people with complex health needs. Consideration of the transitions and care planning should consider issues around accommodation and housing.
   e. Young people leaving the care system. Care orders end at 18. Care leavers may need additional support to manage their own health needs. There is also evidence of young people leaving care at 16.
   f. One-to-one sexual health interventions for high-risk young people. National Institute of Clinical Health (NICHE) guidelines (2007) recommend that at-risk young people under 18 (e.g. from disadvantaged backgrounds, those in care and/ or those who have low educational attainment) are offered one-to-one sexual health advice.
   g. Young people in contact with the youth justice system. There are school nurses in the country who have a dual role in the youth offending service and in school nursing.
   h. Support and advice for parents and carers.

The HCP is recommended in government policy but is not mandatory for NHS delivery. This presents challenges to commissioners who may have to make difficult decisions about the health and well-being of children and young people. Health and Well Being Boards have now been appointed throughout England who will be responsible for identifying local public health needs and for planning effective workforce plans and effective service responses/strategies. The HCP has encouraged service commissioners to:

> Identify evidence-based interventions to address local needs (bearing in mind that implementing a programme well may be as important as choosing the right intervention) and

> Identify currently provided services that are not supported by evidence and decide whether continued investment in these services is justified (Department of Health/Department of Children Schools and Families 2009a, b, p. 7).

The message presented is clear that assessing need is vital and measuring the effectiveness of services is crucial. Supporting children with complex needs in different settings is also a key role for the children's workforce.

The HCP also gives practitioners opportunities to support both children and parents through the key transitions of childhood. This may start in the preconception period, through pregnancy and into childhood. Parents and children and young people need help to face challenges which different stages of their development and social integration bring.

It is clear that to deliver a service which provides the best outcomes for all children, there needs to be an integrated children's workforce and well-developed strategies for interagency working across all sectors. In 2004 the concept of a Common Assessment Framework (CAF) was introduced by the then Labour Government. The aim was to ensure that children and families would receive appropriate services for their needs in a timely fashion. The CAF allows any member of the Children's Workforce to consider, in partnership with parents, appropriate services which may be delivered by health education, social care or voluntary agencies (Universal Partnership Plus). The assessment, carried out by any one professional who knows the family best, has a holistic inter-professional approach that empowers parents to make choices about what they feel their child and the family need for best possible outcomes. Where children present with complex needs, an inter-professional TAC will be formed. A health visitor or school nurse may often be the lead professional, and they will be charged with coordinating and communicating between professionals, the children and families. Evaluations show that this supports good practice in interagency working practice.

The practitioner's role in safeguarding and child protection

Safeguarding is recognised as a key theme throughout the HCP. Health visitors and school nurses are the universal contact for children, young people and their families. They need to have good understanding of how to identify children at risk of harm and know the referral processes: access to appropriate multi-agency training is essential to ensure that they practise safely. This mandatory training enables practitioners to develop understanding of the professional roles and responsibilities of all those involved in the care of children. Previous reports about child protection from Laming (2009) and Munro (2011) continue to highlight the importance of good communication between agencies and that early identification and intervention ensures optimum outcomes for children and young people. This area of practice is the most challenging and emotionally charged, and therefore, practitioners need to access good supervision and support for their role.

High-profile child protection cases in recent years have led to increasing numbers of children identified at risk of harm across caseloads, for both health visitors and school nurses. Reduced numbers of practitioners in recent years have led to an increased percentage of time being allocated to these cases. The health visitor implementation plan hopes to address these shortfalls in the early years and improve the chances for identification and intervention (DH 2011a). In the older age group, it is hoped that the School Nurse Implementation Plan will mirror this aim.

Although child protection processes have improved over the last few years, research still shows that in some areas, thresholds for accepting referrals by social care remain high, especially in the category of neglect (Community Care 2012). Health visitors and school nurses need to be able to articulate their specific concerns competently and with confidence in order to ensure appropriate action is always taken. Understanding child development and the factors that will impact on physical and emotional health needs to be an essential component of SCPHN programmes. This knowledge and key skills should be reflected in the quality of practitioners' referrals and report writing. To protect children, they need to be fully aware of their accountability to maintain currency in this area of practice, and ongoing training should be identified as part of their annual appraisal.

The social framework of peoples' lives is constantly changing, and health visitors and school nurses need to be aware of the risks associated with the specific communities and age groups within their caseloads. This will vary hugely across the country and sensitivity to cultural differences will be important when protecting children from risk of significant harm. Building trusting relationships with individuals and groups enables effective working practices.

The practitioner role in improving emotional health and well-being

The HCP provides the framework for the assessment of need and for delivery of services. Health visiting and school nursing teams need to be aware of the evolving problems which face children, young people and their families in the changing society within which they live. Acknowledging the continuing growth of understanding of early brain development and the impact of experience in utero and the first years of life (Center on the Developing Child [CDC] 2009) gives validity to early preparation for parenthood. Evidence exists to suggest that this should start in primary education when children should be supported to develop empathy and caring skills. A study by the NSPCC in 2009 found that 25% of teenage girls and 18% of boys had reported physical violence in relationships and emotional violence was reported at the even higher rate of 59 and 50%, respectively (NSPCC 2009). This confirms the need for good education to be provided in schools to support young people to develop healthy relationships. The impact of stress and raised cortisol levels on the developing fetus (Gerhardt 2003) and on the architecture of the brain through the early years of development (CDC 2009) means that prospective parents have to understand the impact of behaviour on their child. In Birth and Beyond (DH 2011b) the need for preparing parents to adapt their relationships and have realistic expectations of early parenthood is recognised. Integrated working between maternity services and health visiting teams should ensure parents who are vulnerable and are in need of further support are identified.

Practitioners are aware that Child Protection is a core theme throughout their daily work. Munro (2011) points to an upstream approach which not only strives to identify abuse but seeks to put in place measures which prevent it happening. A better resourced service (DH 2011a, b) not only will allow involvement with families where children are subject to a child protection plan but will provide early intervention services to foster better parenting and build resilience within the developing child. Barlow and Calum (2011, p. 252) call for a public health approach to safeguarding and child protection. In so doing they envisage:

> a public health, population-based strategy that is aimed at ensuring all parents are able to develop the skills they need to parent effectively, and as part of an integrated tiered approach in which multidisciplinary teams of workers are able within community and primary care settings to both intervene with families and also use existing policy frameworks (e.g. CAFS) to move children on to higher levels of service provision where necessary

In 2007 UNICEF published the report 'An overview of child well-being in rich countries'. The United Kingdom was placed at the bottom in the league table, below substantially poorer countries, such as Greece and Poland. The three dimensions where the United Kingdom rated lowest were 'family and peer relationships', 'behaviours and risks' and 'subjective well-being'. Further research (UNICEF 2011) concluded that the focus on materialism and living in a consumerism-based society continued to have a detrimental effect on the emotional well-being of children. In the United Kingdom, unlike other countries children still spend less time with family and feel less secure about themselves rather than their possessions. The Children's Society (2012) identified six key priorities for promoting children's well-being:

- Have positive relationships with family and friends
- Have enough of what matters
- Have the conditions to learn and develop
- Have a positive view of themselves and an identity that is respected
- Have a safe and suitable home environment and local area
- Have opportunities to take part in positive activities to thrive

These are key messages for the children's workforce as they seek to work effectively and responsively with families and communities to improve children's well-being.

Conclusion: future development and challenges for practice

The importance of early intervention work has been clearly identified in government policy in recent times and, in particular, a commitment to increasing the health visiting workforce. Given the historical lack of attention on children's and young people's services, this must be a positive step forward. However, the importance of working across and between the full range of agencies who are working in this sector is vital. The role and contribution of other community practitioners such as school nurses is also being reviewed and more integrated and responsive service models being developed. Resources need to follow these developments, as have been advocated in the health visitor plan to enable the delivery of successful and improved outcomes for children, young people and their families. The context in which services are delivered is the subject of an ever-changing environment, but positive outcomes for children and young people should always remain the central focus of everyone's agenda. The key skills and knowledge that are needed across sectors should be co-ordinated so that the right person for the right job, with the right skills, is clearly identified. The deployment of effective leadership and management skills are crucial and need to be evidenced within community nursing to motivate teams to accept and to respond proactively to change within the context of a constantly evolving public health service. A key to achieving this will be through the provision of robust educational programmes and by engaging in practice-related professional development learning activities.

References

Barlow, J. & Calum, R. (2011) A public health approach to safeguarding in the 21st century. Child Abuse Review, **20**, 238–255.

BBC Two (2010) *The British Family*. BBC Two, April 2010, April 16, Episode 4.

Center on the Developing Child (CDC) (2009) *Excessive Stress Disrupts the Architecture of the Developing Brain*, CDC, Harvard, Cambridge, MA.

Change4life. (2012) Available from http://www.nhs.uk/change4life/Pages/change-for-life.aspx. Accessed on 12 December 2012.

Community Care (2012) Thresholds for accepting child protection referrals 'too high'. Available from http://www.communitycare.co.uk/articles/31/07. Accessed on 3 January 2013.

Council for the Education and Training of Health Visitors (1977) *An Investigation of the Principles of Health Visiting*, CETHV, London.

Coram, T. (2012) *The Foundling Museum – History – The Story of London's Abandoned Children* Available online from: http://golondon.about.com/od/londonmuseums/a/foundlinghist.htm Accessed 24 May 2012.

Cowley, S. & Frost, M. (2006) *The Principles of Health Visiting: Opening the Door to Public Health Practice in the 21st Century*, CPHVA, London.

Cribb, J., Joyce, R. & Phillip, D. (2012) *Living Standards, Poverty and Inequality in the UK: 2012*, E.S.R.C – Economic and Social Research Council – IFS/JRF, London.

Department for Children, Schools and Families (DCSF) (2010) *Working Together to Safeguard Children: A Guide to Interagency Working to Safeguard and Promote the Welfare of Children*, DCSF, London.

Department for Communities and Local Government (2012) *Listening to Troubled Families*, DCLG, London.

Department for Education (DE) (2012) *The Statutory Framework for Early Years Foundation*, DE, London.

Department of Health (DH) (2004) *The National Service Framework for Children Young People and Maternity Services*, DH, London.

DH (2011a) *The Health Visitor Implementation Plan 2011–2015: A Call to Action*, DH, London.

DH (2011b) *Birth and Beyond*, DH, London.

DH (2012a) *Getting it right for children, young people and their families. Happy, healthy children and young people: maximising the contribution of the school nursing team.* DH London.

DH (2012b) *The Maternal Mental Health Pathway.* DH, London.

DH (2012c) *Immunisation Against Infectious Disease. (The Green Book).* TSO, London.

DH/Department for Education and Skills (2004) *Every Child Matters.* DH/DfES, London.

DH/Department of Children Schools and Families (2009a) *The Healthy Child Programme: Pregnancy and the First Five Years of Life*, DH/DCSF, London.

DH/Department of Children Schools and Families (2009b) *The Healthy Child Programme: From Five to Nineteen*, DH/DCSF, London.

Field, F. (2010) *The Foundation Years: Preventing Poor Children Becoming Poor Adults*, HM Government, London.

Gerhardt, S. (2003) *Why Love Matters*, Routledge, London.

Hall, D. & Elliman, D. (2006) *Health for All Children Revised*, 4th edn. Oxford University Press, Oxford.

Heywood, C. (2001) *A History of Childhood*, Polity Press, London.

Hislop, I. (2010) *Suffer the Little Children*, BBC – first broadcast, December 2010.

HM Government (1989) *The Children Act*, HMSO, London.

HM Government (2004a) *The Children Act*, HMSO, London.

HM Government (2004b) *The Common Core of Skills and Knowledge for the Children's Workforce.* TSO, London.

Hough, D. (2012) *Youth unemployment statistics.* House of Commons Library, London.

Kirby, P. (2003) *Child Labour in Britain 1750–1870*, Palgrave Macmillan, London.

Laming, W. (2003) *The Victoria Climbie Inquiry*, The Stationery Office, London.

Laming, W (2009) *The Protection of Children in England: A Progress Report.* The Stationery Office, London.

Munro, E. (2011) *The Munro Review of Child Protection. Final report. A Child-Centred System*, Department of Education, London.

National Institute Clinical Health Excellence (2007) *Prevention of sexually transmitted infections and under 18 conceptions (PH3).* Available from http://guidance.nice.org.uk/PH3. Accessed on 13 December 2012.

NSPCC (2009) *Partner Exploitation and Violence in Teenage Intimate Relationships*, NSPCC, London.

Nursing and Midwifery Council (NMC) (2004) *The Standards of Proficiency for Specialist Community Public Health Nurses*, NMC, London.

The Children's Society (2012) *The good childhood report 2012 a review of our children's wellbeing.* The Children's Society, London.

The Factory Act 1833 Available from http://www.nationalarchives.gov.uk/education/lesson13.htm. Accessed on 24 May 2012.

Tickell, C. (2011) *The Early Years: foundation for life, health and learning*, DE, London.

UNICEF (2007) *Child poverty in perspective: an overview of child well being in rich countries.* UNICEF report card, 7. UNICEF, New York.

UNICEF (2011) *Children's well being in the UK, Sweden and Spain: The role of inequality and materialism*, UNICEF, New York.

7

Community Children's Nursing

Mark Whiting

West Herts PCT, Peace Children's Centre Watford, Watford, UK

Introduction

In 1994, as the first edition of this text was being prepared for publication, the provision of CCN services in the United Kingdom was very different to the situation which is to be found as this fifth edition of the text is being written, in 2012.

In 1994, almost two thirds of the children in the United Kingdom lived in an area where there was no CCN service at all. Although some parts of the United Kingdom were relatively well provided for, with a range of both generalist and specialist CCN services, in other areas, particularly those whose populations were quite widely dispersed, community children's nurses were a 'rare breed'. The whole of South-Western England NHS Region, for instance, contained only two generalist CCNs; a total of five nurses were employed (all in specialist roles) to provide a community nursing service for children in Wales; there was not a single CCN in the whole of Northern Ireland (RCN 1994). This situation led the 1997 House of Commons Health Select Committee to conclude:

> It is a cause for serious concern that only 50% of health authorities purchase CCN services and that only 10% of the Country's children have access to a 24-hour CCN service (para. 48).

In the 19 years that have passed since the publication of the first edition of this text, the provision of CCN has shown a dramatic expansion, to the extent that there are very few areas of the United Kingdom which are not covered by a CCN service

Community and Public Health Nursing, Fifth Edition. Edited by David Sines,
Sharon Aldridge-Bent, Agnes Fanning, Penny Farrelly, Kate Potter and Jane Wright.
© 2013 John Wiley & Sons, Ltd. Published 2013 by John Wiley & Sons, Ltd.

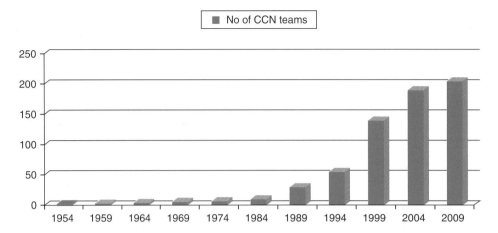

Figure 7.1   The growth of CCN provision in the United Kingdom between 1954 and 2009

(Whiting *et al.* 2009; Royal College of Nursing 2010a) (Fig. 7.1). However, CCN has a rather longer history than this text book, and therefore, before examining current arrangements for provision of community nursing support to children, it may be helpful to reflect briefly on the origins and evolution of services within the United Kingdom.

Early days

In 1874, Charles West and Dame Catherine Wood, respectively the Senior Consultant Physician and Lady Superintendent at the Hospital for Sick Children in Great Ormond Street, London, proposed the development of a private domiciliary nursing service which was intended to both provide care for children in home settings and enhance the experience of nurses in training. However, the proposal, which was largely supported by the hospital medical officers, did not go ahead at this time, because the lay members of the hospital committee 'were unanimously opposed to the extension of the work of the hospital beyond the walls' (THFSC 1874). Some 6 years later, however, the hospital's 28th annual report recorded that:

> A scheme is in preparation … to supply skilled nurses for children, for service outside its walls, thereby satisfying a demand that is undoubtedly greatly needed. (THFSC 1880)

By 1888, a 'Private Domiciliary Nursing Service' was established, based at the Great Ormond Street Hospital and staffed by nurses who had completed at least 3 years of training in the medical and surgical care of children in a hospital of not less than 60 beds. Training in tracheostomy nursing was considered to be particularly important at this time in respect of the care of children who were recovering from diphtheria. The Community Children's Nurses, for that is surely the correct term for this pioneering team, also provided care for children experiencing a range of medical conditions including orthopaedic problems such as cervical curvature and hip disease; post-operative care following surgical treatment for phimosis, abdominal abscess and peritonitis; and acute paediatric conditions including whooping cough, scarlet fever, scarlatina, malnutrition and marasmus (Hunt and Whiting 1999). The service was very popular and expanded rapidly over the course of the next 50 years. At its peak, in 1938, 30 nurses were employed within the Private Domiciliary Nursing Service, providing full-time care for 30 children, often on a 'living-in' basis.

Great Ormond Street was not alone in providing such a service. Lomax (1996) records that a number of the early specialist children's hospitals offered some sort of a domiciliary care provision including both visiting physicians and outreach nursing support. However, these services were generally only available on a fee-paying basis, and Lomax observes that many hospitals were forced to abandon these arrangements because of the 'expense involved and opposition from both hospital and general physicians' (Lomax 1996, p. 12).

The NHS

The introduction of the NHS in July 1948 was swiftly followed by the closure of the small number of hospital outreach nursing services for children, which had survived up to this time. The Private Nursing Service which operated out of Great Ormond Street was afforded special dispensation to continue to provide care for two children with long-term conditions (LTCs). However, on 14 March 1949, the final member of the Service returned to work in the hospital wards.

The first recorded appointment of a nurse within the NHS to provide care for sick children in the community was in Rotherham in 1949 (Gillett 1954). This scheme was initially staffed by a single Queen's Nursing Sister who had undertaken a postgraduate course covering 'children's diseases'. The establishment of this pioneering scheme arose as a result of concerns relating to a high rate of infant mortality in the Rotherham area during the course of the preceding winter, including hospital deaths arising from cross infection within the local children's ward. The work of the community nurse included a particular focus upon the care of children with acute infectious diseases, notably pneumonia, bronchitis, measles and gastroenteritis. Avoidance of unnecessary hospital admission was highlighted as a major benefit of this initiative (Gillet 1954).

In 1954, as a result of a collaborative venture between the Birmingham Health Committee, the Local Medical Committee and the Local Executive Council, a CCN service was introduced in Birmingham. Initially staffed by two district nursing sisters who had undertaken an orientation programme in the care of sick children at the Birmingham Children's Hospital, this scheme, much like the initiative in Rotherham, also focused upon the care of children with acute infectious disease. From the outset, close working relationships were established with the local general practice population, and Smellie (1956) reports that the work of the nursing sisters supported both avoidance of hospital admission and facilitation of early discharge. Evening visits by the nurses were identified as being the 'most important in allaying the worries and anxieties of the mothers so that there have been very few emergency calls during the night' (Smellie 1956, p. 256). Over the course of the next 20 years, however, the 'Children's Home Nursing Service' in Birmingham shifted its emphasis significantly away from the care of children with acute illness towards those with more long-standing nursing care needs. In addition, whilst in 1960, 92% of referrals to the service were made by general practitioners (GPs), by 1973 this figure had reduced to 43% (Howells 1974).

A 'home care scheme' for children was introduced in Paddington, North West London, in 1954. In addition to a team of three nurses 'with paediatric training' (Lightwood 1956, p. 13), the scheme also employed trained paediatricians. Lightwood and colleagues describe the motivation behind this initiative thus:

> ...nearly a quarter of the children in hospital during the review period were admitted for conditions which could have been managed at home if the doctors (GPs) had possessed the facilities and experience required, and that there were other children whose stay in hospital could have been shortened (Lightwood *et al.* 1957, p. 313).

The work of the home care team was a unique collaboration between paediatricians, GPs and community children's nurses, often involving joint home visits between all three. In the first 10 years that the service operated, it received a total of 2923 referrals of which 1882 (64%) were made by GPs. Two thousand four hundred and ninety-seven children were nursed at home following assessment by the paediatrician, with only 165 admitted to hospital. As with the schemes in Rotherham and Birmingham, acute infections of the respiratory and gastrointestinal tracts and 'contagious diseases' formed a major part of the caseload in Paddington (Bergman *et al.* 1965).

In 1969, two very different CCN services were established. The first involved the appointment of two nurses who were qualified as both Queen's Nurses and Registered Children's Nurses and whose role was specifically intended to support the establishment of a new Regional Centre for Paediatric Surgery at Southampton Children's Hospital (Atwell *et al.* 1973). The work of this nursing team focused particularly upon the care of children undergoing day surgery – often involving surgical procedures which in many other units required a stay of one or more nights in hospital. By 1980 Gow and Atwell reported that the nursing team were supporting 10-day surgery lists per week as well as providing care to children who had required a formal inpatient stay care for a range of medical and surgical problems. In addition, the team were taking direct referrals from GPs, health visitors and social workers (Gow 1976).

An outreach service was established from the outpatient department of the Royal Hospital for Sick Children in Edinburgh in 1969. The work of the nursing sister who was appointed to the service was concerned with providing support to the parents of children with a range of LTCs including diabetes mellitus and coeliac disease as well as congenital abnormalities such as cleft lip (Hunter 1974). In 1970 a second community nursing service was introduced at the hospital, involving the attachment to the hospital of a district nursing sister who had previously trained as a children's nurse. This initiative was focused upon children who were referred to the hospital either for inpatient care or for outpatient review of a range of predominantly acute problems. Hunter (1974) records how in the year leading up to the introduction of this new service only four children in total had been seen by the local district nursing teams, but in the first year of operation of the new service, 2400 visits were made to children in the community, increasing to 5700 home visits the following year.

Each of the services described earlier provides a particular insight into the somewhat eclectic history of the emergence of CCN services within the United Kingdom. More detailed examination of the schemes reveals how a range of local circumstances, clinical imperatives and professional interests (of both nursing and medical staff) prompted the introduction and development of community nursing services for children during the first 40 years of the NHS.

In 1988, a national 'census' review of CCN service provision in England identified a total of 23 services (Whiting 1988). Although there was a considerable variation between the services, for instance, in terms of where they were based (18 hospital outreach and 5 community-based services), NHS organisations within which teams were managed (11 within hospital service providers and 10 within community service providers) and numbers of staff within the teams (11 teams with only 1 member of staff, 11 teams with between 2 and 4 staff members and 1 team of 7 nurses), a consistent pattern of clinical activity was beginning to emerge in the workload of many of the teams (Tables 7.1 and 7.2).

Table 7.1   Which of these following broad categories of nursing care form part of your regular caseload? (Whiting 1988)

Care category	Number of teams (*n*=23)
Care of children with chronic disease	23 (100%)
Management of acute 'medical' problems	23 (100%)
Follow-up of non-day-case surgical patients	19 (82.6%)
Care of children with physical and mental disabilities	18 (78.3%)
Follow-up of day cases after discharge	11 (47.8%)

Table 7.2   Which of these following specific clinical conditions form part of your regular workload? (Whiting 1988)

Care category	Number of teams (*n*=23)
Respiratory conditions such as asthma	20 (87.0%)
Children with stomas such as tracheostomies, gastrostomies and ileostomies	18 (78.3%)
Cancer/leukaemia	17 (73.9%)
Congenital orthopaedic problems	17 (73.9%)
Eczema and other skin disorders	15 (65.2%)
Enuresis/encopresis	15 (65.2%)
Congenital heart disease	15 (65.2%)
Acute medical conditions such as non-specific infections and gastroenteritis	14 (60.9%)
Diabetes mellitus	14 (60.9%)
Renal problems such as nephrotic syndrome	10 (43.5%)
Blood dyscrasias such as sickle cell disease	9 (39.1%)

During the course of the past 20 years, CCN provision across the United Kingdom saw a dramatic expansion to the extent that by 2010 a directory of CCN services produced by the Royal College of Nursing (RCN) listed over 200 such services throughout the United Kingdom (RCN 2010a, Fig. 7.1). Whilst this clearly represents a very significant improvement in the situation which had been reported to the House of Commons Health Select Committee in 1997, many of the services listed in the RCN directory were either of 'teams' consisting of only one nurse or were of services that were clearly identified as being of a 'specialist' nature, providing care only to groups of children with particular medical conditions (such as diabetes) or who required quite specific nursing support (for instance, children with life-limiting or life-threatening conditions).

This expansion in provision has been supported by a succession of government reports dating back to the seminal review of the Welfare of Children in Hospital, the Platt Report in 1959 (Ministry of Health 1959; Department of Health and Social Security 1976; DH 1991, 2004a, 2010a; NHS Executive 1996; House of Commons Health Select Committee 1997).

NHS at home: Community children's nursing services

In 2009, the Department of Health (DH) convened an expert working group whose purpose was to identify and share local good practice in CCN services. This led to the publication of a report (*NHS at home: community children's nursing services* DH 2011a) whose target audience was those responsible for both the commissioning and provision of children's services and which was intended to inform:

> Quality, Innovation, Productivity and Prevention (QIPP) plans to reduce hospitalisation, and should be seen alongside the requirement set out in paragraph 4.34 of the Operating Framework for the NHS in England 2011/2012 for 24/7 community services to improve end-of-life care, and the Palliative Care Funding Review Interim Report (p. 2).

The executive summary to the report began with the following words:

> Currently, few local community children's nursing (CCN) services are able to meet the needs of all ill and disabled children and young people (DH 2011a, p. 3).

The report went on to identify four particular groups of children whom the DH believed should form the basis for the work of CCN services:

• Children with acute and short-term conditions.
• Children with LTCs.
• Children with disabilities and complex conditions, including those requiring continuing care and neonates.

- Children with life-limiting and life-threatening illness, including those requiring palliative and end-of-life care.

The report noted that 'Community children's nursing services are the bedrock of the pathway of care for these groups of children' (DH 2011a, p. 4). In the remainder of this chapter, consideration will be given to the ways in which CCN teams are addressing the needs of children in each of these care categories.

Children with acute and short-term conditions

The DH (2011a) identifies a number of possible roles which CCNs might play in respect of children with short-term care needs, including follow-up of children who have already been assessed by another professional, acting as advanced nurse practitioners, assessing acutely ill children in a range of settings, assessing children with acute exacerbations or complications of LTCs in order to prevent admission and facilitating early discharge from hospital in order to reduce length of stay. Many children, particularly infants, are receiving care in hospital for episodes of acute ill health when evidence suggests that admissions can often be avoided if appropriate assessment, treatment, management and support are available to families in the community (DH 2012a, b).

In 2010 there were 20.6 million emergency department attendances in England, a quarter of these were of infants, children and young people. Analysis of hospital admission statistics following these attendances identifies that 50% were for six high-volume conditions:

- Abdominal pain
- Asthma/wheeze
- Bronchiolitis
- Feverish illness
- Gastroenteritis
- Accidental head injury

In 2008–2009, these conditions accounted for over 420 000 hospital admissions for children in England under the age of 19 years, with an associated cost of £327 million (NHS Institute 2011; Right Care 2012).

When a child becomes unwell, parents want competent assessment, management, treatment and advice from skilled professionals who are experienced in meeting the unique needs of their child (Neill 2008; Carter *et al.* 2009; Parker *et al.* 2011). They may however be faced with a wide range of options and a multiplicity of potential providers of advice and/or clinical care (RCGP/RCN/RCPCH/CEM 2011) (Fig. 7.2, NHS Institute 2011).

It is hardly surprising that parents find local health services to be complex and confusing. This is complicated by the fact that many services are staffed by clinicians who

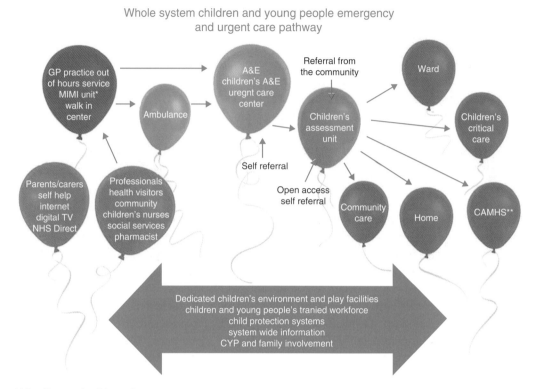

Whole system children and young people emergency and urgent care pathway

* Minor illness, minor injury unit
** Child and adolescent mental health service

Figure 7.2 Whole system children and young people emergency and urgent care pathway. (NHS Institute 2011)

have no specific training in either children's nursing or the medical care of children – for instance, fewer than half of all GPs have been formally trained in child health (RCN 2010b; DH 2012a, b; RCPCH 2012a).

There is an ever-increasing demand upon emergency departments and reliance on hospitals in respect of the care of children who are acutely unwell (RCPCH 2011). This is neither desirable nor sustainable. Work undertaken by the NHS Institute for Innovation and Improvement (NHS Institute 2011; National Health Service Institute for Innovation and Improvement 2012. Personal Communication. (Kath Evans, Programme Lead – Children & Young People Emergency Care Pathway, NHS Institute for Innovation and Improvement)) has highlighted how commissioners and clinicians are progressively recognising the potential of CCN services to deliver high-quality expert acute nursing care in nonhospital settings. The RCPCH review 'Facing the future' published in 2011 identifies the need to increase the number of children's nurses working in community-oriented roles as one of five interlocking levers that will be required to work together in order to deliver future health services for children that are fit for purpose and that will help to reverse this trend. The other four key levers are:

* Reduction in the number of hospital sites providing inpatient care for children.
* Increase in the number of paediatric consultants.
* Expansion in the number of GPs trained in paediatrics.
* Decrease in the number of paediatric trainees.

In 2010, Sir Ian Kennedy's review of services for children and young people (DH 2010a) reported that CCN services offer the potential to provide an alternative to emergency department attendance and hospitalisation. It is important, however, to recognise that this will depend on effective integration with other services in the urgent care system, including GPs, out-of-hours GP services, walk-in centres, emergency departments and observation and assessment units. Local partnerships are essential (DH 2011a; Parker *et al.* 2011).

A recent study by Kyle and colleagues (2012) which compared the experiences of two CCN teams in North West England provided a clear illustration of how the provision of acute care is dependent on integration and robust governance infrastructures within local services which ensure that children are only cared for at home with the support of CCN teams, when it is clinically safe and appropriate to do so. The study reinforced the view that acute and community care provider organisations need to work together to develop care pathways for common conditions in order to facilitate this.

Within the NHS in England, a variety of innovative models are evolving related to the care and management of children who are experiencing acute ill health. These focus upon the provision of a coordinated and systematic approach to both the commissioning and delivery of care pathways with a clear emphasis upon the need to maximise the choices which are available for families whilst aiming to keep care closer to home. Box 7.1 provides three short vignettes illustrating innovative practice in CCN which have been supported through the NHS Institute for Innovation and Improvement.

There is a growing recognition within the field of CCN that the care needs of this particular group of children need to be matched by the development of equivalent skill sets within the nursing team. Community children's nurses are registered children nurses. In addition, many CCNs have completed the post-registration specialist practitioner qualification in CCN. A number of teams are also employing nurses who have completed paediatric advanced nurse practitioner programmes or are supporting the development of team members to acquire skills in assessing acutely ill children, in making diagnoses and in the ordering of investigations and treatments including non-medical prescribing. In Greater Manchester, the development and reconfiguration of children's community nursing and ambulatory care services, including a very significant investment in the development of enhanced/advanced clinical skill sets within the nursing workforce, has been fundamental to the whole-system redesign of children's services centred around the building of the new Manchester Children's Hospital (www.makingitbetter.nhs.uk/index.php/childrens-community-teams).

Innovation within Community Children and Young People's Nursing services: Meeting acute care needs of children, young people and their families

In **Luton** a small team of paediatric nurse practitioners have been employed as part of a Rapid Response Community Children's Nursing Team which works in an integrated and collaborative way across acute and community provider organisations.

A series of 'acute care whole-system pathways' have been developed, supported by patient information resources which are used by all providers, including GPs, ambulance service, emergency department, assessment and inpatient areas and the community nursing service, to ensure consistency in care for children and their families.

The Community Children's Nursing services in **Portsmouth** have adopted a 'health-care system-wide' approach, with a particular focus upon keeping care closer to home. Key to the success of this innovative scheme is the establishment of strong links with local general practitioner services, including the establishment of clear referral criteria and agreed pathways of acute care.

The team have established a staff-rotation programme, which allows community nurses to work flexibly across primary and secondary care settings: within the acute children's assessment unit and emergency department as well as in the community, ensuring that the skills of the workforce are maintained in caring for children who are acutely unwell.

The Community Children's Nursing Team in **South of Tyne and Wear** are active participants in the 'whole-system' approach to reforming children and young people's care. Collaborative working across three Foundation Trusts has resulted in the growth and development of assessment and short stay services whilst supporting a reduction in inpatient-bed capacity. The Community Nursing Team have embraced this opportunity, by developing service specifications, agreeing referral and care pathways to support acute care at home in collaboration with commissioners and clinicians.

A key feature within each of these exemplars is the role of Community Children's Nurse Leaders who have articulated the needs of children, young people and families, whilst embracing the changing landscape within the NHS and maximising these opportunities.

They have engaged, influenced and collaborated with commissioners, clinicians and users. They have encouraged people to think differently to progress local services, and they have also taken time to learn from others to build on success and opportunities to enhance outcomes for children and young people.

Parker and colleagues undertook a detailed review of the role of community children's nurses in supporting care closer to home. They concluded that this approach 'can provide safe and effective care for a wide range of children who would previously have been in hospital, and may do so with reduced costs to the health service, and to families too' (Parker *et al.* 2011, p. 16). The interventions of Community Children's Nurses to support acute care can enable admission avoidance and facilitate timely discharge from a variety of urgent and emergency care settings including GP practices. This supports the delivery of care closer to home for children with acute episodes of ill health, significantly reducing costs of hospital admission and ultimately delivering safe, high-quality care at home in collaboration with and through the empowerment of families. In 2012, the Children and Young People's Health Outcomes Forum recommended:

> Acutely ill children and young people need access to specialist knowledge, rapid assessment of treatment, admission avoidance, shorter length of stay, with community children's nursing teams managing acutely ill children (DH 2012b, p. 5).

Children with LTCs

The DH (2011a) identifies several key roles played by community children's nurses in supporting children with LTCs including:

- Improved management of LTCs, supporting a reduction in hospital admissions/inpatient care.
- Education of children and families in order to enable them to better manage their illness and its treatment.
- Teaching families how to recognise early signs of exacerbation or deterioration of a long-standing illness.
- Providing specialist knowledge and skills for children with specific conditions, including epilepsy, asthma, diabetes, eczema or cancer.
- Provision of nurse-led clinics in community settings as a viable alternative to hospital-based, consultant-led outpatient services.

A number of authors have considered in some detail the role of the community children's nurse in the provision of care to children with a range of LTC (Whiting 1998; Eaton 2000; Parker *et al.* 2002; Myers 2005). Myers (in Whiting *et al.* 2009) provides an insightful account of the care of children with eczema in Islington, North London, detailing how the introduction of a community children's nurse consultant-led clinic has resulted in the provision of greater consistency of care, higher level of parental compliance and understanding, improved outcomes for children and reduction in referrals to secondary care.

The Kennedy Review (DH 2010a) highlighted the provision of specialist community nursing support to children with asthma, epilepsy and diabetes, going so far as to suggest that these conditions may be 'managed by a children's community nurse specialist, with contributions and support from paediatricians, the school health team and their GP' (p. 63). These three particular conditions were recently highlighted in the NHS Outcomes Framework 2012–2013 (DH 2011b) as accounting for around 94% of unplanned admissions to hospital occurring as a result of an exacerbation of pre-existing long-standing illness for young people under the age of 19 years. The extent to which CCN services are contributing to the care of children with established LTCs is however unclear. A major review undertaken by Parker and colleagues in 2011 offered little evidence of the systematic engagement of CCN teams in supporting children with either asthma or epilepsy, though the community nursing care of children with diabetes did seem to be rather more well established. The review team offered an additional challenge to the potential contribution of CCNs to this group of children:

> Whilst home-based support for children with long-standing conditions such as diabetes or asthma is increasingly popular, the systematic review concluded that 'there seems relatively little evidence to suggest whether or not it improves outcomes or reduces costs, for children themselves, their families or the health service' (Parker *et al.* 2002, pp. 71–72).

Specialist roles related to a number of LTCs have become established within CCN services. In addition to asthma, diabetes and epilepsy, CCNs have also developed a particular focus on conditions such as cystic fibrosis, sickle cell disease and thalassaemia, eczema and cancer and leukaemia. However, this specialisation is somewhat patchy and inconsistent, perhaps developing out of the particular interest of a member of the CCN team or paediatric medical colleague, rather than as a result of a systematic assessment and delineation of clinical needs within the local child population.

In 2011, the DH confirmed that it planned to introduce a Best Practice Tariff in children's diabetes care (DH 2011c). Included within the tariff is a requirement that:

> On diagnosis, a young person is to be discussed with a senior member of the paediatric diabetes specialist team within 24 hours and seen by a member of the team on the next working day. A senior member is defined as a doctor or paediatric specialist nurse with appropriate training in paediatric diabetes (p. 58).

The RCN (2011) identifies the key role played by nurses working within CCN teams as part of the paediatric diabetes specialist team.

The number of children with diabetes has increased dramatically in the past two decades in particular. A national audit of paediatric diabetes in 2011 has provided significant insights into the clinical care needs of this population, including a clear delineation of measures which provide useful information related to the impacts and outcomes of care provision for children with diabetes (RCPCH 2012b). It may well be that this approach has a wider applicability across a range of LTCs.

If community children's nurses are to establish themselves in the pivotal role in which the Kennedy Review suggested was potentially available to them in supporting children with LTCs, then it is of critical importance that they begin to establish the necessary evidence base to demonstrate the specific interventions, impacts and outcomes which relate to their work with such children. As noted earlier, a number of relatively common clinical conditions, namely, asthma, diabetes, epilepsy, eczema, cystic fibrosis, sickle cell disease and thalassaemia and cancer and leukaemia, contribute significantly to the work of CCN teams. It is important that those teams now take the opportunity to clearly set out:

- The expert care that they are providing to these children.
- The knowledge and skills that underpin that expert care.
- The impact of this care for children and their families, in particular in preventing admission/readmission to hospital and in facilitating early hospital discharge.
- The improvement in both short- and long-term outcomes for children and families arising as a direct result of the care which CCNs are providing.

Children with disabilities and complex conditions, including those requiring continuing care and neonates

The DH (2011a) highlights several specific areas of work for community children's nurses related to this group of children:

- Enabling care at home – reducing length of stay and costs.
- Safe governance arrangements/supervision of carers/support workers providing complex packages of care including training and ensuring ongoing competence of parents/carers/non-registered staff.
- Coordination of a multi-agency package of care – acting as the lead professional.
- Neonatal care.

However, this particular grouping of children within the DH report is somewhat arbitrary, and in many ways both the children themselves and their care needs overlap significantly with each of the other three groups identified within the report. There can be little doubt, however, that the provision of support for children with disabilities presents significant challenges not only for CCNs but also for the large number of health, education and social care staff who may be involved in this area of work.

Historical surveys of both the prevalence and nature of disability in childhood have lacked clarity, and this creates difficulties for both commissioners and providers of children's services. In the mid-1980s, the Office of Population Censuses and Surveys (OPCS) undertook a survey of the prevalence of disability amongst children. Based upon data collected from 80 000 households, OPCS estimated that there were likely to be between 338 000 and 382 000 children with a disability in Great Britain (OPCS 1989). The figure most often quoted is 360 000 (320 000 in England), just under 3% of the child population. This figure was used as the basis for service planning for almost 20 years; however, in January 2005 an interdepartmental review 'Improving the life chances of disabled people' which was published by the Prime Minister's Strategy Unit (PMSU) and based upon data derived from the General Household Survey (ONS 2004) stated:

> There are currently around 11 million disabled adults and 770000 children in the UK, equivalent to 24% of the adult population and 7% of all children. One in twenty children under 16-years old is disabled and there are increasing numbers of children with complex needs (p. 27).

Subsequent research, undertaken by Blackburn and colleagues from the University of Warwick (Blackburn *et al.* 2010) and based upon a detailed secondary analysis of the Family Resources Survey, reinforced the PMSU survey, noting that around 7.3% of children were reported as with disabilities according to the Disability Discrimination Act (1995) definition:

> A person has a disability for the purposes of this Act if he has a physical or mental impairment which has a substantial and long-term adverse effect on his ability to carry out normal day-to-day activities. (Part 1, Section 1(1))

> The effect of an impairment is a long term effect if it has lasted 12 months; the period for which it is lasts is likely to be at least 12 months or it is likely to last for the rest of the life of the person affected. (Scheduled 1, 2(1))

The PMSU figure of 770000 children with disabilities effectively doubled the number of children with disabilities in the population overnight and informed a number of national policy initiatives, the 'Children's National Services Framework' (DH 2004b), 'Every Child Matters' (DfES 2003) and 'Aiming High for Disabled Children' (Her Majesty's Treasury/DfES 2007). Over the course of several years, a clear focus upon the need to provide coordinated care for children with disabilities emerged, at the heart of which was a recognition of the need to ensure that:

> Children and young people who are disabled or who have complex health needs received coordinated high-quality and family centred services which are based on assessed needs, which promote social inclusion and, where possible, which enable them and their families to live ordinary lives (DH 2004c, p. 5).

It is important to acknowledge that in relation to this group of children, the focus of CCN activity is primarily upon children with physical health care needs. Relatively little of the work of CCNs is concerned with the care of children with mental health problems, those with learning disabilities or children with communication disorders (including autism spectrum disorders). In large part CCN work is concerned with the provision of expert clinical care to children in the context of a physical health care need. This work is, however, holistic in nature and encompasses several elements:

- Offering practical advice to children and their families including problem-solving/ troubleshooting issues related to clinical care.
- Coordinating care (sometimes as a formally designated key worker or lead professional), including advocating for and networking on behalf of families.
- Empowering children and families to promote independence and self-sufficiency in taking responsibility for their own care.
- Teaching and training children, their parents and other carers.
- Provision of equipment, including electrical equipment, disposable supplies, continence products and items not available on GP prescription.

- Provision of emotional and psychological support to children and their families.
- Promotion of health and prevention of ill health both in the context of the child's existing LTC, complex health need or disability and more generally.

Technology dependence

One particular group of children who feature significantly in the work of children's community nursing teams are those who might be described as technology dependent. Although prevalence data are somewhat elusive, there is strong evidence that the number of children whose care in the community is supported by a range of medical technology is growing year-on-year. This is in no small part because of the success of heroic medical intervention in keeping alive many babies and infants born prematurely or with complex inherited conditions, congenital abnormalities or perinatal pathology who might previously have died without ever leaving the hospital (Jardine & Wallis 1998; Ludvigsen & Morrison 2003; Kirk & Glendinning 2004; Lenton *et al.* 2004). In addition, through the long-term use of technology such as assisted ventilation, tracheostomy, home oxygen therapy, enteral and parenteral nutrition and peritoneal/renal dialysis, children who, in the past, were unlikely to survive infancy and early childhood are now surviving for many years, often into adulthood (Glendinning *et al.* 1999; Heaton *et al.* 2003).

As part of a wider study of families caring for technology-dependent children funded by the DH and undertaken by the National Primary Care Research and Development Centre at Manchester University, Glendinning and colleagues (1999) undertook a review which drew upon a range of data sources including material derived from the Family Fund Trust and the Norah Fry Research Centre. The review team estimated that there were around:

- 2500 children receiving artificial feeding
- 1000 children with tracheostomies
- 1000 children on intravenous infusions
- 150 on peritoneal dialysis
- Over 1000 receiving oxygen at home
- 93 on long-term ventilation at home

(Glendinning *et al.* 1999, p. 17)

This data has not been 'refreshed' and it is now significantly out of date. By way of illustration, Wallis *et al.* 2010 reported a 600% increase in the number of long-term ventilator-dependent children in the United Kingdom between 1998 and 2010. If CCN teams are to provide the necessary support to the technology-dependent child population, then a clearer understanding of the needs of these children, in particular of the number of children who require such support within the local population, will need to be more fully understood.

Continuing care

In recent years, CCN services have contributed significantly to the delivery of NHS continuing care for children. This area of work (whose origins lie in the introduction of continuing care for adults during the mid-1990s (DH 1995) evolved during the first decade of the twenty-first century in a somewhat piecemeal fashion but has developed rather more consistently following the publication in 2010 by the DH (England) of a 'National framework for children and young people's continuing care'. Children's continuing care is based upon:

> an equitable, transparent and timely process for assessing, deciding and agreeing bespoke packages of continuing care for those children and young people under the age of 18 who have continuing care needs that cannot be met by existing universal and specialist services alone (DH 2010b, p. 2).

The care packages which are provided for children generally take the form of home-based respite care, though may include support to access education or out-of-home respite. Such packages are often assessed, coordinated and delivered by local CCN teams.

Neonates

The DH (DH 2011a) recognises that a growing number of sick and very premature babies require long periods of specialist intervention and support resulting in prolonged hospitalisation. The DH suggests that many such babies could be safely cared for at home by their families with appropriate support from community-based or hospital outreach nursing teams. This can promote family-centred care, facilitate early discharge, reduce length of hospital stay and cost of in-hospital care and continuity of care and provide social, economic and psychological benefits for families.

This aspect of CCN activity involves particularly close working with colleagues such as neonatal paediatricians, hospital-based neonatal nursing teams and a small but growing number of community neonatal nurses. Specific areas of clinical focus for this work include supporting babies with long-term oxygen dependency and babies who require support with feeding (including short-term nasogastric feeding), the management of neonatal jaundice and neonatal palliative care.

Children with life-limiting and life-threatening illness, including those requiring palliative and end-of-life care

In the United Kingdom, at the turn of the twenty-first century, death in childhood is considered to be an infrequent occurrence. However, a major review of children's palliative care undertaken on behalf of the DH in 2007 by Sir Alan Craft and Sue Killen reported that each year approximately 20,100 children (0–19 years, including neonates,

2005 data) were living with conditions that were likely to require palliative care (DH 2007a). A detailed statistical analysis to accompany the DH review (DH 2007b) found that between 2001 and 2005, approximately 4000 children under 19 years of age died each year (including around 2100 neonatal deaths p.a.) from causes likely to have required palliative care. This represents around 50% of all deaths in childhood in the United Kingdom (Hain *et al.* 2011). Based upon the NHS commissioning arrangements that were in place at the time of the DH review, the authors estimated that Primary Care Trusts might expect there to be between 35 and 448 children living with such conditions within their commissioning locality at any one time, of whom between 1 and 55 children might be expected to die each year.

A more recent study by Fraser and colleagues, based upon a robust analysis of hospital episode statistics data, has estimated that there were more than 40000 children (0–19 years, including neonates) in England in 2009/2010 who were living with a life-limiting condition (Fraser *et al.* 2012).

CCN teams have been identified as one of the cornerstones of support for children with life-limiting and life-threatening conditions, particularly those children who require palliative care including end-of-life care (DH 2007a, 2008, 2010a, 2012a; ACT 2009; CLIC Sargent 2009). Much of this work is focused upon supporting children and their families towards the achievement of a 'good death' in the child's own home. However, the DH review in 2007 found that only 19.2% of all deaths for children who required palliative care occurred at home, whereas almost three quarters of all deaths (74.2%) were in hospital, with very high numbers of all child deaths in hospital occurring in intensive care settings (Ramnarayan *et al.* 2007).

Community Children's Nurses including staff based in both 'generic' CCN teams and those whose role has a specific focus upon children with life-limiting and life-threatening conditions contribute significantly to supporting this group of children and their families. In addition to the previously identified elements of holistic care provided by CCNs, a number of specific care roles have been developed to support these children:

- Symptom care, including the management of complex medication regimes, working alongside GPs, paediatricians and specialist palliative care doctors (ACT 2011).
- Out-of-hours care, including 24-hour care, particularly when supporting children and families at the end-of-life.
- Emotional and psychological support including bereavement care to the family.
- Counselling and support of siblings.

The overall expansion in CCN provision that was described earlier in this chapter (Fig. 7.1) has included a number of significant developments in the provision of support for children with life-limiting and life-threatening conditions. Box 7.2 sets out summary details of six specific funding initiatives related to this group of children and each based upon a broad acceptance that for many children the preferred place of death is at home, with their family.

BOX 7.2   Funding initiatives related to CCN support of children's palliative care

- 1992: £1.8 million 'Pilot projects for children with life threatening illnesses' to support a range of initiatives with a particular focus upon Community Children's Nursing (NHSE 1998a).
- 1999: £2 million to support the establishment of 'Diana Nursing Teams' within each of the Regions in NHS England – this funding was renewed for a further 3-year period from 2002 (NHSE 1998b).
- 2003: New Opportunities Fund investment in 135 grant schemes to support children's community-based palliative care services (£30.7 million) and children's hospice care (£15.3 million) in England (Carter & Petchey 2007).
- 2006: £27 million funding by the DH to support children's hospices in England (DH 2006). This is now established as a £10 million annual grant to support children's hospice and hospice at home care.
- 2007: specific targeting of children with palliative care needs as a subset of children with disabilities within the £340 million investment for 'Aiming High' (HM Treasury/DfES 2007).
- 2010: £30 million made available to fund a range of children's palliative care projects www.dh.gov.uk/en/Publicationsandstatistics/Publications/Publications PolicyAndGuidance/DH_117172.

As was noted earlier, in spite of this very significant investment to support the provision of palliative and end-of-life care for children in the community, most children with life-limiting and life-threatening conditions die away from home, sometimes in a children's hospice but more often than not in hospital. The provision of care and support to children and their families throughout the 24 hour day, and particularly at the very end of a child's life, remains a major challenge for CCN teams. In the summer of 2010, the DH agreed to fund a major independent review of the funding of palliative care for both children and adults. The review team published its final report in July 2011 in which it highlighted 'a stunning lack of good data surrounding costs for palliative care in England' (DH 2011d, p. 9) and has recommended the introduction of a per-patient tariff for the provision of community-based palliative care for both adults and children. A pilot-study-based review of funding is currently in progress. This pilot review is scheduled to be completed in 2013 and will hopefully support the provision of enhanced palliative and end-of-life care for both children and adults in the community in the future.

Conclusion

In this chapter, a brief synopsis of the historical emergence of a community nursing service for children in the United Kingdom has been followed by a detailed examination of the multifarious roles currently played out by Community Children's Nurses.

Although this examination has drawn significantly upon a DH (England) report focused upon NHS provision in England, the principles may be applied to settings throughout the United Kingdom.

This chapter has demonstrated that CCN has a rich history, a sophisticated present and an exciting future.

References

ACT (2009) *A Guide to the Development of Children's Palliative Care Services*, 3rd edn. ACT, Bristol.

ACT (2011) *Basic Symptom Control in Paediatric Palliative Care: The Rainbows Children's Hospice Guidelines*, 8th edn. Together for Short Lives, Bristol.

Atwell, J., Burn, J.M.B., Dewar, A.K. & Freeman, N.V. (1973) Paediatric day case surgery. *Lancet*, 2 (7834), 895–897.

Bergman, A.B., Shrand, H. & Oppe, T.E. (1965) A pediatric home care program in London – ten years' experience. *Pediatrics*, 36, 314–321.

Blackburn, C.M., Spencer, N.J. & Read J.M. (2010) Prevalence of childhood disability and the characteristics and circumstances of disabled children in the UK: secondary analysis of the Family Resources Survey. *BMC Pediatrics* 10, 21. Available from www.biomedcentral. com/1471-2431/10/21. Accessed on 24 October 2012.

Carter, Y. & Petchey, R.P. (2007) Evaluation of the big lottery fund palliative care initiative: final report. Available from www.biglotteryfund.org.uk/er_palliative_care_eval_summary.pdf. Accessed on 24 October 2012.

Carter, B., Coad, J., Goodenough, I., Anderson, C. & Bray, L. (2009) *Community Children's Nursing in England: An appreciative review of CCNs*, Department of Health in collaboration with the University of Lancashire and the University of the West of England, London.

CLIC Sargent (2009) *"More Than My Illness": Delivering Quality Care for Children with Cancer*. CLIC Sargent, Bristol.

Department for Education and Skills (2003) *Every Child Matters*, The Stationery Office, London.

Department of Health and Social Security (1976) *Fit for the future. The report of the committee on child health services*, HMSO, London.

Department of Health (DH) (1991) *The Welfare of Children and Young People in Hospital*, HMSO, London.

DH (1995) *NHS Responsibilities for Meeting Continuing Health Care Needs. HSG(95)8*. The Stationery Office, London.

DH (2004a) *National Service Framework for Children, Young People and Maternity Services: The Ill Child*. The Stationery Office, London.

DH (2004b) *National Service Framework for Children, Young People and Maternity Services: Core Standards*. The Stationery Office, London.

DH (2004c) *National Service Framework for Children, Young People and Maternity Services: The Disabled Child*. The Stationery Office, London.

DH (2006) *Funding for Children's Hospices and Children's Hospice at Home Grant for Voluntary Organisations in England*. DH, London. Available from http://www.dh.gov.uk/en/ Publicationsandstatistics/Publications/PublicationsPolicyAndGuidance/DH_4138727. Accessed on 24 October 2012.

DH (2007a) *Palliative Care Services for Children and Young People in England*. The Stationery Office, London.

DH (2007b) *Palliative Care Statistics for Children and Young Adults*. DH, London. Available from www.dh.gov.uk/en/Publicationsandstatistics/Publications/PublicationsStatistics/DH_074701. Accessed on 24 October 2012.

DH (2008) *Better Care: Better Lives. Improving Outcomes and Experiences for Children, Young People and Their Families Living with Life-Limiting and Life-Threatening Conditions*. The Stationery Office, London.

DH (2010a) *Getting it right for children and young people: overcoming cultural barriers in the NHS so as to Meet Their Needs*. Available from www.dh.gov.uk/en/Publications andstatistics/Publications/PublicationsPolicyAndGuidance/DH_119445. Accessed on 24 October 2012.

DH (2010b) *National Framework for Children and Young People's Continuing Care*. The Stationery Office, London.

DH (2011a) *NHS at Home: Community Children's Nursing Services*. Available from www.dh.gov.uk/en/Publicationsandstatistics/Publications/PublicationsPolicyAndGuidance/DH_124898. Accessed on 24 October 2012.

DH (2011b) *The Operating Framework for the NHS in England 2012/13*. Available from www.dh.gov.uk/en/Publicationsandstatistics/Publications/PublicationsPolicyAndGuidance/DH_131360. Accessed on 24 October 2012.

DH (2011c) *Payment by results guidance for 2011–12*. Available from www.dh.gov.uk/prod_con sum_dh/groups/dh_digitalassets/documents/digitalasset/dh_126157.pdf. Accessed on 24 October 2012.

DH (2011d) *Funding the right care and support for everyone. Creating a fair and transparent system; the final report of the palliative care funding review*. Available from www.dh.gov.uk/en/Publicationsandstatistics/Publications/PublicationsPolicyAndGuidance/DH_133100. Accessed on 24 October 2012.

DH (2012a) *Report of the children and young people's health outcomes forum*. Available from www.dh.gov.uk/health/files/2012/07/CYP-report.pdf. Accessed on 24 October 2012.

DH (2012b) *Children and young people's health outcomes forum: report by the acutely ill themed group*. Available from www.dh.gov.uk/health/files/2012/07/CYP-Acutely-Ill.pdf. Accessed on 24 October 2012.

DH (2012c) *Children and young people's health outcomes forum: report of the long term conditions, disability and palliative care subgroup*. Available from www.dh.gov.uk/health/files/2012/07/CYP-Long-Term-Conditions.pdf. Accessed on 24 October 2012.

Fraser, L.K., Miller, M., Hain, R., et al. (2012) Rising national prevalence of life-limiting conditions in children in England (online). *Pediatrics*, 123 e923. Available from http://pediatrics.aappublications.org/content/129/4/e923.full.html. Accessed on 24 October 2012.

Eaton, N. (2000) Children's community nursing services: model of care delivery. A review of the United Kingdom literature. *Journal of Advanced Nursing*, 32 (1), 49–56.

Gillett, J. (1954) Domiciliary treatment for sick children. *The Practitioner*, 172, 281–283.

Glendinning, C., Kirk, S., Guiffrida, A. & Lawton, D. (1999) *The Community-Based Care of Technology-Dependent Children in the UK: Definitions, Numbers and Costs*, Manchester, National Primary Care Research and Development Centre.

Gow, M.A. (1976) Domiciliary paediatric care in Southampton. *Queen's Nursing Journal*, 192, 205.

Gow, M.A. & Atwell, J. (1980) The role of the children's nurse in the community. *Journal of Pediatric Surgery*, 15 (1), 26–30.

Hain, R., Heckford, E. & McCulloch, R. (2011) Paediatric palliative medicine in the UK: past, present, future (Online). *Archives of Disease in Childhood*. Available from http://adc.bmj.com/content/early/2011/10/28/archdischild-2011-300432. Accessed on 24 October 12.

Heaton, J., Noyes, J., Sloper, P. & Shah, R. (2003) *Technology and time: home care regimens and technology dependent children*, University of York, Social Policy Research Unit, York.

Her Majesty's Treasury & Department for Education and Skills (2007) *Aiming High for Children: Supporting Families*, The Stationery Office, London.

Howells, M. (1974) *Domiciliary Care of Children in Birmingham its History and Development.* Presented to the Annual Conference of the National Association for the Welfare of Children in Hospital, NAWCH, London.

House of Commons Health Select Committee (1997) *Health services for children and young people in the community, home and school.* Third Report. The Stationery Office, London.

Hunt, J. & Whiting, M. (1999) A re-examination of the history of children's community nursing. *Paediatric Nursing*, 11 (4), 33–36.

Hunter, M.H.S. (1974) *A programme of integrated hospital and home nursing care for children.* Presented to the Annual Conference of the National Association for the Welfare of Children in Hospital, NAWCH, London.

Jardine, E. & Wallis, C. (1998) Core guidelines for the discharge home of the child on long term assisted ventilation. *Thorax*, 153 (9), 762–767.

Kirk, S. & Glendinning, C. (1999) *Supporting Parents Caring for a Technology Dependent Child.* National Primary Care Research and Development Centre, Manchester.

Kyle, R., Banks, M., Kirk, S., Powell, P. & Callery, P. (2012) Integrating community children''s nursing in urgent and emergency care: a qualitative comparison of two teams in North West England. *BMC Pediatrics*, 12 (1), 101. Available from www.ncbi.nlm.nih.gov/pubmed/22799532. Accessed on 24 October 2012.

Lenton, S., Franck, L. & Salt, A. (2004) Children with complex health needs: supporting the child and family in the community. *Child: Care, Health and Development*, 30 (3), 191–192.

Lightwood, R. (1956) The home care of sick children. *The Practitioner*, 177, 10–14.

Lightwood, R., Brimblecombe, F.S.W., Reinhold, J.D.L., Burnard, E.D. & Davis, J.A. (1957) A London trial of home care for sick children. *Lancet*, 9, 313–317.

Lomax, E.M.R. (1996) *Small and Special: The Development of Hospitals for Children in Victorian Britain.* Wellcome Institute for the History of Medicine, London.

Ludvigsen, A. & Morrison, J. (2003) *Breathing Space: Community Support for Children on Long Term Ventilation*, Barnardo's, Illford.

Myers, J. (2005) Community children's nursing services in the 21st century. *Paediatric Nursing*, 17 (2), 31–34.

Ministry of Health (1959) *The Welfare of Children in Hospital. Report of the Committee*, HMSO, London.

National Health Service Executive (1996) *Child Health in the Community: A Guide to Good Practice*, The Stationery Office, London.

National Health Services Executive (1998a) *Evaluation of the Pilot Project Programme for Children with Life Threatening Illnesses.* The Stationery Office, London.

National Health Services Executive (1998b) *Diana Children's Community Nursing Teams. (HSC 1998/201).* The Stationery Office, London.

National Health Service Institute for Innovation and Improvement (2011) *A Whole System Approach to Improving Emergency and Urgent Care for Children and Young People.* Available from www.institute.nhs.uk/index.php?option=com_joomcart&Itemid=194&main_page=document_product_info&products_id=762&Joomcartid=4p6p553p1t895lv9ovh8v86e86. Accessed on 24 October 2012.

Neill, S. (2008) *Family management of acute childhood illness at home: a grounded theory study.* Unpublished PhD thesis. King's College, London.

Office for National Statistics (2004) Living in Britain: Results from the 2002 General Household Survey. The Stationery Office, London.

Office of Populations Censuses and Surveys (1989) *OPCS surveys of disability in Great Britain Report 3: The prevalence of disability among children.* (Compiled by Bone, M. & Meltzer, H.) HMSO, London.

Parker, G., Bhakta, P., Lovett, C.A., et al. (2002) *A systematic review of the costs and effectiveness of different models of paediatric home care.* NHS R&D HTA Programme, Health Technology Assessment, London, 6, 35.

Parker, G., Spiers, G., Gridley, K., *et al.* (2011) *Evaluating models of care closer to home for children and young people who are ill: main report.* Social Policy Research Unit, University of York, York.

Prime Ministers Strategy Unit (2005) *Improving the Life Chances of Disabled People.* The Stationery Office, London.

Ramnarayan, P., Craig, F., Petros, A. & Pierce, C. (2007) Characteristics of deaths occurring in hospitalised children: changing trends. *Journal of Medical Ethics*, 33 (5), 255–260.

Right Care (2012) *NHS Atlas of Variation in Healthcare for Children and Young People.* Available from www.rightcare.nhs.uk/index.php/atlas/children-and-young-adults/. Accessed on 24 October 2012.

Royal College of General Practitioners, Royal College of Nursing, Royal College of Paediatrics and Child Health, College of Emergency Medicine (2011) *Right Care, Right Place, Right Time.* Available from www.rcpch.ac.uk/news/right-care-right-place-first-time. Accessed on 24 October 2012.

Royal College of Nursing (1994) *Directory of Paediatric Community Nursing Services*, 11th edn. RCN, London.

Royal College of Nursing (2010a) *Directory of Community Children's Nursing Services.* Available from www.rcn.org.uk/development/communities/rcn_forum_communities/children_and_young_people_field_of_practice/cyp_continuing_care/resources. Accessed on 24 October 2012.

Royal College of Nursing (2010b) *Maximising Nursing Skills in Caring for Children and Young People in Accident and Emergency Departments*, RCN, London.

Royal College of Nursing (2011) *Children and Young People with Diabetes: RCN Guidance for Newly-Appointed Nurse Specialists.* RCN, London.

Royal College of Paediatrics and Child Health (2011) *Facing the Future: A Review of Paediatric Services.* RCPCH, London.

Royal College of Paediatrics and Child Health (2012a) *Standards for Children & Young People in Emergency Care Settings.* Intercollegiate Committee for Standards for Children and Young People in Emergency Care Settings. Available from http://www.rcpch.ac.uk/emergencycare. Accessed on 24 October 2012.

Royal College of Paediatrics and Child Health (2012b) *National Paediatric Diabetes Audit Report 2010–11.* RCPCH, London.

Smellie, J.M. (1956) Domiciliary nursing service for infants and children. *British Medical Journal*, 1, 256.

The Disability Discrimination Act (1995).

The Hospital for Sick Children (1874) *Medical Committee Minutes: Volume 6 'Special meeting of the joint committee'.* March 18th. The Hospital for Sick Children Archives. London.

The Hospital for Sick Children (1880) *The 28th Annual Report of the Hospital for Sick Children.* Folkard & Sons, Bloomsbury, UK.

Wallis, C., Paton, J.Y., Beaton, S. & Jardine, E. (2011) Children on long-term ventilatory support: 10 years of progress. *Archives of Disease in Childhood*, 96 (11), 998–1002.

Whiting, M. (1988) *Community paediatric nursing in England in 1988.* Unpublished MSc Thesis, University of London.

Whiting, M., Myers, J. & Widdas, D. (2009) Community children's nursing. In*Community Health Care Nursing*, (4th edn) (Sines, D., Saunders, M. & Forbes-Burford, J. (eds)) Blackwell Publishing Ltd. Chichester, pp. 148–171.

8

Public Health Nursing (Adult): A Vision for Community Nurses

Jane Wright and Kate Potter

Faculty of Society and Health, Buckinghamshire New University,
High Wycombe, UK

Introduction

This chapter identifies the emerging public health challenges for communities now and in the future, and in particular, it will explore the role of community nurses within the new public health agenda. It will outline the vision for public health improvement in England introduced by the coalition government in 2010 (DH 2010a). The public health outcomes framework was published in January 2012 and emphasised the renewed focus on achieving positive health outcomes for the population and reducing inequalities in health – specifically 'increased healthy life expectancy, reduced differences in life expectancy and healthy life expectancy between communities' (DH 2012a, p. 5). These objectives are not new and the fundamental causes of ill health have remained the same throughout history: infection, the environment, lifestyle choices, genetics and biology. However, as societies have evolved, illnesses arising out of environmental conditions and poorly understood disease processes have, arguably, been replaced with those problems associated with modernity. Capitalism, globalisation and the technological revolution have changed the way we live, work and communicate with each other, and this has a profound effect on the population's physical and mental health and well-being (Kerr *et al.* 2005).

Across the world, the pattern of disease is changing and in middle- and high-income countries, nine out of ten leading causes of death are non-communicable.

Community and Public Health Nursing, Fifth Edition. Edited by David Sines,
Sharon Aldridge-Bent, Agnes Fanning, Penny Farrelly, Kate Potter and Jane Wright.
© 2013 John Wiley & Sons, Ltd. Published 2013 by John Wiley & Sons, Ltd.

These include ischaemic heart disease, stroke, chronic obstructive pulmonary disease and cancer (WHO 2010a). The pattern, however, is also changing in low-income countries with the development of better health-care systems and improving environmental conditions; life expectancy is increasing. In countries such as Chad, with the lowest life expectancy in the world, average life expectancy has increased to 49 years in 2012 (WHO 2012). Ischaemic heart disease and cerebrovascular disease now feature in the top five causes of death in low-income countries according to the World Health Organisation (WHO 2012). In 2000, the World Health Organisation adopted a tool to measure the overall burden of disease: Disability-Adjusted Life Year (DALY). DALY has become common both in public health and also in health impact assessments, and it effectively combines mortality and morbidity measurements into one metric tool. One DALY is defined by the WHO as one lost year of 'healthy' life. The sum of DALYs across a population (the burden of disease) can be described as a 'measurement of the gap between current health status and an ideal health situation where the entire population lives to an advanced age, free of disease and disability' (WHO 2012).

Long-term conditions arising out of infectious diseases such as HIV/AIDs, human papillomavirus (HPV) and Helicobacter pylori have provided a paradigm shift in our understanding of disease processes, morbidity and mortality (Halpin *et al.* 2010). People are surviving much longer than has been predicted and preventable chronic conditions look set to become a huge challenge for society in terms of health and social care now and in the future (Kerr *et al.* 2005). In addition, people with other, non-infectious, life-limiting conditions such as cystic fibrosis are living much longer, and the life expectancy continues to increase year on year as health-care systems improve (Harrop 2007). Mental health problems are also highlighted as a burgeoning area of concern across the world, and Alzheimer's, dementia and suicide are featuring in the top ten burden of disease in high-income countries (WHO 2010a). Mental health problems can affect the whole population, and postnatal depression, dementia and self-harming behaviours are particularly highlighted in *No Health Without Mental Health: Implementation Framework* (DH 2012a). This document is a cross departmental consultation that has been jointly developed by the DH, Mind, Rethink Mental Illness, Young Minds, the Royal College of Psychiatrists and the Mental Health Foundation. This is reflective of the concerns in that area of public health.

Perhaps an even bigger question for the future is the impact that humans have on the world around them (WHO 2010b). The use of natural resources, population growth, the overuse of antibiotics and climate change impact on the health of populations in the long term and raise questions about the concepts of utilitarianism. The tenets of public health practice have always battled with balancing the rights of humans to self-determination against the collective benefit; do the needs of the many outweigh the needs of the few? Successive governments have struggled with providing the conditions in which individuals and groups can remain healthy and make sensible personal choices without blaming individuals for their own health problems. Poverty, vulnerability and inequality remain major determinants of health, and the Marmot Report confirms that, in the United Kingdom, there remains a significant gap between the rich and the poor (Marmot 2010).

The Nuffield Council on Bioethics (NCB 2007) describes a ladder of public health interventions where at one end of the scale, society does nothing, allowing people to make their own choices, whatever the consequences, while at the other end choice is taken away from individuals in order to protect their health. Community nurses need to consider appropriate actions along this continuum:

1. Do nothing or monitor current situation
2. Provide information
3. Enable choice
4. Guide choices through incentives
5. Guide choices through disincentives
6. Restrict choices
7. Eliminate choices

There are few examples of taking away people's ability to choose for themselves but the smoking ban introduced in England in 2007 is one. Smoking was prohibited from all public places and advertising banned (HM Government 2006). There has been an overall fall in smoking rates since the link between smoking and lung cancer was made over half a century ago. Further evidence of the harmful effects of second-hand smoke influenced this particular piece of legislation. According to the Office of Online Statistics, the level of adult smoking in England has remained at around 21% since 2007 (Office of National Statistics 2011). However, the more long-term effect of the smoking ban on related long-term conditions and the impact on long-term care remains to be seen. The effect of second-hand smoke in confined spaces such as cars is under debate in 2012, particularly the harmful effect on children and babies (Ribeiro 2012).

Health care is expensive and there have been examples of individuals being refused treatment unless they change their health behaviour. For example, refusal to operate unless a patient gives up smoking or drinking or loses weight. These are real ethical dilemmas as one could argue that if you refuse treatment for these people, then you should refuse treatment for anyone who has taken a risk with their health: played rugby, ridden a horse or climbed a mountain. However, resources are finite and with increasing costs, the NHS must look to prevention to find a way to reduce the ever-expanding health needs of the population (Wanless 2002). Measuring the outcomes of preventative work has always been problematic, but it is an essential part of the public health agenda.

This chapter will examine the current public health issues that have driven the policy agenda on the population's health and well-being. The focus will be on how community nurses work within public health principles and how they contribute to the key objectives of reducing health inequalities and enabling people to live as healthy a life as possible given their individual circumstances.

The vision for health reform: the policy context

Since devolution in 1999, the four governments of the United Kingdom have determined their own health policies on the basis of what is considered best to meet the needs of each country and fits with their political ideology. Any government faces huge challenges in prioritising the allocation of funds across public services, particularly in a time of global economic slowdown. However, promoting and protecting health are an essential part of sustaining economic and social development and crucial to human welfare (WHO 2010b). With rising costs of health care provision and widening inequity, ensuring the health of the population through timely access to health services which balance health promotion, prevention, treatment and rehabilitation is difficult. Derek Wanless in 2002 was asked to make an independent report on the financial situation in the NHS by the Labour Party in power at the time. It was an independent enquiry from the King's Fund into the predicted technological, demographic and medical trends for the following two decades which are likely to affect the health service in the United Kingdom as a whole. *Securing our future health: taking a long term view* (Wanless 2002) looked at the resources that would be required to ensure that the NHS could provide a publicly funded, comprehensive, high-quality service available on the basis of clinical need and not ability to pay. The key findings were that there needed to be increased productivity in the NHS and, in relation to public health, that there should be improved health promotion initiatives and disease prevention. In addition to this, the report suggested that there should be more clearly identified outcome measures to monitor progress and plan effective services.

In all countries, public health policy over history has been successful; we have an ageing population, average life expectancy has increased in all parts of the world, premature babies are surviving at an earlier age, and there are curative treatments for many life-threatening conditions. These changes have been achieved through successful public health interventions, which include vaccinations that have eliminated infectious diseases such as smallpox, improvements in the environmental conditions that cause disease, better health care systems, advances in surgery and germ theory development. The biggest changes have emerged through the determined efforts of many pioneering individuals across the world, not just those involved in health care but also the social reformers who linked disease to the social conditions of their times.

Following World War II, the Welfare State evolved following the Beveridge Report. Beveridge identified five 'giant evils' which needed to be tackled in order for Britain to fully recover from the effects of war. These giants were want, disease, squalor, ignorance and idleness (Beveridge 1942). There were a number of outcomes from this report including the establishment of the National Health Service (NHS) in 1948 and the expansion of the National Insurance Act (Beveridge 1942). Improvements in the population's health rely on many things: the political will to drive change, the behaviour of groups and individuals in making healthy choices and a workforce which is committed to improving the health of the nation. Traditional public health services have not always acknowledged nursing as part of the public health workforce, and the sphere of influence that community nurses have can be debated. However, there are many areas in which they can directly impact on the health of individuals or groups and influence policy at a high level. Green Papers are consultative documents which enable governments to obtain the views of a wide range of experts in the field before a White Paper goes through parliament to become an Act. Anyone can contribute to the consultation, and nurses should be aware of what is in the public domain and understand that they can contribute as individuals as well as professional groups.

The new coalition government in 2010 produced a White Paper, *Equity and excellence: Liberating the NHS* (DH 2010b), without a preceding Green Paper. The White Paper set out the government's aims to reduce the central direction of the NHS, to engage doctors in commissioning health services and to give patients greater choice (House of Commons Library (HCL) 2011). It was reported as the biggest NHS reform since its creation in 1948. As part of the proposed reforms, public health was embedded through the White Paper *Healthy Lives, Healthy People* (DH 2010a) with a public health outcomes framework published in 2012 (DH 2012c).

In 2011, the proposed Health and Social Care Bill was stalled as it went through parliament because influential pressure groups questioned many of its proposals. This demonstrated the power of user groups to hold governments to account for their plans and ensure that the voice of the population is heard. The main changes in the Health and Social Care Act (HM Government 2012) in relation to community health were to abolish Primary Care Trusts and Strategic Health Authorities and create GP consortia run, in the main, by general practitioners. The key concerns surrounding the Bill were around the accountability and governance arrangements for commissioners and providers of health services and the role of competition in the NHS (HCL 2011). An NHS Future Forum was appointed to listen to concerns and report back to government. The eight-week listening exercise was completed on 31 May 2011, and the final report made a number of detailed recommendations for change. These included a change of the name 'GP consortia' to Clinical Commissioning Groups (CCGs) to reflect a recommendation that there should be a much wider membership of these groups, including multi-professional members. Specifically, at least one nurse, a specialist doctor from secondary care and other lay members were recommended in order to improve the accountability. CCGs will also be required to hold public meetings and publish data from the meetings to ensure transparency.

Acknowledgement that the health sector cannot work in isolation to improve the health of the nation has been clearly articulated throughout policy documents for some time, and both a top-down and bottom-up approach is essential to successful public health policy (DH 2010a). The key to success hinges on building healthy public policy, creating supportive environments, strengthening community involvement, developing personal skills and reorientating health services. These goals have been both implicit and explicit in public policy since the *Ottawa Charter for Health Promotion* in 1986 (WHO 1986). There have been different approaches to achieving these goals, and successive governments have used different languages to describe these aims. The current coalition government has emphasised measuring outcomes, building community capacity, devolving responsibility to local communities and commissioning services locally according to need (DH 2012b). The new structure for the NHS was outlined in the Health and Social Care Bill 2012, and public health is structured within the Department of Health with local public health services provided locally within local authorities. As Public Health England will be an executive agency of the Department of Health, its Chief Executive will be accountable to the Secretary of State for Health.

The commissioning framework will focus on the productivity of services, and productivity may be defined as the 'measure of the efficiency of the production'. The 'product' in the NHS, one could argue, is improved health outcomes for individuals. The overarching aims of the public health outcomes framework (DH 2012b) are to increase healthy life expectancy and reduce the differences in healthy life expectancy across communities (i.e. reduce inequalities).

The public health outcomes framework (2012)

The public health outcomes framework is the key government policy driving the public health agenda. The operational framework will rely on the roles of three key partners: the NHS, local government and Public Health England. Public Health England will sit within the Department of Health and have the broad population health protection responsibilities. Responsibilities for local populations will be devolved to local authorities where services will be commissioned according to local health needs assessments. A common theme running through national policy in health, public health, education and social care is the devolvement of responsibility for services to local areas (DH 2012b). This has both positive and negative consequences. It enables local areas to interpret guidelines according to the needs of the local population, but it also means that 'standardised services' are less likely across the country. The coalition government promotes the notion of outcomes and performance indicators, and results will be accountable to central government through Public Health England. Measurable outcomes are an essential part of the commissioning agenda and in relation to public health; indicators are divided into four domains:

- Improving the wider determinants of health
- Health improvement
- Health protection
- Health care public health and preventing premature mortality

Improving the determinants of health

Michael Marmot's report *Fair Society, Healthy Lives* reported a continuing gap between the richest and poorest in our society (Marmot 2010). The report found that people living in the poorest neighbourhoods in England will, on average, die seven years earlier than those living in the richest neighbourhoods. He suggests that they will also spend more of their lives with a disability, an average total difference of 17 years. Health inequalities are complex and arise from an interaction of many factors including income, education, social isolation and disability. However, they are largely preventable with a concerted political will, community co-operation and a multi-agency approach. Marmot argues that there is a strong economic case for addressing health inequalities; it is estimated that the annual cost to society is between £36 and £40 billion. This is through lost taxes, welfare payments and costs to the NHS (Marmot 2010). Amongst the indicators for the determinants of health are:

- Children living in poverty
- Pupil absences
- 16–18-year-olds not in education, employment or training (NEETs)
- People in prison who have a mental illness
- Sickness absence rate
- Violent crime (including sexual violence)
- Domestic abuse

Health improvements

The objective of improving the health of the nation is to support people in the lifestyle choices that they make. Through history, there have been unpopular or unfashionable messages: that smoking causes lung cancer, that alcohol destroys lives, that eating too much makes you ill, that living in crowded conditions spreads disease or that it is not the fault of the poor that they are poor. The growth of the term 'nanny state' has arisen out of the balance of having healthy public policy which attempts to achieve sensible, achievable health outcomes for individuals and populations against the right to choose how we live our lives. Amongst the indicators for health improvements are:

- Low-birth-weight term babies
- Breastfeeding rates
- Under 18 conceptions
- Excess weight in 4–5- and 10–11-year-olds
- Hospital admissions as a result of self-harm
- Proportion of physically active and inactive adults
- Alcohol-related admissions to hospital
- Self-reported well-being
- Falls and injuries in the over 65s

Health protection

This domain has a focus on protecting the general population from major threats such as climate change, pollution and contagious diseases such as influenza. Locally, public sector organisations are expected to have board-approved sustainable development management plans and comprehensive agreed interagency plans to respond to a public health incident. An example would be contaminants in the water supply, outbreaks of specific diseases such as Legionnaire's disease or a gas explosion. The measures of success in this domain include measurements of:

- Air pollution
- Chlamydia diagnoses (15–24)
- Population vaccination coverage
- People presenting with HIV at a late stage of infection
- Treatment completion for TB

Healthcare public health and preventing premature mortality

The aim of this domain is to reduce the number of people living with preventable ill health and people dying prematurely whilst reducing the gap between communities. Improvements in this area will be co-ordinated across the whole public health system. The three partners, the NHS, Public Health England and the local authorities, will need to work together with other professionals to address these issues. The indicators in this domain have been mapped to the NHS outcomes framework and are directly measurable:

- Infant mortality
- Tooth decay in children aged 5
- Mortality from cardiovascular disease, cancer, liver disease and respiratory disease
- Excess under 75 mortality in adults with a serious mental health illness
- Suicide
- Excess winter deaths
- Dementia and its impact

The issue of preventable ill health is highlighted throughout policy documents. It is clear that there has to be a combined approach to improving the conditions that would enable people to make healthy choices and reduce inequalities. The efforts that society makes to improve public health need to include policymakers in government through to those working directly with individuals and groups. Supporting people to make healthy life choices is a crucial aspect of public health but not an easy one. Entrenched behaviour is hard to change and there has been, in recent years, an emphasis on social marketing strategies. *Changing Behaviour, Improving Outcomes* (DH 2011) is a document which highlights an approach to changing behaviour which borrows concepts and techniques from the commercial sector. In public health care, there has been a paradigm shift away from a professional-led, adult to child information exchange towards a more customer-led, adult to adult communication strategy (French 2012). The National Social Marketing Strategy (NSMS) highlights how people gain information about their health, how they react to information and how they view their own ability to change their behaviour (NSMS 2012). Public health professionals need to understand why people behave the way they do and what competition there is for people's attention, particularly in a climate of global communication, and have a clear focus on achieving specific behavioural goals.

The key points to social marketing are

- Understand the 'customer' using a variety of customer and market research – identifying individual needs in different communities and settings.
- Develop insight into why people behave the way they do: what makes people change their behaviour?
- Use 'exchange' concepts and analysis – what benefit does the customer see in any behaviour change and can you utilise that to change behaviour?
- Assess need and adjust health messages according to that need.
- Use a mix of interve\ntions – multifocal approaches have been shown to be more effective than a single method.

Health promotion versus public health

Defining public health and what it means for both policymakers and practitioners is key to supporting all community nurses to understand their own specific contribution to the health of the communities in which they work. The concept, however, remains difficult to encapsulate but Acheson (1988) provides a well-used definition:

> The science and art of preventing disease, prolonging life and promoting health through the organised efforts of society.

It is clear from this definition that public health practice is broader than practising purely within a framework based on scientific and epidemiological principles. Delivering public health requires an approach which is considered in the context of a wide range of social, cultural and political issues (Reading 2008). An effective approach to improving the health of individuals and communities through a public health approach requires the main determinants of health to be the central focus (see Fig. 8.1).

WHO (1986) defined health promotion as the process of enabling people to increase control over, and to improve, their health. It moves beyond a focus on individual behaviour towards a wide range of social and environmental interventions.

Revisiting the Ottawa Charter for Health Promotion (WHO 1986), it suggested five key themes for promoting health are seen to be:

- *Build public health policy* – the changes in health care delivery and more decisions at a local level for commissioning services will provide opportunities for community nurses to be proactive in local policy development.
- *Create supportive environments* – the need to be aware of the impact of both working and living environments on both physical and emotional health and well-being.

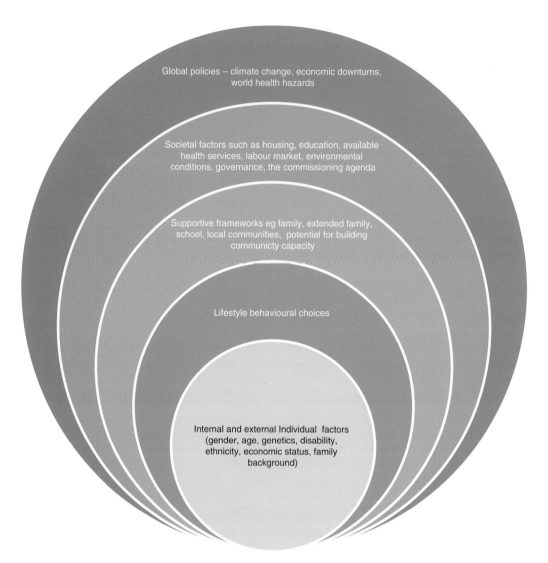

Global policies – climate change, economic downturns, world health hazards

Societal factors such as housing, education, available health services, labour market, environmental conditions, governance, the commissioning agenda

Supportive frameworks eg family, extended family, school, local communities, potential for building communicty capacity

Lifestyle behavioural choices

Internal and external Individual factors (gender, age, genetics, disability, ethnicity, economic status, family background)

Figure 8.1   Factors influencing health

- *Strengthen community action* – empowering communities to set their own priorities and work together to plan and implement strategies to improve health.
- *Develop personal skills* – people need to be facilitated to develop life skills across the lifespan to gain more control over their own health and the environments in which they live and work. Helping people to develop these skills requires collaborative working within schools, the workplace, children centres as well as health care settings.
- *Reorientation of health services* – policy is gradually moving health workers from their responsibility for providing clinical services to prevention and early intervention.

An upstream approach

McKinlay (1975) developed the analogy of a river as illness. He saw the medical model of health care concentrating all efforts to rescue people from drowning downstream whilst no one was trying to investigate why they were falling in the water in the first place. This echoes a much earlier vision of a social model of public health articulated in a poem by Joseph Malins, a temperance activist, in 1875 entitled 'A fence or an ambulance' (Malins 1932). This shows clearly that there was an early recognition that the determinants of health were not just biological but that primary prevention is more cost effective. In the current climate of economic austerity, there is a need to find ways to reduce the burgeoning spending on care in the NHS. The concept of focusing on an upstream approach in which decisions are made by wider society rather than just 'knowledgeable professionals' working in the clinical field is essential.

Health protection

Health protection is part of the delivery of public health. It aims to provide public protection by preventing or limiting exposure to hazards which are harmful to health; this includes

* Prevention, investigation and control of communicable diseases.
* Ensuring the quality of air, water and food is maintained at a safe level.
* Dealing with outbreaks and incidents which are likely to have a severely negative impact on public services; this would include pandemics and bioterrorism.

These functions are currently carried out by the Health Protection Agency (HPA) in England; the National Public Health Service Wales; Health Protection Scotland (HPS); and the Department of Health, Social Services and Public Safety, Northern Ireland. From April 2012, the HPA in England will sit in Public Health England (HM Government 2012). The aim is to devolve more responsibility to protecting the health of the public to a more local level.

Local authorities (and directors of public health acting on their behalf) will have a critical role in protecting the health of their population, both in terms of helping to prevent threats arising and in ensuring appropriate responses when things do go wrong. They will need to have available to them the appropriate specialist health protection skills to carry out these functions.

The scope and scale of work by local government to prevent threats to health emerging, or reducing their impact, will be driven by the health risks in a given area.

Understanding and responding to those health risks will need to be informed by the process of Health and Wellbeing Boards developing joint strategic needs assessments (JSNAs), joint health and well-being strategies and commissioning plans based upon them. Local government will work with local partners to ensure that threats to health are understood and properly addressed (DH 2012b).

This will hopefully allow for better development of services which are responsive to local need and will improve working together across agencies. As stated earlier in the chapter, the concern could be less standardised services and a 'postcode lottery' impact on local communities.

The Public Health Framework (DH 2012a) identifies two overarching outcomes to which all who have a public health remit should be working towards:

- Increased healthy life expectancy. This should include taking account of health quality as well as the length of life.
- Reduced differences in life expectancy and healthy life expectancy between communities (through greater improvements in more disadvantaged communities).

Measuring the outcomes of public health policies will always be challenging. Timescales for gaining evidence that policy has improved life expectancy are considerably longer than a term of office for a government. The framework identifies that measurement has to be by researching indicators across the lifespan. Evaluation, however, is an essential process which has now become part of service delivery across the public, private and voluntary sector. Wanless *et al.* (2007) still believe that there is a need to gain more evidence of the effectiveness of public health practice.

Much has been written on the process of evaluation, and it is important for practitioners to recognise that it is a necessary and important part of implementation of any programme. Douglas *et al.* (2007) identify three approaches to evaluating public health interventions:

1. Formative: assessing the process, planning and development of an intervention
2. Process: assessing the implementation and including the number of participants and their satisfaction level
3. Outcome evaluation: assessing to what extent it has reached its intended purpose

Ideally, all these approaches should be taken to ensure that practitioners are providing services which are of a high quality, cost effective and acceptable to the client group.

Community nursing and public health

There has not always been a link made between the prevention of illness and nursing practice. However, the NHS by its very title is there to promote health rather than illness. One could argue of course that the NHS uses most of its resources to treat the sick whilst paying lip service to preventative work (Wanless *et al.* 2007). Historically, the NHS has developed public health specialist nurses. Indeed, Florence Nightingale (1860) was a keen advocate of promoting public health and also community nursing. In her 'Notes on Nursing' (Nightingale 1860), she outlines the need to consider both the 'well and the sick' and:

...how to put the constitution in such a state that it will have no disease or that it can recover from disease takes a higher place... (Nightingale 1860, Preface)

She was, therefore, concerned with the living conditions of people and not just the disease processes and suggested that building hospitals to tend sick children was not the answer to the high child mortality rates at the time (reflecting her ability to assess need).

...now, instead of giving medicine, of which you could not possibly know the proper amount or indeed its application, nor all its consequences, would it not be better if you were to persuade your poorer neighbour to remove the dung hill from before the door, put in a window that opens and to cleanse and lime wash the cottages?... (Nightingale 1860, p. 78)

With this she describes the early influences of community nurses and health visitors by saying that nurses should be involved within the home to help to educate families on ways to improve their health and well-being. Interestingly, her notes also describe the same issues that we have today around nutrition, a clean environment, hygiene and the benefits of good mental health, and she suggests that the education of all women will go some way to improve the overall health of the population, indicating again a need for early intervention and family support.

The continuing challenge, however, is for community nurses to consider the importance of their public health role and what scope of activities they can and should undertake to improve the health of the communities which they serve. Within their daily work the majority of nurses use health education and health communication strategies to improve outcomes for their clients (Laverack 2005).

The Nursing and Midwifery Council states that

All nurses must support and promote the health, well-being, rights and dignity of people, groups, communities and populations. These include people whose lives are affected by ill health, disability, ageing, death and dying. Nurses must understand how these activities influence public health (NMC 2010, p. 1).

Introduced to the importance of educating patients and clients on an individual basis in their preregistration education, nurses are aware of their responsibility in providing advice on subjects such as diet and exercise or alcohol consumption. Their advice is usually respected by their clients. Nurses and midwives also are often working with clients who are very open to making lifestyle changes, for instance, in pregnancy or following a stroke or heart attack. However, considering the broader range of activities encompassed within health promotion requires a more strategic approach and the willingness to work closely with other agencies.

Community nurses (district nurses, community mental health nurses, community children's nurses, school nurses and health visitors) should not only have an in-depth knowledge of the individual lifestyles of their clients but tacit knowledge of the social and community networks of their practice area. Compiling a community profile provides both a resource for the teams in which they work and also develops deeper knowledge of the main issues impacting on the health of the local community.

This profile should include both the health needs of the area which can be found from the Network of Public Health Observatories (http://www.apho.org.uk/resource/view). It should also include an audit of the services available to meet these needs.

The Royal College of Nursing (RCN) has over the last decade shown a great commitment to developing the role of nurses in public health. In 2007 it (RCN 2007) produced a report recognising the skills nurses have in working with the public to influence behaviour change for the improvement of health both at an individual and community level. In *Pillars of the community* (RCN 2010) and *Health visiting and public health nursing* (RCN 2011), they continue to emphasise this important aspect of the role.

Going Upstream: nursing's contribution to public health (RCN 2012) revisits the challenges in the light of the changes within the devolved governments of the United Kingdom and the evolving public health problems. They envisage a framework for 'upstream working' by nurses, where promotion, protection and prevention are undertaken, supported by partnership working with key agencies at local level.

They identify the following core principles for all nurses to follow:

- Understanding the needs of their local population
- Identifying defined populations who would most benefit from upstream approaches
- Working in partnership with other members of health and social care organisations to influence the work on tackling the wider determinants of health
- Engaging local people and groups, including those who are workless, in upstream awareness and action
- Being informed, aware and responsive to disease outbreaks and other threats to health
- Utilising public health evidence in everyday practice and not just evidence for treating illness
- Nurses working to a public health knowledge and skills framework based on the 'novice to expert' criteria (RCN 2012, p. 4.)

This is a clear mandate for all nurses to be aware of their responsibilities in promoting health as well as supporting those who are suffering from illness whether physical or mental. For nurses whose environment of working is within the community, this framework is especially relevant. The Standards of Proficiency for Specialist Community Public Health Nursing (NMC 2004) ensure that health visitors, school nurses, occupational health nurses and sexual health advisors have the required knowledge and skills to work as competent public health nurses. All nurses need to be aware of the following evolving public health problems:

- An ageing population
- Coronary heart disease
- Reoccurrence of infectious childhood diseases such as whooping cough
- Cancer
- Respiratory disease

- Type 1 and type 2 diabetes
- Influenza
- Sexually transmitted infections
- Accidents/injuries
- Substance misuse including drugs and alcohol
- Risk to vulnerable groups (a safeguarding agenda)
- Community disintegration
- Mental health including dementia and self-harming behaviours
- Climate change

Conclusions: the future

The basic principles of public health have remained the same through history: to improve the health of populations through the combined efforts of society and individuals. Undoubtedly, the new structure of the NHS in 2012, with a change of emphasis towards applying business models to care, will impact on community nursing practice. Social marketing theories have been applied that community nurses have not necessarily been trained in. New skills in managing and leading teams and utilising social enterprise techniques will need to be embedded in community courses across the country. Higher education institutions are recognising this and validating their courses with this new emphasis on brokerage principles. Private enterprise is competing to provide care and nurses will need to consider how they can influence commissioning to ensure the needs of their population are effectively met. Alongside this, there is a drive towards a model of nursing which considers a return to some basic core principles of care, compassion, courage, commitment, competence and communication (Cummings 2012).

These can be applied equally to public health practice as they reflect public health principles. Added to these six 'C's, collaboration could be added as a key part of public health practice. Achieving a healthy nation depends upon working together across disciplines and agencies with co-operation and a common aim.

References

Acheson, D. (1988) *Public Health in England*, HMSO, London.
Beveridge, W. (1942) *The Beveridge Report*, HSMO, London.
Cummings, J. (2012) *Our Commitment to Improve*. Available from http://www.commissioning-board.nhs.uk/2012/07/30/commitment-to-improve/. Accessed on 11 November 2012.
Department of Health (DH) (2010) *Healthy Lives, Healthy People*, London, DH.
DH (2010) *Equity and Excellence: Liberating the NHS*, DH, London.
DH (2011) *Changing Behaviour, Improving Outcomes*. DH, London.
DH (2012a) *No Health without Mental Health: Implementation Framework*, DH, London.
DH (2012b) *Improving Outcomes and Supporting Transparency: Part One A Public Health Outcomes Framework for England 2013–16*, DH, London.

DH (2012c) *Health Protection and Local Government*, DH, London.

Douglas, J., Sidell, M., Lloyd, C. & Earle, S. (2007) Evaluating public health interventions. In: *Theory and Research in Promoting Public Health* (eds S. Earle, C. Lloyd, M. Sidell, & S. Spurr). Sage, London.

French, J. (2012) *Social Marketing and Public Health Theory and Practice*, Oxford University Press, Oxford.

Halpin, A., Morales-Suarez, M. & Martin-Moreno, J.M. (2010) Chronic disease prevention and the new public health. *Public Health Reviews*, 32 (1), 120–154.

Harrop, M. (2007) Psychosocial impact of cystic fibrosis in adolescence. *Paediatric Nursing*, 19 (10), 41–45.

HM Government (2006) *The Health Act*. The Stationary Office, London.

HM Government (2012) *The Health and Social Care Act*. HM Government, London.

House of Commons Library (2011) *The Health and Social Care Bill*, 132 of 2010–2011 RESEARCH PAPER 11/11. House of Commons Library, London.

Kerr, J., Weitkunat, R. & Moretti, M. (2005) *ABC of Behaviour Change: A Guide to Successful Disease Prevention and Health Promotion*, Elsevier, London.

Laverack, G. (2005) *Public Health: Power Empowerment and Professional Practice*, Palgrave, London.

Malins, J. (1932) *The Life of Joseph Malins*, Templar Press, New York.

Marmot, M. (2010) *Fair Society, Healthy Lives*. The Marmot Review, HMO, London.

McKinlay, J. (1975) cited in Earle, S., Lloyd, C., Sidell, M., & Spurr, S. (2007) *Theory and Research in Promoting Public Health*. Sage, London.

National Social Marketing Strategy (2012). Available from http://www.thensmc.com/. Accessed on 8 November 2012.

Nightingale, F. (1860) *Notes on Nursing*, Harrison, London.

NMC (2004) *The Standards of Proficiency for Specialist Community Public Health Nursing*. NMC, London.

NMC (2010) *Competencies for Entry to the Register*. NMC, London.

Office of National Statistics (2011) *Smoking and Drinking among Adults, 2009* Office of National Statistics, London.

Reading, S. (2008) Research and development: analysis and interpretation of evidence. In: *Public Health Skills* (eds L. Coles, & E. Porter). Blackwell, Oxford.

Ribiero, L. (2012) *Smoke-free Private Vehicles Bill [HL] 2012–13*. Available from http://services.parliament.uk/bills/2012-13/smokefreeprivatevehicles.html. Accessed on 11 November 2012.

Royal College of Nursing (RCN) (2007) *Nurses as Partners in Delivering Public Health*, RCN, London.

RCN (2010) *Pillars of the Community*, RCN, London.

RCN (2011) *Health Visiting and Public Health Nursing*, RCN, London.

RCN (2012) *Going Upstream: Nursing's Contribution to Public Health*, RCN, London.

The Nuffield Council on Bioethics (NCB) (2007) *Public Health: Ethical Issues*. NCB, London.

Wanless (2002) *Securing Our Future Health: Taking a Long Term View*. DH, London.

Wanless, D., Appleby, J. & Harrison, A. (2007) *Our Future Health Secured*, Kings Fund, London.

World Health Organisation (WHO) (1986) *The Ottawa Charter for Health Promotion*, WHO, Geneva.

WHO (2010a) *The Top Ten Causes of Death*. Available from www.who.int/mediacentre/factsheets/fs310/en/index.html. Accessed on 11 November 2012.

WHO (2010b) *Climate Change and Human Health*. Available from www.who.int/globalchange/wha_plans_objectives/en/index.html. Accessed on 11 November 2012.

WHO (2010c) *The World Health Report: Financing for Universal Coverage*. WHO, Geneva.

WHO (2012) *Metrics: Disability-Adjusted Life Year (DALY) Quantifying the Burden of Disease from Mortality and Morbidity* Available from http://www.who.int/healthinfo/global_burden_disease/metrics_daly/en/. Accessed on 25 May 2013.

9

Caring for the Adult in the Home Setting

Sharon Aldridge Bent

Faculty of Society and Health, Buckinghamshire New University, High Wycombe, UK

It is a privilege to be invited into someone's home as a guest to deliver care. As health and social care professionals we need to be able to acknowledge that building trust and promoting patient choice is important. There is an increasing pressure to keep people in their own homes no matter how complex or serious their condition is (O'Brien 2012). The location in which care is delivered is significant as home can provide the security for the patient as they are on familiar territory (Wilson and Miller 2012). This chapter aims to explore the challenges faced by health and social care professionals in caring for the adult in the home setting and will provide an overview of the Government's agenda for moving care closer to home and will be framed around the new Department of Health (DH) strategic vision for nursing and midwifery in England 2012 (DH 2012a).

The Kings Fund reported on the need to place integrated care at the heart of the NHS reforms (King's Fund 2011) and advised that caring for people with complex needs will require services to reconfigure to ensure that care is well coordinated and integrated between a range of care providers.

There is no recognised single model of 'best practice' and care coordination may become complex when trying to involve a number of different professionals and organisations (Curry & Ham 2010). The inherent benefits of integrated care need to be promoted to all involved so that significant improvements can be made on a daily basis to unify professionals to collaborate to deliver against a single care plan (Thistlewaite 2011). That aim must be to put patients first, improve health outcomes and empower health professionals to lead, direct and deliver effective care to their patients (DH 2012b):

Community and Public Health Nursing, Fifth Edition. Edited by David Sines,
Sharon Aldridge-Bent, Agnes Fanning, Penny Farrelly, Kate Potter and Jane Wright.
© 2013 John Wiley & Sons, Ltd. Published 2013 by John Wiley & Sons, Ltd.

> The prize to be won is a health and social care system centered on the needs of individuals and patients and delivering the best possible outcome (King's Fund 2011, p. 16).

It is recognised that a wide range of professionals care for adults at home, for example, general practitioners (GPs), occupational therapists, social workers and social carers, physiotherapists, specialist nurses and voluntary organisations. Other teams that have been developed to care for the adult at home include palliative care teams, outreach teams in mental health and rapid response or intermediate care teams (Cook 2008). The main focus of this chapter will be to consider the complexities involved in the delivery of healthcare to adults at home and the specialist skills required of the district nurse. It will draw upon the recent strategy for nursing based on the six fundamental values: care, compassion, competence, communication, courage and commitment (DH 2012a). A new strategy for district nursing is planned in 2013 which will aim to maximise the unique district nursing service contribution to high-quality, compassionate and excellent health and well-being outcomes for all people cared for in their own home setting. Special concentration will be given to the six areas of action noted earlier to support professionals and staff to deliver excellent care in the community setting (DH 2012a).

End of life

This chapter will not discuss caring for those requiring palliative and terminal care in the home since these matters and advanced care planning are discussed further in Chapter 17. The district nurse will need to liaise with and refer to a wide range of practitioners from the multidisciplinary team to ensure that the Gold Standards Framework and End of Life Strategy (DH 2008a) is appropriately adhered (Thomas 2011).

The policy context

The NHS faces a period of unprecedented change both in terms of demographic profile and the shifting burden of disease requiring the reassessment of the more traditional hospital-based model of care (House of Commons of Health Select Committee 2012). The DH's Structural Reform Plan recognised the shift of resources and emphasised care out in the community, and it also highlighted the need to adjust working practices and roles to promote better healthcare outcomes (DH 2010a). This redistribution from hospital-based provision represents a need to enhance the delivery of care in the community setting. The need to make long-term cost savings whilst attempting to maintain and enhance the quality of services is paramount, and the reconfiguration of the workforce by altering the point of service delivery is essential (Holland & McIntosh 2012). This expansion of community services and the emphasis of care closer to home resonate in many recent government and policy reports and emphasise the need to engage with the complexities of caring for people at home. There is some evidence to suggest that community nurses can provide care more effectively for people with longer-term needs than their hospital colleagues, thus promoting commissioners to increase the number of community nurses in the current workforce configuration with the aim of enhancing service efficiency and to meet the economical challenges faced by the NHS (Spilsbury *et al.* 2009).

The increase in demand for healthcare quality and output strongly relates to staffing, and in particular improved outcomes and quality are associated with higher levels of registered nurse staffing (Pronovost *et al.* 2002). Newbold (2008) however suggests that fewer staff could be employed but there is a need for them to be better qualified. This means training district nurses to a highly specialised level and in particular developing their skills at leadership and management. The RCN believes strongly that a renewed investment in the community nursing workforce is essential to people's health and is also affordable. They postulate that if the nation fails to invest in community nursing, the long-term costs of health care are likely to increase (RCN 2010a).

The Government's 'Equity and Excellence' White Paper outlined significant changes in the way in which services will be delivered in the NHS with a call to remove Primary Care Trusts and strategic health authorities and develop GP consortia and commissioning groups (DH 2010b). With an ageing population and increased prevalence of disease, there will need to be a move away from the current emphasis on acute and episodic care towards prevention, self-care and the realisation of more consistent standards of primary care that is well co-ordinated and integrated (King's Fund 2011).

In 2011 the Government published a report – 'Close to Home' (DH 2011) – which focused on the results of an inquiry into older people and their human rights in home care (Equality and Human Rights Commission 2011). It was the first inquiry of its kind, and it uncovered some real concerns about the treatment of some older people, especially when examining how some services were commissioned. Its key findings highlighted neglect around the delivery of care packages, financial abuse and a chronic disregard for older people's privacy and dignity. Whilst this report concentrated on older people's experiences of receiving social care at home, its findings were far reaching in terms of the infrastructure and systemic problems related to promoting human rights in the home care setting.

The Queen's Nursing Institute (QNI) undertook an extensive survey of patient's and carer's experiences of being cared for in the home in 2011, which resulted in the report 'Nursing People at Home – the issues, the stories' (QNI 2011). The findings highlighted three things that patients said they wanted from community nurses: they want them to be competent, confident and caring. This theme was the start of the larger DH strategy launched in December 2012 (DH 2012a).

The case for integrated care has never been stronger with the ageing population and with an associated increased prevalence of chronic diseases. Care for people with complex health and social care needs must be made a real priority with commissioners and providers (King's Fund 2011). The new model of integrated community care that focuses on prevention of ill health as opposed to treating people when they become ill has been viewed as forward thinking. This integrated model will require all key stakeholders to work in partnership in the coordination of this care. A network of primary care providers is required therefore that promote and maintain continuity of care and act as links for the provision of chronic disease management and generalist care (Holland & McIntosh 2012).

District nurses work in partnership with other health and social care professionals to provide care to people in their own homes. However, it has been estimated that 35% are eligible to retire within the next 10 years (DH 2009); this has implications for the future district nursing workforce and will impact on the drive for more care closer to home. The QNI (2006) predicts an increase in national demand on the district nursing service in the future. The potential future problem is exacerbated by the projected growth of the UK population to over 70 million in the next 20 years (ONS 2011).

Additional figures supplied by the Health and Social Care Information Centre (HSCIC) show that there were 6937 full-time equivalent district nurses in England in September 2011, 922 fewer than the previous year and down from 10526 in 2001 (Duffin 2012). This has been recognised as a 'creeping tragedy' for patients and in particular the increasing number of older people living at home with complex long-term conditions (LTCs) (Duffin 2012, p. 7). Duffin (2012, p. 6) suggests that

> we are reaching the point where the district nursing service will not be able to regenerate because the workforce will be 'out of sight' and subject to different educational approaches of a variety of new and inexperienced providers.

Managing LTCs in the community

The issue of LTCs has been at the top of the Government's health agenda for many years. It is estimated that 15.5 million people in the United Kingdom have an LTC (DH 2008b). The cost of this presents as phenomenal with people with LTCs accounting for a large proportion of the NHS budget (Darzi 2007).

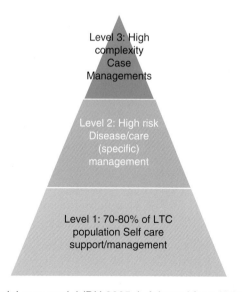

Figure 9.1   Health and social care model (DH 2005a). Adapted from Kaiser Permanente Triangle

Health policy in the United Kingdom has been shaped to an extent by American policy on LTCs, and no explanation of this policy would be complete without reference to the Kaiser Permanente triangle (see Fig. 9.1) (DH 2005). This model acknowledges that people affected or potentially affected by LTCs have differing and complex needs. Level one refers to 70–80% of the population that self-manage their own condition and may require advice on health promotion. Level two are those with a disease-specific unstable LTC; this is the level at which district nurses are mostly likely to be involved. Level three are those with highly complex multiple conditions that require intense case management. The role of the community matron was first introduced in *Liberating the Talents* (DH 2002) as the professional to case manage the level one group of patients (Billingham 2004).

Ongoing debate is currently focused around levels two and three of the triangle in relation to who is best placed to care for these patients. District nurses would indentify that the core focus of their work is with older people in the home with disease-specific case management. They may also acknowledge that their role is not always fully recognised or valued (Pratt 2006). The idea of deploying highly skilled clinicians to deliver complex care was supported by the work of Mckenna and Keeney (2004) who also highlighted that those district nurses who acquired additional skills and experience would have the most impact on the management of people with LTC.

Case Study based upon complexities of patient care in the home setting

---

Geraldine Conway (72-year-old woman)

Geraldine has lived alone following the death of her husband nine years ago. She has one daughter that lives in Australia. Geraldine has said she feels lonely as unable to go out and meet people.

Geraldine has a past medical history of mature onset diabetes controlled on insulin with twice daily injections. She has poor circulation with peripheral neuropathy. She is a heavy smoker 30 cigarettes daily and has severe shortness of breath that prevents her going out.

She has home carers visiting twice daily to assist her with hygiene and to prepare her breakfast, cooked lunch and evening packed lunch.

Recently Geraldine has developed two small ulcers on her legs that require dressing twice weekly. She has also needed more help to manage her diabetes.

The district nurse has visited and performed a holistic assessment and has identified the following ongoing needs:

- Major review of medications as Geraldine seems to have many medicines in her cupboard, but is unable to determine recent medications. D/N to liaise with GP and monitor any changes in medication.

- Educate Geraldine to change lifestyle to adopt healthier changes e.g. smoking cessation and nutrition and exercise.
- Adhere to advice provided by the Diabetic Specialist nurse to better manage her diabetes.
- Monitor leg ulcer treatments and refer to specialist for advise if wounds continue to deteriorate
- Liaise with social carers in order to co-ordinate and inform of any changes in Geraldine's condition.
- Liaise with voluntary organisations to attempt to engage Geraldine with a local social group e.g. day centre or activity group.
- Maintain comprehensive records and care plans of all care provided.

Over recent years there has been a sense that district nursing had been forgotten and even neglected in terms of direction and strategy, prompting Professor James Buchan, a nursing workforce expert at Queen Margaret College, University of Edinburgh, to comment: 'The question for the Government is why there is no policy direction for district nursing' (Duffin 2012, p. 6). It was therefore uplifting and encouraging when the DH and the NHS Commissioning Board, with input from the QNI, commissioned a consultation and subsequently a report into the vision and future strategy of community nursing.

This comprehensive report was part of the wider national vision and strategy, for nursing, midwifery and caregivers. It is widely acknowledged that nurses, midwives and caregivers are in a powerful position to influence the quality of care and play a major role in improving health and well-being outcomes. The aim of this report was to examine the work of a well-equipped community workforce and to identify who would deliver the public health and healthcare support to service users. Its focus was to particularly highlight the support of older people being cared for at home and improve the management of LTCs (DH 2013). The success will be measured by

- Establishing a clear vision of service
- Articulation of the vision to service users and partners
- Ensuring that outcomes contribute to and feed into major policies including mental health and quality forum
- Ensuring that the service vision is robust enough to support the Health and Wellbeing Boards in their commissioning decisions

The nursing profession has had to evolve in line with changing disease patterns, new treatments and different service delivery. There has been a need to develop new knowledge and skills, accept more responsibility and accountability and create robust

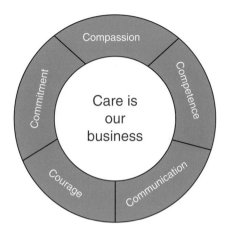

Figure 9.2   Care is our business (DH 2013)

Table 9.1   Maximising the contribution of the district nursing service

Maximising the unique district nursing service contribution to high-quality, compassionate and excellent health and well-being outcomes for all people cared for in the home setting:

Care – Providing high-quality care nearer to home, within community settings. Ensuring care is centred on the patient's own environment.

Compassion – Providing care with dignity and respect. Acting as an advocate for patients and always with integrity. Encouraging patients to be active participants in care and decision making.

Competence – Competent, capable staff, who can influence the lifestyle of individuals, families and communities. Specialist practitioners using their accountable role to drive service improvements and support the educational needs of the workforce.

Communication – Providing information and guidance to support patients whilst communicating with other agencies to provide a seamless approach to care.

Courage – Ensuring patients' best interest at the centre of service delivery and providing challenge to others when services are not meeting the needs of patients and when things go wrong.

Commitment – Delivering and designing ongoing support and quality services within patients own environment, with a commitment to improving health outcomes.

Adapted from the Department of Health (DH 2012a) – Ensuring' patients best interest

education opportunities. However, there has also been a need to return to the fundamentals of nursing, which have been characterised in the 6 'C's that formed the baseline for the CNO's nursing strategy (Fig. 9.2 and Table 9.1) (DH 2012a).

As part of the vision for the report, six areas of action were identified that underpinned the six 'C's, and these will now be discussed in the context of the community setting and describe how district nurses might take the lead in these areas to maximise care for the adult at home.

Maximising health and well-being: helping people to stay independent

The DH's overarching aim is to enable people to live better for longer by improving the health and care outcomes that matter to people (DH 2012a). Historically within primary care, measuring outcomes have been problematic with district nurses at times struggling to be able to identify and indeed quantify their role within the public health arena. The extent to which district nurses influence public health has been much debated, and the challenge will be to articulate their contribution to promoting health and well-being, not just to other professionals but also to the commissioners of community services (Rawlinson *et al.* 2012). As far back as the Audit Commission (1999) report, there has been criticism that district nurses have been unable to define their role, as the majority of their work is carried out in the home setting and could be described as 'invisible'. It has always been part of the district nurse's role to have the ability to examine the wider determinants of health and to have skills to perform health needs analysis (Audit Commission 1999). District nurses have always assessed a need but often this is associated with individual needs rather than population needs profiling or analysis. District nurses are well placed to promote health and well-being as they are in a unique situation to influence the care received by individuals in the home setting. They do this by managing and being accountable for an active caseload and providing population interventions to improve community health and well-being. This will include working with a range of health and social care partners (including GPs, voluntary sector and community health and social care services) to provide services for adults and their carers, at home and in other community settings. They achieve this by providing support and care so that people can stay well and remain at home independently (Holland & McKintosh 2012). In 'Improving health and care: the role of the outcomes frameworks', clearer direction is provided for public health, which also promotes high levels of improvement and performance of practitioners (DH 2012b). There is a call for all professionals to work together, integrate care and co-ordinate services to achieve success in areas such as dementia, prevention of premature death and enhancing the quality of life of people with LTCs (DH 2012b).

Working with people to provide a positive experience of care

This action highlights the need for professionals to be able to identify need swiftly and particularly so when specific health need solutions are required. These may relate to short-term issues or sudden health crises but the ability to determine what is most significant or urgent requires well-honed clinical decision-making skills (Gould 2012).

Within the home setting, building a good therapeutic relationship makes the difference between a patient feeling empowered or not. This relationship must be built upon trust and honesty and mutual respect. The professional must at all times be able to focus on the needs of the patient whilst promoting patient autonomy with the view to providing a positive care experience (Foster & Hawkins 2005).

Adult safeguarding

Within the community setting it can be quite difficult to offer a single definition or concept of vulnerability (Drew & Smith 2012). It is paramount that professionals are aware of both national and local policies for the protection of their patients (Brammer 2009). As practice evolves, so does the need to develop understanding of the terminology around risk and vulnerability. In more recent years the term 'adult at risk' has replaced 'vulnerable adult' for the reason that the term 'vulnerable adult' may wrongly imply that some of the fault for the abuse lies with the abused adult (Social Care Institute for Excellence 2011). Under the new 'Protection of Freedoms Act' (HM Government 2012), the definition of vulnerable has been thus redefined:

> ...adults are considered vulnerable because of their age, behaviour, illness and other characteristics. A person will now be considered vulnerable because of the nature of the regulated activity being provided to them, regardless of where or how often that activity takes place (HM Government 2012, p. 54).

As part of their role and 'duty of care', district nurses are required to be up to date in respect of the current changes soon to be implemented under the 'Protection of Freedoms Act' (2012). The main changes proposed relate to vetting, barring and criminal records schemes and, in particular, redefining 'regulated activity' with vulnerable groups. Any person working within these newly defined staff groups, of which there are several categories, for example, health care, relevant personal care, social work, assistance with finances and/or personal affairs and transportation, will need to be legally vetted. When the scheme comes into force, anyone working in a newly defined area of 'regulated activity', which will include district nurses, must have an enhanced criminal record check together with a barred list check (Griffin & Tengnah 2012).

Following many serious case reviews that examine the shortcomings of safeguarding, the overwhelming majority of recommendations relate to the need to improve multiagency working and communication (Flynn 2007). In a report by Sir David Nicholson (2010), the view was reinforced that collaborative ways of working were essential:

> ...It is critical that in challenging economic times we work more closely with our partners – between primary and secondary care, and between health and social care – rather than retreating within our own organisational boundaries (Nicholson 2010, p. 3).

A further consideration when caring for people at home is the right to dignity and choice and the provision of informed consent to the care being given. Within the primary care setting, district nurses need to be aware that adult patients have the right to refuse treatment even if it maybe to their own detriment as the law recognises that adults have the right to determine what is done to them (Griffith & Tengnah 2012).

Measuring impact of service through patient feedback

> When a person reflects on care received in the community by a professional (district nurses) they consider whether they were treated kindly with respect and dignity. The people that we care for and in many instances their families and carers are our partners in care and our practice must reflect this (DH 2012a, p. 17).

A new initiative to be launched by the DH in the spring of 2013 was announced by David Cameron. The 'friends and family test' will aim to improve patient care and identify good performance. Patients will be asked a simple question: whether they would recommend the service to a friend or relative based on their treatment. The friends and family test will start in the acute setting but has been recommended to be linked to other proposals after consulting frontline nurses, care staff and patients. The answers to the test will then be published and will allow the public to compare health care services and clearly identify the best performers, and the aim is to raise standards of care (DH 2012a). This test will apply equally to community-based service provision.

Delivering high-quality care and measuring impact

This action is concerned with the ability to measure the quality and effectiveness of services that are delivered and to publicise this data to a wider audience to improve health (DH 2012a).

The redistribution of care to the community is a vehicle for enhancing the delivery of treatment and care to people at home. This is now the opportunity for reconfiguration of the workforce to deliver quality care closer to home. There is a need to optimise productivity in community nursing and to demonstrate output, patient outcomes and efficiency (Holland & Mckintosh 2012). One way that this can be measured is by the utilisation of robust data collection that is streamlined, simple and effective in informing practice (DH 2012a). The NHS Commissioning Board will also have to work closely with GPs and local commissioners to influence and develop the provision of local primary care services, which will include the care of adults in their own homes. Within the nursing arena district nurses will need to develop skills in business planning, social innovation and leadership in order to market and promote their services to potential commissioners. This may take the form of developing business plans and service level agreements. The benefits of this approach are seen to be high productivity, greater innovation, better care and greater patent and personal job satisfaction. Team managers should seek to combine these values with business principles, enabling nurses to be autonomous, innovative, flexible and more responsive to patients' needs (Robinson 2010).

Building and strengthening leadership

The emphasis on the importance of effective nurse leadership in the NHS has been well documented over many years and is pivotal to improved patient outcomes (Wong & Cummings 2007). Effective leadership can increase motivation and empower nurses when delivering care and is a prerequisite for the clarification of roles. The DH (2012a) document 'Compassion in Practice' has identified further the importance for our leaders to have leadership skills that include:

> change management skills, building coalitions of support and communications and engagements with staff, patients, service users and other stakeholders (DH 2012a, p. 21).

Leadership has been specifically identified as vital to the development of community nursing as a way of driving the service to become more innovative within the context of the clinical governance agenda (McKenna & Keeney 2004). There is much debate around the qualities needed to lead and district nurse teams but essentially leaders should demonstrate strong clinical leadership to achieve the best outcomes for patients (Cameron *et al.* 2011). The relevance of transformational leadership is particularly key in community nursing as it is concerned with promoting compliant behaviour and the stimulation of employees into positive action. The needs of the organisation and organisational change are of high importance, and it is for the nurse leader to inspire and influence that change (Curtis & O'Connell 2011). Consequently there is a particular drive for community nurses to improve their leadership and management skills, and this has been reinforced by the DH (2012a) calling for community nurse leaders to be supervisory and 'given the time to lead the team' (p. 22) – and these competencies should be built into future workforce development tools. Advanced decision-making skills will also be essential to enable nurses to practise autonomously at all levels of service design and delivery (Dickson 2012).

Ensuring we have the right staff, with the right skills in the right place

The QNI has been campaigning for over 2 years for the right balance of skills in community health care teams. If more care is going to be delivered in the community, including nursing homes, it is essential that more investment is made in procuring well-trained staff, including nurses, who have the time and the expertise to deliver high-quality, compassionate and person-centred care to the most vulnerable members of society (QNI 2012). The complexity of district nursing care is highlighted by the work of the QNI (2011), including examples of engagement with the assessment of complex needs, risk assessment, leadership and management and application of specialist knowledge and skills, with the ability to work collaboratively across organisations. The key skills required for the district nurse are demonstrated in Fig. 9.3.

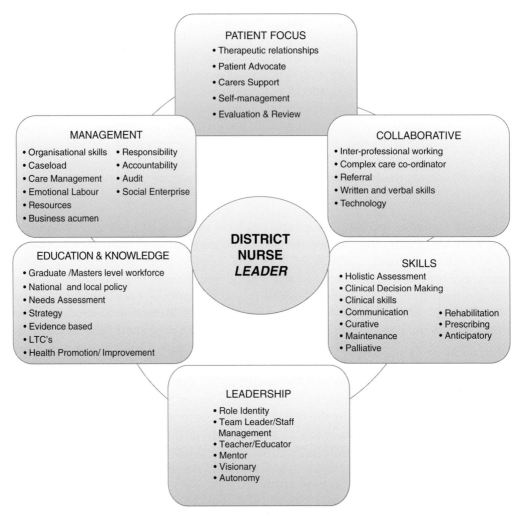

PATIENT FOCUS
• Therapeutic relationships
• Patient Advocate
• Carers Support
• Self-management
• Evaluation & Review

MANAGEMENT
• Organisational skills   • Responsibility
• Caseload   • Accountability
• Care Management   • Audit
• Emotional Labour   • Social Enterprise
• Resources
• Business acumen

COLLABORATIVE
• Inter-professional working
• Complex care co-ordinator
• Referral
• Written and verbal skills
• Technology

DISTRICT NURSE LEADER

EDUCATION & KNOWLEDGE
• Graduate /Masters level workforce
• National and local policy
• Needs Assessment
• Strategy
• Evidence based
• LTC's
• Health Promotion/ Improvement

SKILLS
• Holistic Assessment
• Clinical Decision Making
• Clinical skills
• Communication   • Rehabilitation
• Curative   • Prescribing
• Maintenance   • Anticipatory
• Palliative

LEADERSHIP
• Role Identity
• Team Leader/Staff
  Management
• Teacher/Educator
• Mentor
• Visionary
• Autonomy

Figure 9.3   The role of the qualified district nurse

The qualified district nurse is also professionally responsible and accountable for the quality of care that they provide and is well qualified to assess the needs of individuals and their carers. District nurses also lead and manage a multi-skilled team of nurses and are skilled to work collaboratively with a multiplicity of agencies (statutory, voluntary and private) in order to deliver care to a defined population (Boran 2009). The reality of the level of responsibility and accountability in the qualified nurse is depicted in Fig. 9.4.

The Standards for Specialist Education and Practice (NMC 2002) remain as the sole regulatory competence descriptors for district nursing programmes in the United Kingdom. Specialist practice is the exercising of higher levels of judgment, discretion and clinical decision making in clinical care to enable the monitoring and improvement of standards of care through supervision of practice, clinical audit, the development of

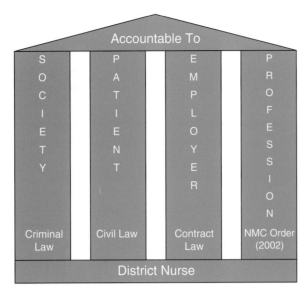

Figure 9.4   The responsibility and accountability of the qualified district nurse. Data from Caulfield (2005) (RCN (2010) Pillars of Community)

practice through research and teaching, the support of professional colleagues and the provision of skilled professional leadership (Boran 2009). In 2004 the NMC (NMC 2004) created a 'third part' of the professional nurse register for all specialist community public health nurses that included school nurses, health visitors and occupational health nurses. This did not include district nurses who remained on the first part of the register with a recordable rather requiring a post qualifying, registerable qualification – Dickson *et al.* (2011). This division within and amongst the family of community nursing has generated much debate around the education of district nurses, and there have been calls for the standards to be revised to meet the needs of contemporary community nursing from organisations such as the Association of District Nurse Educators (ADNE www.adne.co.uk) (Cook *et al.* 2011). The ADNE is committed to raising the profile of district nursing, and its main purpose is to enhance the educational profile of community nurses in the United Kingdom.

There has also been a demand to focus on the educational development of all carers working in the community that provide care to people in the home setting. The health care assistant resource has also grown over the last 10 years, and this body of carers needs to engage in the educational process in order to enhance their practice. Many higher education institutions have introduced Foundation Degrees in health and social care as a pathway towards progression into nursing (Boran 2009).

The qualified Band 5 and 6 practitioners who may not wish to follow a district nursing pathway, preferring to practise in more generalist roles in primary care, are also being encouraged to follow new educational programmes, aimed at enhancing clinical skills, knowledge and competencies of the support staff workforce Boran (2009). For example, since 2011 Buckinghamshire New University has offered a module in 'Transition to Community Nursing' for community staff nurses that acknowledges that practitioners are often working alone in environments with complex client group. These combined factors require nurses from the acute sector to refocus their working methods and skills to equip them to deal with the highly complex collaborative relationships with both clients and families and also with a myriad of disparate health, social and voluntary agencies. Nurses working in primary care settings also need to be able to make more autonomous decisions than their hospital-based colleagues and to engage proactively in clinical decision making and risk assessment. This occurs often in the absence of immediate peer support (Drennan & Davis 2008).

Technology

There has been a dramatic increase in the use of technology in healthcare, and this move is driven by government policy (Carlisle 2012). The Government has dedicated £100 million to support the use of technology in all health care settings and has identified the benefits that technology provides for nursing care staff (DH 2012a). The use of technology could be a viable alternative way of delivering health care in the future (QNI 2012).

In the United Kingdom this move is already underway in the community in the form of the provision of assistive technology and patient-friendly monitoring equipment. This encourages patients to become more autonomous and engaged in managing their own care and could reduce the number of contact visits with healthcare professionals (Carlisle 2012).

The QNI (2012) published the document 'Smart New World' to review the status of technology and 'eHealth' in community nursing practice. It highlighted the need for community nurses to develop an active vision which sees technology as a key enabler. Healthcare provided in the community is ripe for the use of new technologies, allowing patients to take control of their care and bringing nurses closer to patients.

Whilst there may be some reluctance to fully embrace and utilise technology, especially if nurses feel that nothing can replace 'face to face' consultation, there is another school of thought that has seen patients' lives transformed by telehealth systems in the home. It has been said that in order for community nurses to feel confident about the use of technology, they need to be convinced of the benefits (RCN 2010) and for the technology to be embraced fully, time must be taken to invest in the provision of local training to enable district nurses to understand how to operate the equipment (QNI 2012).

Informal carers

When discussing caring for the adult at home, it would be impossible to discuss care without recognising the role of informal carers. Carers provide unpaid care by looking after an ill, frail or disabled family member, friend or partner. Most of us

Table 9.2   Empowering patients

Enhancing the patient experience – promoting a positive patient carer experience

Recognising what is important to the patient and carer

Adapting to the care setting and respecting patients' home

Going the extra mile – flexibility and responsiveness

Making a difference – support and anticipation needs

Advocacy role and managing risk to keep patients safe

Family/home centred

Hands on and highly skilled

will look after an elderly relative, sick partner or disabled family member at some point in our lives. However, whilst caring is part and parcel of life, without the right support, the personal costs of caring can be high financially and emotionally (Carers UK 2012).

Carers act as expert care partners in providing high quality and make valuable contributions to social services and NHS service providers. There are an estimated 6.4 million carers in the United Kingdom today and an expected increase of 40% rise in the number of carers needed by 2037, and the financial impact and value of this care is estimated at £87 billion per year (Carers UK 2012). The informal workforce, who provide significant amount of unpaid care, may not be able to meet the demand, leaving a significant 'care gap' (King's Fund 2012).

It is imperative that important issues such as carer identification, assessment and education and partnership working are acknowledged. Carers have a tendency not to pay attention to their own health needs and are categorised as a high-risk group for health problems (Simon 2011). The role of the health and social care professional is to be able to carry out carer assessments in order to fully understand the carers' experiences and then to implement strategies in order for carers to feel supported in care delivery (Chilton *et al.* 2012).

The DH (2012a) recognises also that by empowering patients it will promote a positive patient and carer experience (see Table 9.2).

Supporting positive staff experience

This action is concerned with supporting the staff who provide the care and emphasises the need to provide supervision and support within a culture of care for all employees. It recognises the fact that care can be emotionally challenging and that the amount of emotional labour that can be devoted to the provision of quality care is immense. Research has proven that there is a direct connection between staff experiences and the delivery of care and interpersonal aspects of the caring relationship should be valued higher (Smith & Gray 2001).

The provision of support for staff needs to be demonstrated clearly within the clinical supervision framework, and community nurses need to be able to embed the concept of support and supervision within the culture of community nursing. In a study performed by Dr Dee Drew, it was discovered that group identity was seen to be key in supporting nurses in difficult times. As much of community nursing is performed in patients' homes in isolation, the study highlighted the handover period as the time when district nurses had the opportunity to explore their thoughts and feelings. The study went on to investigate the 'cultural behaviour, knowledge and cultural artefacts exemplified during community nurses handover sessions' (Drew 2012). The DH (2012a) also discusses the implementation of a cultural barometer in order to help managers, leaders and staff on the frontline to reflect on the culture of their organisation and how to measure the impact that their support services have on the provision of support for their staff.

Conclusion

This chapter has discussed the future for district nursing practice in caring for the adult in the home setting. This is potentially an exciting time for district nurses to embrace change within the context of the health and social care agenda. The nursing strategy (DH 2012a) has provided district nursing with a new lease of life; practitioners now need to fully embrace and make the changes needed to collectively develop the profession at this pivotal point in a long history of community nursing.

References

Audit Commission (1999) *First Assessment: A Review of District Nursing Services in England and Wales*. Audit Commission Publications, London.

Billingham, K. (2004) The rise of the district nursing profession. *British Journal of Community Nursing*, 9 (1), 410.

Boran, S. (2009) Contemporary issues in district nursing. In: *Community Health Care Nursing* (eds D. Sines, F. Appleby & E. Raymond). 4th edn. Blackwell Science, Oxford.

Brammer, A. (2009) Legal developments since no secrets. *Journal of Adult Protection*, **11**, 43–53.

Cameron, S., Harbison, D. J., Lambert, V. & Dickson, C. (2011) Exploring leadership in community nursing teams. *Journal of Advanced Nursing*, 68 (7), 1469–1481.

Carers UK (2012) *Policy Briefing – Facts about Carers 2012*. Carers UK, London.

Carlisle, D. (2012) Remote access to closer care. *Nursing Standard*, 26 (29), 20–21.

Caulfield, H. (2005) Vital Notes for Nurses: Accountability, Blackwell, Oxford.

Chilton, S., Bain, H., Clarridge, A. & Melling, K. (2012) *A Textbook of Community Nursing*. Hodder Arnold, London.

Cook, R. (2008) QNI seek clarity over the future of the specialist practitioner role. *British Journal of Community Nursing*, **11** (6), 241.

Cook, R., Bain, H. & Smith, A. (2011) Educating community nurses. *Nursing Times*, 107 (38), 20–22.

Curry, N. & Ham, C. (2010) *Clinical and Service Integration: The Route to Improved Outcomes*. The Kings Fund, London.

Curtis, E. & O'Connell, R. (2011) Essential leadership skills for motivating and developing staff. *Nursing Management*, 18 (5), 32–35.

Darzi, A. (2007) *Healthcare for London: a framework for action*. NHS, London.

Department of Health (DH) (2002) Liberating the Talents: Helping Primary Care Trusts and nurses deliver The NHS Plan. DH, London.

DH (2005) *National Service Framework for Long Term Conditions*. DH, London.

DH (2008a) *Raising the Profile of Long Term Conditions Care: A Compendium of Information*. DH, London.

DH (2008b) *End of Life Strategy: Promoting high quality care for all adults at the end of life*. DH, London.

DH (2009) *The National Dementia Strategy*. DH, London.

DH (2010a) *Equity and excellence: Liberating the NHS*. DH, London.

DH (2010b) *Structural Reform Plan*. DH, London.

DH (2011) *Care Close to Home*. DH, London.

DH (2012a) *Health and Social Care Act*. DH, London.

DH (2012b) *Compassion in Practice Nursing, Midwifery and Care Staff our Vision and Strategy*. DH, London.

DH (2013) *Care in Local Communities: A Vision and Model for District Nursing*. DH, London.

Dickson, C. (2012) Clinical Leadership and quality care. In: *A Textbook of Community Nursing* (eds S. Chilton, H. Bain, A. Clarridge & K. Melling). Hodder Arnold, London.

Dickson, C., Gough, H. & Bain, H. (2011) Meeting the policy agenda, Part 2: is a 'Cinderella service' sufficient?. *British Journal of Community Nursing*, 16 (11), 540–545.

Drennan, V. & Davis, K. (2008) *Trends over the Last Ten Years in Primary Care and Community Nurse Workforce in England*. DH, London.

Drew, D. (2012) Professional identity and the culture of community nursing. *British Journal of Community Nursing*, 16 (3), 126–131.

Drew, D. & Smith, D. (2012) Managing Risk. In: *A Textbook of Community Nursing* S. Chilton, H. Bain, A. Clarridge & K. Melling. London. Hodder Arnold.

Duffin, C. (2012) 'Creeping tragedy' of decline in district nurse numbers. *Primary Care*, 22 (6), 6–7.

Equality and Human Rights Commission (2011) *Close to Home: An Inquiry into Older People and Human Rights at Home*. Equality and Human Rights Commission, Manchester.

Flynn, M. (2007) *The Murder of Steven Hoskin – A Serious Case review – Executive Summary*. Adult Protection Committee, Cornwall.

Foster, T. & Hawkins, J. (2005) Nurse –patient relationships: dead or merely impeded by technology? *British Journal of Nursing*, 14, 1698–702.

Gould, L. (2012) Organisation and management of care. In: *A Textbook of Community Nursing* S. Chilton, H. Bain, A. Clarridge & K. Melling. Hodder Arnold, London.

Griffith, R. & Tengnah, C. (2012) Protection of Freedoms Act: safeguarding vulnerable groups. *British Journal of Community Nursing*, 17 (8), 393–396.

Holland, A. & McKintosh, B. (2012) Optimising productivity, quality and efficiency in community nursing. *British Journal of Community Nursing*, 17 (8), 390–392.

House of Commons Health Select Committee (2012) *Evidence from the QNI (ETWP 09)*. Parliament, London.

HM Government (2012) *Protection of Freedoms Act*. The Stationary Office, London.

King's Fund (2011) *A Report to the Department of Health and the NHS Future Forum*. King's Fund publications, London.

King's Fund (2012) *Health and Wellbeing Boards: System Leaders or Talking Shops?* King's Fund publications, London.

McKenna, H. & Keeney, S. (2004) Community nursing: health professional and public perceptions. *Journal of Advanced Nursing*, 48 (1), 17–25.

Newbold, D. (2008) The production economics of nursing: a discussion paper. *International Journal of Nursing Studies*, 45 (1), 120–8.

Nicholson, D. (2010) *A letter to NHS Chairs, Chief Executives and Directors of Finance.* p. 3. NHS, London.

NMC (2002) *Standards for Specialist Community Education and Practice*, NMC, London.

NMC (2004) *Standards for Proficiency for Specialist Community Public Health Nursing.* NMC, London.

Office of National Statistics (ONS) (2011) *Population, Social Trends 41.* ONS, London.

O'Brien, L. (2012) *District Nursing Manual of Clinical Procedures.* Wiley-Blackwell, West Sussex.

Pratt, L. (2006) Long term conditions 5: meeting the needs of highly complex patients. *British Journal of Community*, 11 (6), 234–240.

Pronovost, P., Angus, D., Doorman, T., Robinson, K., Dremsizov, T. & Young, T. (2002) Physician staffing patterns and clinical outcomes in critically ill patients: a systematic review, *JAMA.*, 288 17, 2151–62.

Rawlinson, M. Baker, D. & Fergus, M. (2012) Public health and the promotion of wellbeing. In: *A Textbook of Community Nursing* (S. Chilton, H. Bain, A. Clarridge, and Melling. K . Hodder Arnold, London.

Robinson, F. (2010) Social enterprise in primary and community care. *Practice Nurse*, 40 (10), 45–48.

Royal College of Nursing (RCN) (2010) *Pillars of the Community: The RCN's UK Position on the Development of the Registered Nursing Workforce in the Community.* RCN, London.

RCN (2010) Putting Information at the Heart of Nursing. RCN, London.

Simon, C. (2011) Organising your practice to support carers. *InnovAit*, 4 (8), 443–449.

Smith, P. & Gray, B. (2001) Emotional labour of nursing revisited: caring and learning 2000. *Nurse Education in Practice*, 1, 42–49.

Social Care Institute for Excellence (2011) *Keeping Personal Budgets Personal: Learning from the Experiences of Older People, People with Mental Health Problems and Their Carers.* SCIE, London.

Spilsbury, K., Stuttard, I. & Anderson, J. (2009) Mapping the introduction of assistant practitioner roles in acute NHS (hospital) trusts in England. *Journal Nursing Management*, 17 (5), 615–26.

The Queen's Nursing Institute (QNI) (2006) *Vision and Values: A Call for Action on Community Nursing.* The Queen's Nursing Institute, London.

The Queen's Nursing Institute (2011) *Nursing People at Home – The Issues, The stories.* QNI, London.

The Queen's Nursing Institute (2012) Smart New World. QNI, London.

Thistlewaite, P. (2011) *Integrating Health and Social Care in Torbay: Improving Care for Mrs Smith.* The Kings Fund, London.

Thomas, K. (2011) *The Gold Standards Framework in Palliative Care. A Handbook for Practice.* Macmillan Publications, London.

Wong, C.A. & Cummings, G.C. (2007) The relationship between nursing leadership and patient outcomes: a systematic review. *Journal of Nursing Management*, 15 (5), 508–21.

Wilson, P. & Miller, S. (2012) Therapeutic relationship. In: *A Textbook of Community Nursing* (S. Chilton, H. Bain, A. Clarridge & K. Melling). Hodder Arnold, London.

10

General Practice Nursing in Context

Sue Axe and Zoe Berry

Faculty of Society and Health, Buckinghamshire New University, Uxbridge, UK

Introduction

General practice nursing is one of the fastest growing specialities in nursing for a variety of reasons. Traditionally it is suggested that the working hours have been attractive because they may be adapted around family commitments and have tended not to involve shift work. However, its popularity has grown recently because of the opportunities offered to work with individuals and families and to undertake a variety of roles and responsibilities.

In order to better understand the General Practice Nurse (GPN) role and how it has evolved, it is necessary to understand the context of general practice and the history of its development. This is because in the main, GPNs are employed by GPs who are independent contractors to the National Health Service (NHS), and as a result most general practices are run under a small business model. This means that GPNs may not be so constrained by the inevitable bureaucracies of large organisations and may feel more autonomous but conversely are at risk of becoming professionally isolated. General practice, as is the case with many aspects of the NHS, has not been developed in a purposeful way but rather has changed and adapted dramatically over the last 50 years in response to changes in society and political influences that have impacted on the organisation of the NHS.

Community and Public Health Nursing, Fifth Edition. Edited by David Sines,
Sharon Aldridge-Bent, Agnes Fanning, Penny Farrelly, Kate Potter and Jane Wright.
© 2013 John Wiley & Sons, Ltd. Published 2013 by John Wiley & Sons, Ltd.

Origins

General practice finds its roots in the formation of the Society of Apothecaries in 1817, as their licentiateship was the most common qualification to be held by the equivalent to GPs at that time. During the mid-1850s increasing concern about access to healthcare for the general population was accompanied by the need to also improve the regulation of GPs. Following the Medical Act of 1858, the General Medical Council was formed in order to establish a register of approved medical practitioners who in the main were GPs. A division between physicians and surgeons operating within hospitals was beginning to emerge, but the concept of specialist practice was still frowned upon into the late 1800s (Porter 1997).

Nursing had also witnessed a significant landmark as the first nurse training was offered at St. Thomas' Hospital in London. Prior to this time, 'nursing' care was delivered for the most part by women from religious orders who felt a sense of duty in their calling. This feature of nursing, as well as female subordination towards the male medical hierarchy, was to prevail for decades, despite the magnificent achievements of Florence Nightingale (1820–1910) as a statistician and founding director of nursing!

Increasing concern about public health led to the compulsory National Insurance Scheme in 1911 (Parliament 1911) after which workers began to contribute to a government-underwritten insurance scheme to entitle them to receive approved medical care from 'panel doctors' (Porter 1997). This was the origin of a specific funding scheme known as the 'capitation fee' that provided doctors with an annual sum for every insured patient who was registered with them. There were limitations to the scheme as it did not cover hospital stays or extend to the families of contributors. However, the subsequent Dawson Report (1920), widely seen as a precursor to the founding of the NHS, suggested that 'curative and preventive medicine' should be undertaken by district GPs. Interestingly Dawson's vision of primary health centres, where GPs would provide diagnostics and treatment, in some ways mirrors a similar vision outlined by Lord Darzi who more recently advocated the establishment of polyclinics (DH 2008). However, financial constraints prevented Lord Darzi's ideas from coming to fruition.

The formation of the NHS in 1948, following the Beveridge Report in 1942, confirmed GPs as the 'gatekeepers' of access to health care. They were also responsible for delivering primary and personal medical care to all those patients registered with them. GPs had originally expressed concern about the prospect of becoming salaried employees of the NHS and so were appointed as independent contractors who could maintain their private practice. However, there were no additional resources available to enable GPs to support this role. It is no surprise that by the 1950s they were struggling and demoralised. The divide between the hospital surgeons and physicians and GPs had already widened, and the status of GPs was seen to have been diminished further by a range of ensuing problems.

These issues were eventually recognised and, following the formation of the Royal College of General Practitioners in 1952, resulted in the drawing up of the first contract for GPs in 1966 within which additional resources in return for specific returns were agreed (Tait 2002). Nurses employed by practices were included as ancillary staff, but no additional funding was allocated for their training. However, in these early days nurses were generally employed to work in treatment rooms, undertaking basic nursing care tasks.

A small study undertaken in Scotland at this time describes how nurses typically saw patients who were always referred to them by the GP for such procedures as weighing, testing urine, taking specimens, dressings, injections and observations such as temperature and pulse (Cartwright & Scott 1961). Whilst they would often perform simple roles such as chaperoning patients and supervising surgery equipment (including the contents of the doctor's bag), it is interesting to note that they were also giving advice and information on illness and offering 'therapeutic listening' to patients. Indeed the conclusion of this study was that nurses were extending the range of care offered to the patients, although the authors were already voicing a concern about the potential shortage of suitably qualified nurses in the future.

It is interesting to note that at this time, the demands upon nurses employed in general practice were unlikely to exceed the competencies of a registered general nurse. This perception, particularly amongst GPs, that GPNs were unlikely to require further post-registration training or education to competently fulfil the role generally persisted up until the late 1980s.

The new contract for GPs in 1966 introduced the 'Red Book', a system through which GPs continued to receive a capitation fee for each patient registered with them, but additionally they were also able to claim back 70% of staff costs and 100% of their premises costs. At this time GP contracts were to provide general medical services, which were determined by terms and conditions of service laid down for a registered population. It was the GP Principals who held individual contracts with the Secretary of State for Health which were negotiated through collective bargaining between the General Practice Committee of the British Medical Association and the Department of Health (DH). This included responsibility to provide 24-hour care, 365 days a year (www.legislation.gov.uk 1966).

This system remained relatively stable until the 1990s when the Conservative Government of the time introduced the concept of the internal market to the NHS. GPs were given budgets in which to commission services for their practice population; this system was known as GP fundholding. The premise for this system was that internal competition and local commissioning would reduce costs and provide improved local services. Anecdotally this was the case in particular for large well-organised practices, though some smaller and single-handed practices struggled to manage the demands of the new dual role. By the time GP fundholding was disbanded by the Labour Government in 1998, only 33% of practices were participating, and it was argued that this had led to greater inequalities in access to services for some patients (Kmietowicz 2006).

The advent of contemporary general practice nursing

However, it was the changes made to the GP contract in 1989 (implemented in 1990) that had the greatest impact on the rise of the practice nurse role (DH 1989). The changes were designed to shift the emphasis from general practice being curative and reactive to one of being preventive and proactive. The management of long-term conditions and health promotion were generally delegated to the practice nurse. This led to a requirement for nurses to develop specific skills beyond those of registration, in particular in the management of chronic conditions such as diabetes and asthma. The need for further specialised education had been recognised as the case for many years for colleagues such as district nurses and health visitors. However, this rapid expansion highlighted the existence of a fragmented approach to education and training for practice nurses. Despite this, practice nurses developed their own informal networks to support and disseminate good practice, and through the Royal College of Nursing (RCN), the practice nurse forum lobbied for specialist practitioner recognition from the United Kingdom Central Council (UKCC), which was achieved in 1994 (UKCC 1994).

Whilst there have been inevitable tensions as practice nurses have struggled to achieve recognition of their specialist practice status and to secure funding for education, it is important to acknowledge also that the complexity of managing the day-to-day running of general practice had also increased. By 1995 the number of practice nurses employed had risen to 18 000 in England alone, and practices were employing a variety of managers and administrative staff in order to cope with the changes. Whilst remaining generalists, the role of the GP has extended beyond that of the gatekeeper to managing far more complex care than would have been anticipated previously.

In 1997 the NHS (Primary Care Act) was passed which introduced alternative service delivery models for primary care; these included Personal Medical Service (PMS) schemes, Alternative Provider Medical Services (APMS) and Primary Care Trust Medical Services (PCTMS). The aim was to enable a wider variety of services that could respond flexibly to the needs of local populations and to improve services for some groups who had difficulty accessing traditional general practice, for example, homeless people and travelling communities (National Health Service (Primary Care) Act c 46, Parliament 1997).

These models provided the opportunity for nurses to assume leadership roles because PMS could be provided by individual GPs, a practice, a Primary Care Trust (PCT) or a group of practitioners, including nurses and doctors. It was envisaged that these service options would enable PCTs to provide a wider range of services and expand primary care capacity and patient access to services.

Further, it was determined that new contracts for general practice would be drawn up and negotiated locally between the health authority (subsequently PCTs) and the primary care provider, which would be the practice, rather than the GP as an independent contractor. This gives GPs the opportunity to take up salaried posts within provider teams, which for some offers a more flexible option. The consequence of this for the patient, however, has been that the traditional notion of the named family doctor caring for their patients across the lifespan of their patients has been eroded.

The NHS Plan published in 2001 stated clearly that the 'future of the NHS rests on the strength of its primary care service'. The plan envisaged that a wider range of services would be provided within the community and emphasised the importance of flexible multidisciplinary teamworking (DH 2001). The plan also acknowledged that a review of the primary care workforce and an expanded role for GPNs would be necessary for this to happen, partly in order to reduce or spread the workload of GPs. A subsequent report 'Liberating the Talents' (DH 2002) further reinforced this idea and built upon the ten key roles for nurses that had been identified by the Chief Nursing Officer as a strategic framework that would enable nurses to help deliver the NHS Plan. These key roles, which included ordering diagnostics such as X-rays and to make and receive direct referrals, sent out a clear message as to how all nurses, including GPNs, could extend and advance their clinical roles. This led to the development of a diversified skill mix within the multidisciplinary team, including a wider use of health care assistants (HCAs) and the expansion of the role of the nurse practitioner in general practice.

By 2002 PCTs had been founded across England, and all health care services were commissioned or provided directly by these organisations. In order to emphasise the key role anticipated for nurses and to promote further clinical involvement in decision making, all PCTs were encouraged to appoint nurses to their Professional Executive Committees. For the first time, targets for performance and service delivery were set, and an emphasis on greater accountability and clinical governance within GP organisations was laid down. These changes led to improvements in the provision of employment contracts and training opportunities for GPNs.

The General Medical Services contract was renewed in 2004, which gave GPs the option to opt out of providing out-of-hours services and introduced the Quality and Outcomes Framework (QOF), a voluntary scheme offering additional financial rewards to GPs for extra services and standards of care offered. Practices are still required to provide 'essential services' funded through a 'global sum payment'; these services include the:

- Management of patients who are ill or believe themselves to be ill with conditions from which recovery is generally expected
- General management of patients who are terminally ill
- Management of chronic disease

Practices were also given a preferential right to provide additional services which attract further funding:

- Cervical screening
- Contraceptive services
- Vaccinations and immunisations

- Child health surveillance
- Maternity services
- Minor surgery services

The QOF contains four domains covering the following areas of general practice: clinical care, organisational, patient experience and additional services. Each domain is worth a fixed number of points and practices score points according to the level of achievement within each domain. The higher the number of points achieved, the higher the financial reward to the practice. The stated aim of QOF is to improve standards of care, provide information and to enable practices to benchmark themselves against local and national achievements (The Health and Social Care Information Centre 2012). General practice has been very successful in delivering the requirements of the QOF, and this has been in no small part due to the broad range of skills and care delivered by GPNs. This success has served to highlight to primary care organisations the value of providing training, education, clinical supervision and appraisal support to GPNs (Tinson *et al.* 2011).

Practice nursing roles and functions

The role of the practice nurse can vary considerably depending on several factors. Patient demographics, the size of the practice and the skill set of the individual nurse will all influence the range of functions undertaken. However, all GPNs are expected to possess and deploy a range of core skills such as those listed later.

Core skills for the GPN

- Immunisation and vaccination
- Cervical cytology
- Venepuncture
- Wound care
- Ear care
- Basic IT skills
- Health education/promotion
- Chronic disease monitoring

With the growth of the practice nursing role, these core skills have expanded rapidly, which has provided opportunities for practice nurses to develop special interests within the generalist setting, for example, family planning and chronic disease management. These changes in function have been accompanied by a rapid expansion of skill mix in recent years and may now include the employment of HCAs, treatment room nurses, minor illness specialist nurses and nurse practitioners. In some localities however, there may be a single practice nurse or a small team who may job share. In these situations the practice nurse may work in isolation and not benefit from the support and expertise of an effective larger nursing team. In such circumstances a practice nurse facilitator can be a valuable resource to aid with networking with other practice nurses within the context of a local geographical area. In such situations health visitors and district nurses looking after the same local population can also provide support to local practices.

Education

The majority of skills required by the practice nurse are not all taught or developed as part of preregistration nurse training or acquired through post-qualification hospital-based experience; additionally the skills are not generally found in nurses working in other clinical fields. This can be a real challenge as a newly employed practice nurse is often expected to be competent at the outset; any gaps in knowledge need to be addressed once they are working in practice which has implications for both individual accountability and governance. This can also have financial implications for the employing practice, and there may be particular difficulties in accessing appropriate training programmes which in turn can lead to a wide variation in the skills and knowledge base of GPNs (Tinson *et al.* 2011). The Working in Partnership Programme (WIPP 2008) developed a range of core principles to support the GPN. The aim was to reduce anomalies in roles, skills, competence variation and pay. The programme also provided advice for employers and educators as well as nurses. This toolkit has helped educators and commissioners to standardise practice nurse education through the development of accredited modules as well as addressing core clinical skills such as chronic disease management and to accommodate to a rapidly changing set of new demands in general practice. In some areas the NHS funding has been secured to enable suitable candidates to undertake training prior to being engaged as practice nurses. In such schemes the students undertake a vocational training scheme, similar in concept to the way that GPs are trained.

In many practices, HCAs are employed and are a highly valued resource within the general practice team. The support role and function of the HCA is recognised by the RCN who have published a position statement offering guidance on the best practice in relation to the education and training of HCAs in the United Kingdom (RCN 2012). Core competencies may include many treatment room tasks such as venepuncture, BP measurement and recordings, pulse rates, pulse oximetry, temperature, respiratory rates, peak flow rates, height, weight, BMI, urinalysis and ECGs. Some HCAs are also expanding their skill into other areas, for example, influenza immunisation and ear care. Due to the expanding and extending role of the qualified practice nurse, they may not be able to perform all the tasks required within the practice and as such will delegate some to an HCA. The HCA must be competent to undertake such delegated tasks and accept the responsibility to do so (but always under the overall direction of a qualified practitioner). In order to provide safe practice, such delegated tasks should be governed within the context of practice/clinical protocols and policies and identified within job specifications and competence evidenced and recorded in personal training records to provide endorsement and authorisation (RCN 2012). The registered nurse should ensure that the HCA is competent, capable and confident to carry out their instructions and ensure that the outcome of the delegated task meets the required standards and that everyone they are responsible for is supervised and appropriately supported and their performance monitored (RCN 2012).

There are three key aspects of the role of the practice nurse which the following section will focus on:

1. Scheduled care
2. Unscheduled care
3. Long-term conditions

Scheduled care

This role is often undertaken by a 'treatment room nurse' who may be supported by an HCA. Pre-booked appointments allow the practice population to access a variety of services to both promote and protect health. These two key concepts are forming the focus of the practice nurse ethos emphasising a collective responsibility for health, its protection and disease prevention. Examples include cervical cytology screening, immunisations, smoking cessation advice and advice about healthy eating. In addition other functions include venepuncture, ear care and acute and chronic wound care and management. Many patients will be regular attendees at their local practice requiring long-term management of health issues, for example, regular injections and wound care interventions and treatment. During an episode of care, the practice nurse is in a unique position to form a therapeutic relationship with the patient and sometimes in partnership with their carers or other family members. This provides an ideal opportunity to promote health. This might take the form of promoting individual lifestyle changes such as exercise and healthy eating or address public health issues through the provision of immunisations and disease prevention advice. This role requires excellent communication skills and an understanding of the factors that influence an individual's behaviour. These will include cultural aspects of health and illness, the patient's health belief and understanding of the socioeconomic influences that impact on health. Whilst there is no universally accepted model of health promotion, there are three main types of approach: individual focused, group focused and community focused (Drennan & Goodman 2007). The individual-focused approach can include the provision of educational advice by giving the patient/carer information or helping them interpret this knowledge so that they can make lifestyle choices. Nursing and behavioural interventions may also be provided, such as immunisations to assist in disease prevention and the amelioration of disease presentations and symptoms (Drennan & Goodman 2007).

An example of a group-focused approach is the DESMOND approach for diabetes, which is an NHS organisation that supports the delivery of patient education to people with type 2 diabetes or those at risk of diabetes. DESMOND is also a research organisation, which draws on the expertise of colleagues, academics and the NHS to develop and test the effectiveness of the educational programmes provided (DESMOND 2008).

Community-focused approaches could involve examining prevalence or incidence of a condition within a geographical area, for example, TB, and include campaigns and preventional strategies that respond effectively to local population trends, for example, the need to tackle obesity rates and the manifestation of diabetes (often conditioned and influenced by rapid societal changes in behaviour and diet). The practice nurse has a key role in all such approaches as a key function of the practice.

Examples of scheduled care interventions include the following.

Cervical cytology

Cervical cancer accounts for 2% of all female cancers and is diagnosed in 11 per 100 000 women in the United Kingdom with over three quarters occurring in 25–64-year-olds (Cancer Research UK 2009). The majority of cervical screening is carried out in the primary care setting, and in England the national screen programme offers triennial screening for women aged between 25 and 64. A key role of the practice nurse is to undertake this screening, and specific training in liquid-based cytology is a prerequisite. The introduction of liquid-based cytology in recent years has significantly reduced the numbers of erroneous smear results.

Immunisations

In addition to childhood immunisation programmes, most practices offer travel vaccinations for both adults and children. Most vaccinations given in general practice are provided under the umbrella of a patient group direction (PGD). A PGD is a written instruction for the supply and administration of medicines to groups of patients who may not be individually identified before presenting for treatment (NMC 2006). They are developed at organisational level by a senior doctor, nurse and pharmacist, and the practice nurse is required to sign up to them before commencing immunisations. They have been developed to cover most of the vaccinations commonly administered in primary care, for example, influenza vaccinations, baby immunisations and most vaccinations for travel health. There is a charge for some travel vaccinations, and some, such as yellow fever vaccinations, can only be given at designated centres. The demand for travel health advice is growing with the increase in global communication links and is now regarded as a subspeciality for practice nurses due to complicated travel itineraries. Private travel health clinics are also available and provide a comprehensive range of services that are provided to the fee-paying public. Specialist advice centres have been developed to aid health professionals to make informed safe clinical decisions-making process, for example, the National Travel Health Network and Centre (NaTHNac) www.nathnac.co.org and Travax www.travax.scot.nhs.uk. These services provide an advice on vaccination and public health issues and offer a comprehensive range of travel-related information.

Wound care

Wound management in primary care includes suture removal, minor dressings and short-term care as well as the more demanding leg ulcer management. The prevalence of leg ulcers is between 1 and 2% of the adult population increasing with age and with healing rates ranging from 45 to 80% at 24 weeks (Drennan & Goodman 2007).This can mean that the demand for regular dressings can be high particularly in an area with a high elderly population. Some areas provide dedicated ulcer clinics where Doppler tests are carried out and wound care specialist nurses are employed to care for the practice population. Wherever ulcer dressings are undertaken, teamworking between the district nurse and practice nurse is often required to provide a service for housebound patients or for those requiring dressings at the weekend.

Unscheduled care

Practice nurses are in a unique position to influence the health of the population given that there are nearly a million consultations taking place in primary care every working day (DH 2009). Many patients who are seen regularly by the practice nurse for routine care, for example, for dressings, screening or blood pressure checks, often ask for an advice or treatment for an unscheduled episode as 'they do not want to bother the doctor'. This combined with the extra demand placed on GPs has meant that many practice nurses develop skills in triage and minor illness management and undertake advanced courses to enable them to acquire new clinical competencies, for example, nurse practitioner programmes and Independent and Supplementary Prescribing courses in order to meet patient demand for more localised specialist service delivery. Government policy has provided both challenges and opportunities for nurses to expand their role and undertake some of the traditional functions of a doctor (Wanless 2002; DH 2008a, 2008b). Good consultation skills are of paramount importance for nurses seeing patients with undifferentiated problems, and whilst GP registrars are trained and assessed in consultation skills, this may not be the case with other practitioners (Courtney & Griffiths 2010). These important skills are developed as part of advanced practitioner programmes including programmes for Independent and Supplementary Nurse Prescribing that result in the award of a recordable qualification where the practitioner is accountable for the assessment and management of patients with diagnosed and undiagnosed conditions (NMC 2006). In addition to these skills, advanced practice courses encompass the scope and context of autonomous practice and the accountability issues of expanding and extending practice.

In addition to history-taking skills, nurses seeing patients for the first point of contact care require expertise in physical assessment skills in order to examine patients. An appropriate physical examination plus a focused comprehensive history will foster accurate clinical decision making enabling effective case management or referral of the patient as necessary.

Patients have been found to value the caring aspects of consulting with nurses in addition to the accessibility and time spent with the nurse (Reveley 1998). Kinnersley *et al.* (2000) found that consultations with nurses offered opportunities for the provision of more advice on self-care and management, reinforcing the value of the provision of holistic nursing care.

From 2006 Independent and Supplementary Nurse Prescribers have been able to prescribe anything from the British National Formulary within their scope of competence with the exception of some controlled drugs (NMC 2006). From April 2012 changes in legislation mean that Independent Nurse Prescribers will be enabled to prescribe controlled drugs in schedules 2, 3, 4 and 5 with restrictions on treating addiction (The Royal Pharmaceutical Society 2012). This move has been eagerly awaited by nurses and allows for the holistic management of patients in all care settings where nurses hold prescribing rights.

Depending on the requirements of the GP practice and the skill set of the nurse, unscheduled care may be a role in itself or may be integrated across the practice team and their associated clinics. Other avenues where these skills may be utilised include telephone triage where the nurse will undertake a telephone consultation and assess the need for face to face interview and management.

Just as the demands on doctors are growing in primary care, so are those on the nurses. The government policy that is increasingly moving care to primary care has led to a requirement to assess the capacity, capability and competence issues within and across the workforce in primary care, resulting in the breakdown of traditional boundaries between primary, secondary and community care. The impact this will have on workload is not without its challenges and requires careful consideration in order to employ the appropriate skill mix to meet the needs of the practice population.

Chronic disease management

This is an area of practice nursing that has expanded over recent years. Since the early 1990s, practice nurses have undergone specific training to equip themselves to deal with a variety of chronic disease including asthma, chronic obstructive pulmonary disease (COPD), hypertension, congestive cardiac failure, coronary heart disease and arthritis. The expertise developed has resulted in the instigation of specialist clinics run by experienced and knowledgeable practitioners. In relation to the adult population, the need for these will increase not only due to the move from secondary care management to primary care management for many chronic diseases but also because we are witnessing an increasingly aging population. The fastest growing age group in the United Kingdom are those aged 80 and over, who made up 4.5% of the UK population in 2007. There are now more adults of pensionable age than children (Gosney & Harris 2009). Eighty-five per cent of individuals over 65 years of age have one chronic condition, and 50% have more than one chronic condition (Swonger & Burbank 1995). Primary care is therefore expected to deal with the complex health needs of an increasing elderly population including issues around polypharmacy and increasingly complex drug interactions, fall prevention and issues of social isolation. This care cannot be delivered in isolation; it requires a problem-based approach supported by an inter-professional response including engagement with other nursing specialities such as district nurses and community matrons and members of the allied health professions.

Two examples of chronic disease management are illustrated later. Other chronic disease conditions the practice nurse may be involved in might include diabetes, coronary heart disease, heart failure and arthritis depending on the needs of the practice population.

Asthma management

Asthma management in primary care has been undertaken since the early 1990s as part of the General Medical Service contract attracting financial rewards through the Quality and Outcomes Framework (QOF). The quality indicators include targets for the percentage of patients aged 8 years and older diagnosed from April 2006 with measurement of reversibility or variability (NHS Evidence 2011) resulting in the fact that many practice nurses now undertake spirometry to measure lung function, a skill that was traditionally the remit of secondary care. Other quality indicators focus on smoking status and on the management of asthma. The framework for treating asthma is the British Guidelines on the Management of Asthma (British Thoracic Society & SIGN 2012), which provides an evidence-based care pathway for asthma of varying degrees of severity covering the lifespan. Opportunistic monitoring of peak flow measurements and inhaler technique may be undertaken by the treatment room nurse; however, practice nurses contributing to or running asthma clinics should have attended approved asthma training courses in order to equip them with a broader range of specialist skills, including the rationale for the adjustment of medication doses and addressing patient education (e.g. education for appropriate inhaler technique). Education for health (www.educationforhealth) runs a variety of training courses at diploma and degree level (accredited by the Open University), and study days and workshops in respiratory health suited to nurses working in primary care are provided locally in many areas. In more recent years the management of COPD has also fallen increasingly within the portfolio of an appropriately trained practice nurse.

Hypertension

Hypertension is usually asymptomatic and is often detected during routine clinical screening by the doctor or practice nurse. Regular recording of blood pressure for certain patients is part of the QOF targets set for payment thresholds. These targets for 2013/2014 include recommendations for targets for patients aged both under and over 80 (NICE 2012). The incidence of hypertension increases with age due to structural changes in the vessel walls along with other contributory factors such as obesity, alcohol intake, ethnicity, gender and lack of exercise (Gosney & Harris 2009).The practice nurse is in an ideal position to not only monitor the blood pressure of the practice population but also provide health education relating to lifestyle advice. Blood pressure monitoring may be undertaken in an opportunistic way but may be part of a nurse-led hypertension clinic where bloods are monitored and medications are adjusted. Nurses that run clinics and work in an extended role should ensure they have the expertise and skill required. Monitoring of blood pressure will also be an important function of other chronic disease clinics, for example, coronary heart disease and diabetes.

The future

More recently the Coalition Government has continued to reorganise primary care services since the *Health and Social Care Act* 2012 (Parliament 2012). These changes continue to emphasise the central role that general practice plays in commissioning services such as clinical commissioning groups (CCGs) of practices taking over the former role of the PCTs. It is difficult to anticipate the effect that these changes will have, but many CCGs are making nurse appointments to their Boards. In addition direct ownership of responsibility for workforce planning and clinical governance may result in a greater awareness of the need for sustained and increased funding for GPN training and education. Clinical skills are an essential element of the general practice role; however, development of non-clinical skills must also be a priority. Nurses should be encouraged to contribute to a multi-professional approach to primary care education, enhance leadership in practice nursing and contribute to the development of standards and quality in the practice setting (Tinson *et al.* 2011). Experienced GPNs should be encouraged and supported to develop in a mentorship role which will enhance the scope and development of the GPN and could lead to the further expansion of the role, skill mixing and breaking down of traditional boundaries across the workforce. This must take into account that holistic patient care is not to be viewed as a series of tasks at the lowest cost but a cohesive care package within which practice nurses can make a significant contribution.

References

British Thoracic Society; Scottish Intercollegiate Guidelines Network (SIGN) (2012) *British Guideline on the Management of Asthma* (Online). Available from http://www.brit-thoracic. org.uk/Portals/0/Guidelines/AsthmaGuidelines/sign101%20Jan%202012.pdf. Accessed on 19 November 2012.

Cancer Research UK (2009) *Cervical Cancer – UK Incidence Statistics* (Online). Available from www.infocnacerresearchuk.org/cancerstats/types/cervix/incidence/uk-cervical-cancer-incidence-statistics. Accessed on 3 August 2012.

Cartwright, A. & Scott, R. (1961) The work of a nurse employed in a general practice. *British Medical Journal,* **March**, 807–813.

Courtney, M. & Griffiths, M. (2010) *Independent and Supplementary Prescribing: An Essential Guide.* Cambridge University Press, Cambridge.

Dawson, L. (1920) *Interim Report on the Future Provision of Medical Services and Allied Services Report of Consultative Council on Medical and Allied Services CMD 693.* HMSO, London.

Department of Health (DH) (1989) *Working for Patients. White Paper.* HMSO, London.

DH (2001) *Primary Care, General Practice and the NHS Plan: Information for GPs, Nurses Other Health Professionals and Staff Working in Primary Care in England.* HMSO DH, London.

DH (2002) *Liberating the Talents: Helping Primary care Trusts and Nurses to Deliver the NHS Plan.* DH, London.

DH (2008a) *High Quality Care for All: NHS Next Stage Review Final Report.* The Stationary Office DH, Norwich.

DH (2008b) The Wanless Report: Securing Good Health for the Whole Population. DH, London.

DH (2009) *Primary Care and Community Services: Improving Access and Responsiveness.* HMSO DH, London.

The DESMOND Collaborative (2008) (Online). Available from http://www.desmond-project.org.uk/. Accessed on 25 September 2012.

Drennan, V. & Goodman, C. (eds) (2007) *Oxford Handbook of Primary Care and Community Nursing.* Oxford University Press, Oxford.

Gosney, M. & Harris, T. (eds) (2009) *Managing Older People in Primary Care.* Oxford University Press, Oxford.

Kinnersley, P., Anderson, E., Parry, K., *et al.* (2000) Randomised controlled trial of nurse practitioner versus general practitioner care for patients requesting 'same day' consultations in primary care. *British Medical Journal,* 320, 1043–1048.

Kmietowicz, Z. (2006) A century of general practice. *British Medical Journal,* 332, 39–40.

National Institute for Health and Clinical Excellence (NICE) (2012) *Indicator Recommendations 2013/14* (Online). Available from www.nice.org.uk/aboutnice/qof/Recommendationsindicator retirement.jsp. Accessed on 25 September 2012.

NHS Evidence (2011) *Asthma Goals and Outcome Measures: QOF Indicators* (Online). Available from http://www.cks.nhs.uk/asthma/goals_and_outcome_measures/qof_indicators. Accessed on 19 November 2012.

Nursing and Midwifery Council (NMC) (2006) *Standards of Proficiency for Nurse and Midwife Prescribers.* Nursing and Midwifery Council, London.

Parliament (1911) *National Insurance Act (1911c).* HMSO, London.

Parliament (1997) *National Health Service (Primary Care) Act c 46 .*

Parliament (2012) *Health and Social Care Act.* HMSO, London.

Porter, R. (1997) *The Greatest Benefit to Mankind: A Medical History of Humanity from Antiquity to the Present.* HarperCollins, London.

Reveley, S. (1998) The role of the triage nurse practitioner in general medical practice: analysis of the role. *The Journal of Advanced Nursing,* 28 (3), 584–91.

Royal College of Nursing (RCN) (2012) *Position Statement on the Education and Training of Health Care Assistants* (Online). Available from http://www.rcn.org.uk/__data/assets/pdf_file/0003/441912/Position_statement_-_HCAs_Final_V3.pdf. Accessed on 19 November 2012.

Royal Pharmaceutical Society (2012) *Changes to the Professional Use of Controlled Drugs by Pharmacists and Nurses (Including Independent Pharmacist Prescribing of Controlled Drugs)* (Online). Available from www.rpharms.com/support-alert-article.asp?id=505. Accessed on 7 August 2012.

Swonger, A.K. & Burbank, P. (1995) *Drug Therapy and the Elderly*. Jones and Bartlett, London.

Tait, I. (2002) *History of the College* (Online). Available from http://www.rcgp.org.uk/about-us/history-heritage-and-archive/history-of-the-college.aspx. Accessed on 29 October 2012.

The Health and Social Care Information Centre (2012) *Quality and Outcomes Framework: Online GP Practice Results Database* (Online). Available from http://www.qof.ic.nhs.uk/. Accessed on 12 November 2012.

Tinson, S., Axe, S. & Zoe, B. (2011) General practice nurse education: introducing mentorship. *Education for Primary Care*, 22 (4), 219–22.

UKCC (1994) *The Future of Professional Practice – The Council's Standards for Education and Practice Following Registration*. UKCC, London.

Wanless, D. (2002) *Securing Our Future Health: Taking a Long Term View* (Online). Available from http://webarchive.nationalarchives.gov.uk/+/http://www.hm-treasury.gov.uk/consult_wanless_final.htm. Accessed on 19 November 2012.

www.legislation.gov.uk (1966) *National Health Service Act 1966 c8* (Online). Available from http://www.legislation.gov.uk/ukpga/1966/8/pdfs/ukpga_19660008_en.pdf. Accessed on 29 October 2012.

www.wipp.nhs.uk (2008) *Working in Partnership Programme: Creating Capacity in General Practice* (Online). Available from http://www.wipp.nhs.uk/. Accessed on 20 November 2012.

11

Occupational Health Nursing

Anne Harriss

Faculty of Health and Social Sciences, London South Bank University, London, UK

OHNs provide specialised nursing care in a specific public health-care setting – the workplace. The National Health Service (NHS) makes occupational health provision for their staff, and many OHNs practise in settings outside of the NHS. The International Labour Organisation (ILO) and the World Health Organization (WHO) are two international institutions that regularly comment on both health and health and safety at work. They have defined the aims and objectives of an occupational health (OH) service. One of the ILO's recommendations, Recommendation 112, highlights that the aim of an OH service is to protect workers against health hazards arising out of their work, or their working environment, and adapting work processes so that optimum physical and mental health of the worker can be achieved (ILO 1959). The WHO takes a similar stance but also comments on the identification and control of all 'chemical, physical, mechanical, biological and psychosocial agents that are known to be or expected to be very hazardous' (WHO 1973).

OHNs as specialist practitioners

This chapter provides an overview of the role of the OHN as a specialist public health practitioner promoting health, safety and welfare in the workplace. In order to give the reader an understanding of contemporary OH nursing practice, a historical perspective, which outlines the influencing factors and domains of OHN practice, is explored.

Community and Public Health Nursing, Fifth Edition. Edited by David Sines,
Sharon Aldridge-Bent, Agnes Fanning, Penny Farrelly, Kate Potter and Jane Wright.
© 2013 John Wiley & Sons, Ltd. Published 2013 by John Wiley & Sons, Ltd.

Historical perspective

An appreciation of the effect of work on health is not new. Indeed, more than 300 years ago, Ramazzini, a professor of medicine at Padua, Italy, acknowledged that work impacts on health. Ramazzini is widely considered to be the father of occupational medicine, and his practice involved looking after the health needs of artisans and labourers. He stressed the importance of asking patients this question: 'What is your occupation'? This question is often forgotten by many medical (and nursing) practitioners of today but is not forgotten by nurses working in OH as they appreciate the possible adverse effects of work on health and health on work performance.

OH nursing has a long history in the United Kingdom. The first nurse working in the industrial setting is reputed to be Phillipa Flowerday who was employed in the late nineteenth century in the Coleman's mustard factory in Norwich. Her role was innovative at that time and encompassed a public health dimension as she offered a treatment service in the factory during the morning and then spent the rest of her working day working with sick employees and their families in their own homes. Contemporary OHN practice has evolved from such a treatment-based approach to one that is both evidence-based and proactive and has a preventative focus.

OH services of the twenty-first century are directly involved in employee health management, and they work towards reducing employee exposure to health risks and preventing illnesses associated with occupation. This is congruent with the ILO/WHO's stance that OH services aim to promote and maintain the highest degree of physical, mental and social well-being of workers in all occupations. It involves controlling risks and adapting work processes to workers.

In order to accomplish this aim, OHNs must have an understanding of the factors impacting on the health of workers and be innovative in their approach to the client care offered by them to all strata within the organisation. They have an understanding of how organisations function and an appreciation of the social influences on health status. The Acheson report (DH 1998) indicated that poverty continues to exert a negative effect on health with the gap between the social classes widening. Wilkinson and Pickett (2010) referred to earlier in this chapter take a similar stance. OHNs are able to work with employees at all levels and within all social groups. Consequently, they contribute to the improvement of the health of all strata of the workforce and are able to focus on particularly vulnerable groups. One such group are people, often low-paid unskilled workers, employed to operate hazardous processes. These people are already disadvantaged, and such exposure to workplace hazards has the potential to further contribute to the health divide between the social classes.

Lewis and Thornbory (2006) comment that 'Occupational health nurses are probably the largest group of occupational health professional in the UK' (p. 81). OHNs practise within a public health framework and have the potential to make a significant contribution to the health of the working population. Marmot (2005) highlights inequalities in health arise as a result of the complex interplay between employment, socioeconomic status, housing and education. Keeping people economically active has the potential to positively impact on health status. Indeed, Waddell and Burton (2006) refer to the positive benefit to an individual of work and the negative association between unemployment and poor health. Wilkinson and Pickett (2010) take this further high-lighting the influences of socioeconomic status on society as a whole.

It is not an easy task for nurses who practise in other settings to be able to influence these factors, but proactive OHNs do have the opportunity to engage with a workforce that may consist of a 'crunchy social mix' of people of differing ages, cultures, ethnicities and social backgrounds. This engagement can lead to health improvements as not only are OHNs well placed to offer impartial general health advice to employees but they can also assist employers prevent, or at least reduce, the incidence of workplace accidents and work-related ill health, thus meeting the aims proposed by the ILO and the WHO.

OH nursing is a distinct specialty within the family of public health nursing. Its practice is multifaceted utilising a unique blend of specialised nursing skills developed from health needs assessments for their specific client group – people at work. The age range of this client group is wide, ranging from school leavers to those of retirement age and beyond. The OHN is responsible for devising strategies which reduce the potential for work-related ill health and accidental injury. The role of the OHN is diverse and involves working collaboratively with management and a range of other practitioners, both health and non-health professionals, in order to address the health needs of the population for whom they are responsible.

A specialist OHN is a nurse who holds a role-preparation qualification in OH nursing conferring registration with the Nursing and Midwifery Council (NMC) as a specialist community public health nurse (SCPHN). The scope of practice and competencies of an OHN is further described in the RCN document *Occupational health nursing: career and competence development* (Royal College of Nursing 2011). This document highlights the range of skills of a competent OHN including those of risk assessment, health surveillance, health promotion and health protection. It underlines the importance of the role of the OHN in attendance management and the development of strategies that facilitate a successful return to work following an accident or serious illness. Supporting people back into work is a key feature of the role of the OHN and congruent with the Government's welfare reforms and public health strategy.

The NMC set, and the RCN describe, standards for practice. Sadly, there is currently no mandatory requirement for nurses employed to provide care in the workplace to hold a specialist qualification in OH nursing. Unfortunately, many employers do not provide an OH service for their staff. Of those organisations that do, a number do not require the nurses they employ to hold a qualification in the specialty. This is a lost opportunity as an effective OH service adds value to the organisation. Promoting a healthier workforce and assisting people with long-term conditions and disabilities remain at work. OHNs are well positioned to contribute to organisational policy development and advise on compliance with legislation including that covering health and safety and some elements of employment legislation. Their input to their employing organisation is a definite return on investment. There is now a move to employ technicians to support specialist OHNs. Such technicians undertake a task-driven role. Universities are now offering programmes that prepare technicians for this role. The role that technicians undertake is dependant on the needs of the employing organisation. It commonly includes participation in statutory health surveillance programmes such as is required by the Control of Substances Hazardous to Health Regulations 2002.

Technicians are becoming more commonplace in workplace health management but do not operate at the strategic level of the OHN specialist. They may hold a nursing or health qualification but there is no requirement to do so. However, holding an appropriate qualification is essential as this is a very specialist area of autonomous nursing practice and decision-making. It is the role of the OHN specialist practitioner that will be explored in this chapter.

The model of OH service provision is influenced by a multitude of factors including the current state of the economy, legal requirements and the hazards to which employees could be exposed (Smedley *et al.* 2007). OHNs practise nursing in a unique way. Working with specific populations in the workplace, they perform an important public health function. Although their role is diverse and complex, it is primarily concerned with promoting general health status and preventing work-related ill health and accidents. Experienced OHNs play an important part in organisational health policy development and risk and health management. They are thus in a prime position to contribute to attendance management and rehabilitative interventions assisting those with chronic health issues to remain in productive and paid employment. These interventions will be explored later in this chapter.

The Health and Safety Executive (HSE) highlights that in 2010/2011 an estimated 1.8 million people were suffering from a health condition which they believed was caused or exacerbated by their current or previous work (Health and Safety Executive 2011, p. 3). Unfortunately, not every employee in the United Kingdom has access to an OH service; those employed in small- and medium-sized enterprises are less well served than those working in large organisations. These people are missing out on preventative health care and their employers on initiatives which can impact on work attendance and thus organisational productivity (Paton 2012).

An effective OH service adds value to the employing organisation; there are clear benefits to both employee and employer by improving the quality of working life as well as having a positive impact on business productivity. Employer commitment to employee health improvements not only contributes to the long-term health status of the community but also benefits the organisation through an improvement in worker retention, a reduction in sickness absence and accident rates and an increase in productivity. As the HSE has long asserted, 'good health means good business' (Health and Safety Executive 1995). Organisations providing an OH service do so because of the associated benefits. OHNs recognise that well-designed work processes should do employees no harm, and as Manos and Silcox comment, 'good work is good medicine' (Manos and Silcox 2007, p. 17).

There is a paradoxical relationship between work and health; for most people employment is a financial necessity and often socially rewarding. However, it must be acknowledged that under some circumstances work may result in significant adverse health effects.

All occupational groups have the potential to be exposed to a wide range of health hazards associated with the work they undertake. Although the following is not a definitive list, such hazards include:

- *Psychosocial* aspects including work-related stress.
- *Biological materials* involving work with plants, animals or microorganisms including blood and body fluids.
- *Chemical agents* including detergents and other cleaning products that are associated with range of health issues including occupational dermatitis.
- *Ergonomic aspects* resulting in musculoskeletal disorders (MSDs).
- *Physical agents* including high levels of noise and vibration. Noise can result in hearing loss, and working with vibrating tools has the potential to result in disabling vascular and neurological damage to the hand and arm or even the whole body.

Some high-risk work areas such as construction sites have obvious dangers, and construction incidents and accidents result in both morbidity and mortality (Health and Safety Executive 2011). These include working in a hazardous environment, often in adverse climatic conditions, using dangerous machinery and possible exposure to harmful chemicals. It is important to note that in addition to contractors and subcontractors, the construction industry employs a predominantly itinerant workforce. Although many construction industry workers are highly skilled, others are semi- or unskilled employees; a large proportion of these people speak English as a second or subsequent language, and a number may speak no English at all. The combination of these factors results in an increased risk of accidents. Indeed construction sites are probably some of the most dangerous work areas in the United Kingdom with workers at risk of falls during tasks carried out at heights, incidents involving the movement of large vehicles and use of machinery and incidents associated with the lifting of heavy loads. The nature of their occupation results in construction workers being more likely to be involved in serious accidents than people employed in less dangerous work areas. Furthermore, their work is also associated with a range of occupational illnesses. Working with noisy, vibrating tools can result in the development of occupational deafness and hand–arm vibration syndrome (Health and Safety Executive 2005). Their exposure to materials such as oils and cement predisposes them to developing occupational dermatitis and chemical burns. There are now a growing number of OHNs who choose to work in the construction industry as a result of the diversity of the hazards associated with such employment.

Construction is only one of many sectors with associated ill-health effects. Occupational asthma is a work-related condition associated with a number of work processes including exposure to flour in food production, exposure to isocyanates in the two-pack paint spraying of motor vehicles and exposure to dander and body fluids from working with animals. Noise-induced hearing loss is associated with a range of occupations including factory work and the military and amongst professional musicians. Unsurprisingly, a number of high-profile rock musicians are reputed to have developed noise-induced hearing loss. These performers are particularly at risk due to both their ongoing exposure to noise and their probable reluctance to wearing hearing protection.

Members of other performing arts such as actors, singers and dancers are also predisposed to developing occupationally related conditions. Dancers are prone to joint and other MSDs, whilst singers and actors may develop problems with their voice. There is a small group of OHNs working specifically in this highly specialised field of OH practice. Their client group is interesting and unusual as it includes every age range from infant to child to adolescent to adult, including those who have passed what would be considered a normal retirement age for other occupations. Even office work is not without risk; work-related upper limb disorders including repetitive strain injuries are associated with repetitive tasks such as poorly designed work tasks involving extensive keyboard use.

Provision of OH services in the United Kingdom

Unfortunately there is currently no legal requirement in the United Kingdom for employers to provide an OH service for their employees, and this is unlikely to change in the foreseeable future. Large organisations, or those with exposure to workplace hazards such as dangerous chemicals, often choose to provide one. The provision of such a service is not mandatory and is therefore an option for businesses rather than an obligation. The decision whether to provide an OH service is usually a financial one. A consequence of there being no statutory requirement for OH services is that OH provision in the United Kingdom is patchy; in short there is no 'National Occupational Health Service'. A government strategy to promote the health and well-being of working-age people encompassed within the document *Health, work and wellbeing – Caring for our future* (HM Government 2005) could be a small step forward to making this a reality. Central to this strategy was the appointment of a National Director for Occupational Health, Dame Carol Black (Manos & Silcox 2007), and initiatives to help and encourage people to return to the workplace after a period of sickness absence. A proactive OH service is well placed to develop high-quality return to work recovery programmes key to reducing the impact of long-term sickness absence. Important elements of such an initiative include promoting health and assisting people with chronic health problems to stay in work and out of a benefit trap, thus reducing both the financial burden on society and the social exclusion of those living with chronic health deficits. OH services have the potential to promote health, thus reducing health inequalities between the richer and poorer members of the community.

The passing of the Health and Social Care Act (Parliament 2012) underlines the importance of public health to this government. The requirement of this legislation has the potential to impact on health inequalities as it promotes the delivery of public health within the United Kingdom at macro and micro levels. It provides opportunities for a 'joined-up' approach to promoting community health improvement, integrating the responsibilities of the NHS, social care, transport, leisure and environmental health services. Nationally, an executive agency of the Department of Health has been established: 'Public Health England'. The aim is to develop a public health-focused system directly accountable to the Secretary of State.

Local authorities (LAs) will have a more explicit public health remit with the aim of reducing the health inequalities experienced by less affluent members of society. The Health and Social Care Act 2012 established Health and Wellbeing Boards with the aim of providing a forum at which key players can work together with the aim of reducing health inequalities within the populations they serve.

These boards will coordinate Clinical Commissioning Groups and councils, thus facilitating a broader understanding of their community's health and well-being requirements. Although OH services are key to promoting the health of the working population, OH practitioners have not been identified as key members of these boards. This failure to incorporate OH practitioners as key members of Health and Wellbeing Boards is a lost opportunity. It could have resulted in health initiatives delivered in the workplace, health being integrated within a national public health strategy. If OH providers are not seen as integral to this aspect of public health provision, then there is little hope that a national OH service will indeed become a reality in the foreseeable future. The nearest to such a service to date was the establishment in 11 March 2010 of pilot Fit for Work Services (FFWS). These services did not provide a full OH service but were limited to case-managed support for workers in the early stages of sickness absence. The aim was to facilitate an effective return to work for these workers, thus supporting job retention. These pilot services were subsequently evaluated at the end of the first year of operation: those who accessed these services found them to be supportive, most respondents indicating that they would not have received the interventions they had without the support of FFWS (Hillage *et al.* 2012). Unfortunately, the number of people who utilised these services was disappointing and well below the access levels which had been anticipated. A dramatic expansion of such a service at a time of financial austerity is therefore unlikely.

It has been suggested that OH as a specialty has been slow to progress owing to its exclusion from the NHS at its inception in 1948. This omission was probably due to financial reasons resulting from concerns regarding the cost of developing a new NHS. The Government's stance that employers are responsible for OH provision has resulted in this inconsistent approach, and, until recently, there was little collaborative working evident between the NHS and the workplace. NHS Plus, which is discussed later in this chapter, helped to bridge this gap. Dame Carol Black's review of the health of Britain's working population, *Working for a healthier tomorrow*, for the Department for Work and Pensions indicates that detachment of OH from mainstream health care undermines holistic patient care (Department for Work and Pensions 2008).

The changing nature of UK workplaces

The nature of UK workplaces is changing and the role of the OHN is developing to meet the challenges these changes present. Their role can be as diverse as the workplaces in which they are employed. There is now a decline in the number of large manufacturing industries in the United Kingdom, and work is increasingly undertaken within a multicultural context. Non-discriminatory government policy has resulted in employers being required to make arrangements to facilitate the employment of people with a range of physical and mental disabilities. Employers must also offer equality of opportunity for both men and women; women of all ages now form a much larger proportion of the workforce, particularly so in what had previously been occupations dominated by male workers. This raises particular health and safety issues in respect of those who are pregnant or those who have recently returned to work following maternity leave. Pregnant women and new and nursing mothers are at risk from some work processes including exposure to some chemicals or the moving and handling of heavy or cumbersome loads.

The rapid growth of information technology has had a significant influence on work practices. This development has led to a growth of 'call centres' in which people are employed to undertake work that depends on the use of both telephones and computers. On the face of it, this would appear to be a safe place of work. However, on closer inspection there are a number of health problems associated with work of this nature. One of the most significant is voice strain; it is arguable that there is also the potential for some degree of damage to the ear with possible hearing loss associated with loud noise from a poorly adjusted volume control on telephone headsets (Maltby 2005). Other health problems are not specific to workers in call centres but are common to other occupations requiring work with computers such as work-related upper limb disorders. Working in a call centre is generally more stressful than other occupations. Careful work planning and equipment design can alleviate some of this stress, and an OHN can advise on such issues.

OHN practice requires an appreciation of the bio-psychosocial sciences recognising that employment is an integral part of adult life and health should not be harmed as a result of it. The ability to participate productively in workplace activities can, and should, contribute to ongoing physical and psychological well-being. However, not all work is free from risk. Workers of lower social status experience more injuries and work-related ill health than those from the middle classes. The financial circumstances of those living in socially deprived areas, single parents or those without skills or qualifications may be forced into hazardous, low-paid occupations. Cognisance of this situation enables OHNs to focus workplace health promotion activities on this group of workers – people who may not access such information from other sources.

Semi-skilled and unskilled workers frequently undertake tasks on poorly designed production lines predisposing them to MSDs such as work-related upper limb disorders and back pain. An example of a successful initiative put in place by one company is the protection of people working on a poultry processing production line. Their work tasks had hitherto included lifting plucked, semi-processed turkeys from a production conveyor belt located behind them and at waist height. The birds were then lifted onto a hook positioned in front of, and at the shoulder height of, the operatives. Many of these workers subsequently developed a range of work-related MSDs including neck, shoulder and back pain. The design of both the equipment with which they worked and their work tasks predisposed them to such pain due to the resulting repetitive twisting actions of the trunk, lifting a load (the turkeys) away from the body and repositioning and anchoring it at shoulder height. The high-risk operations they were required to undertake included twisting, reaching and handling a heavy load held at a distance from the body. The OH service took a proactive involvement in the redesign of both the work process and work equipment. Risk assessment pro formas were developed in order to identify any future problems associated with the process. The OHNs were able to refer clients with MSDs to a fast-track, in-house, physiotherapy service. These initiatives resulted in a dramatic reduction in MSDs with reduced costs relating to labour relations and turnover, sickness absence and possible future litigation. These employees were fortunate to have access to such a proactive OH service that was funded by their employer. This was possible due to the size and financial turnover of their company. Employees in many other workplaces in similar factories are not so fortunate.

Changing work patterns

It must be acknowledged that the world of work is rapidly changing with fewer large industries and a higher proportion of small- and medium-sized business enterprises. Even in large organisations employment does not always take place in a conventional workplace. 'Hot-desking' and even home working, for example, have been facilitated by developments in information technology. There are benefits and challenges associated with using the home as a workplace. Reduced travel costs with fewer distractions are appealing; however, isolation, the potential for longer working hours and higher levels of stress may result in workers employed in this way experiencing more emotional difficulties than their colleagues employed in a conventional office environment. Home working brings challenges to the OHNs who provide a service for people who work in this way.

Employers have a duty of care under legislation including the Health and Safety at Work etc. Act 1974. They must ensure the health, safety and welfare of their staff no matter where they work. It is also in the employer's financial interest to reduce absences resulting from work-related ill health. OHNs are suitably positioned and experienced to work collaboratively with workers, their representatives, management and other health and health and safety practitioners to improve worker health. Changing work patterns and work requirements and improved control strategies have resulted in a reduction of health deficits linked to exposure to hazardous chemicals. However, there has been an increase in work-related upper limb disorders associated with the use of computers. Likewise, workplace stress seems to be a topical subject of much debate. Work should not lead to mental ill health. There is poorer mental health amongst those who are unemployed compared to those in employment.

Workplace practices

The role of the OHN requires cognisance of the organisational, sociological and psychological factors that affect workplace practices impacting on worker health status. They are able to advise and work with management, employees and their representatives towards ensuring a safe and a health-promoting workplace. OHNs are well placed to influence the health of the community as the workplace provides a captive audience for interventions, which further promote health amongst a group of well adults who are often otherwise difficult to access. The workplace offers the potential for improving the health of the nation, albeit the health of those who are employed. The workplace facilitates ease of access to a large group of workers, and there are established communication channels facilitating the exchange of health-related information. Significant health gain ban be facilitated by an enthusiastic and proactive OH team.

Unfortunately, financial and organisational constraints mean that not all OH departments are able to offer a full OH service. Some OH departments offer a very limited service with an emphasis on attendance management – sadly, this is a lost opportunity and reflects a service which has been unable to move forward. By contrast other services have a much more proactive and holistic approach more closely aligned to a broader public health agenda. Such proactive services provide very much a preventative role integrating the skills of risk and health assessment. Many OHNs are highly experienced in formulating return to work recovery programmes for employees who have been absent from work as the result of accidents or following serious ill health.

The discussion so far has indicated that OHNs are specialist practitioners aware of the effect of work on health and health on work and are able to work with both individuals and groups to improve health. Their advice to all concerned aims to minimise any adverse effects of work on health and assist in reducing accidents. Most OHNs undertake health and risk management to achieve this aim, whilst experienced and more senior OHNs operate at a more strategic level contributing to policy formation and professional leadership in the organisations in which they work.

The domains of OH nursing practice

OHNs face challenges and practise in a way that differs from that undertaken by nurses employed in other community or hospital settings. Although their practice has a different emphasis, OHNs bring with them the values and beliefs developed as a result of having initially qualified as general or mental health nurses. Much, but not all, of what OHNs undertake as part of their practice would be unrecognisable to many other nurses as 'nursing skills', and their role will now be explored.

The role of the OHN incorporates a number of domains including professional, managerial, environmental and educational spheres. How these are applied depends on the OHN's area of practice and the needs of their employing organisation, but there are certain commonalities.

The professional domain

The professional domain is very broad and encompasses the 'nitty-gritty' of practice as nurses in the workplace setting. They must be able to work within the requirements of both legislation and the NMC professional code of conduct. This is often challenging as many of the people with whom OHNs work including managers and human resource professionals do not fully appreciate the implications of their professional code of conduct particularly in relation to client confidentiality.

OHNs have the potential to undertake an important role in research and epidemiology – identifying work-related health issues. They use their nursing skills in the assessment of health in a range of activities including pre-employment health assessments to ensure that prospective employees are fit to take on the requirements of their proposed job. They are involved in providing ongoing health surveillance for workers exposed to workplace hazards such as work involving exposure to a vast array of hazardous chemicals including isocyanates, chrome, lead and solvents. Chemicals used in the workplace can have numerous pathophysiological effects of which the OHN should be aware. They have the potential to impact on a number of organs and body systems including organs such as the skin, liver, and kidneys and the respiratory, reproductive, haematopoietic and central nervous systems. Health surveillance provides an opportunity to identify early changes linked to such exposure in order to identify people at risk.

The focus on promoting health, reducing the number of people on incapacity benefit and effective vocational rehabilitation is central to Dame Carol Black's review of the health of Britain's working population (Department for Work and Pensions 2008). This report emphasises the importance of vocational rehabilitation and multi-disciplinary working. The report highlights the links between health and employment and their effects on productivity. The promotion of health and well-being benefits all as it raises employability and reduces worklessness. These in turn assist in achieving greater social justice, promoting economic growth and reducing poverty, benefiting the individual and the community alike. OHNs are well placed to take a strategic role in this strategy.

The costs of sickness absence are a significant drain on the profitability of many organisations. Over the past few decades, OHNs have increasingly been undertaking a role in attendance management. However, it is essential that they clarify their role to ensure that there is no conflict between maintaining an impartial role as employee

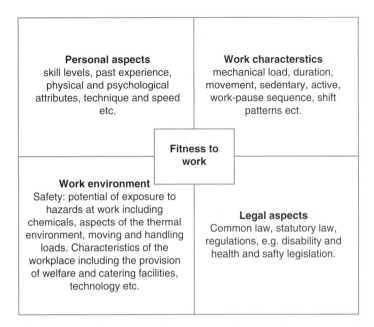

Figure 11.1   The fitness to work framework of assessment. (Source: Murugiah *et al*. 2002. Reproduced with permission.)

advocate and acting as an advisor to management. Part of their contribution to attendance management strategies put in place by organisations is the undertaking of health assessments for employees following periods of repeated short-term or one episode of long-term absence prior to their return to work. This offers an ideal opportunity to identify whether a health problem is caused, or exacerbated, by job requirements. The OHN is then able to devise recovery programmes facilitating a successful and productive return to work, a benefit to all concerned.

It is appropriate that the OHN is asked for an opinion on the health of employees with a tendency to repeated short-term absences as well as those who have had a period of long-term absence, whether or not these are work related. The trigger for an automatic OH review is advisable following a period of long-term sickness absence of, perhaps, three weeks' duration or following a reportable workplace accident as this offers the opportunity to decide whether the person is now fit enough to carry out the full requirements of their job or whether a phased return to work programme should be negotiated with both the client and their manager.

A competent assessment of a worker's fitness to return to work involves consideration of the extent of fitness or any degree of impairment and current health status in the light of their job demands. A skilled and competent assessment requires consideration of aspects of the individual, their job and the hazards to which they may be exposed at work, each considered in the light of a range of legal requirements. These requirements are incorporated into the Murugiah *et al.* (2002) health assessment model: fitness to work (Fig. 11.1). This model, developed by three practising OHN educators, was formulated specifically for use in the OH setting and assists in the decision-making process regarding whether a worker who had previously experienced a significant health deficit is fit to return to work perhaps on a graded return to work recovery programme as part of a vocational rehabilitation strategy. Their return to work may, in the short term, be on modified duties, but the aim is to return them to duties compatible with their ongoing abilities and health status (Murugiah *et al.* 2002).

There are occasions when a return to work following serious illness or injury would be difficult without modifications being made to the work process and/or the equipment used at work. The Equality Act 2010 requires employers to make such reasonable adjustments for people who are disabled, as defined by the Act. In order to do so, they need access to competent and professional advice. The specialist OHN is well placed to do this as they have knowledge of health and illness and the requirements of the worker's job coupled with an understanding of both employment and health and safety legislation. They are able to integrate clinical and problem-solving skills with other expertise such as the skills of risk assessment, problem-solving and multidisciplinary team working.

In order to facilitate a successful return to work programme, it may be necessary for the OHN to make effective links with a range of practitioners including medical practitioners and those who work in the allied health professions such as occupational and physiotherapists and disability advisers. This facilitates them giving the best possible advice to both worker and manager. Although an employee may be fit to undertake work of some type, a multitude of factors, not least continuing health problems, may preclude them from returning to their previous post. Unfortunately under such circumstances, redeployment may be the only option. Occasionally even redeployment is not possible owing to the nature, severity or circumstances of their health status, and the person chooses to retire from work on the grounds of ill health seeing this as a positive step. The OHN can give valuable advice and support at this time.

Senior OHNs manage and lead multidisciplinary teams, a role previously only assigned to a physician. The managerial domain of OHN practice incorporates policy development. The range of health-related policies an organisation may need to formulate is very broad and reflects the type of work they undertake. Some of these include those covering home working, work with computers, moving and handling of loads, food hygiene, waste management and working with chemical and microbiological hazards. OHNs also contribute to the formulation of policies focused on human resources including attendance management policies and strategies as already discussed.

Increasingly many OH services outsource their services; this is particularly the case since the advent of NHS Plus that has facilitated services initially set up for NHS establishments offering their services to businesses leading to valuable income generation. This process must be well managed if it is to be successful. There are commonalities with managing any OH service as both require significant leadership and business acumen. Outsourcing involves the setting and negotiation of service level agreements, effective budgeting and procurement of human and other resources. The final part of the process is the effective management of both these contracts and the staff required to service them.

The environmental domain

The environmental domain is perhaps the aspect that is least recognisable to a 'generalist' as 'nursing care'. This can be the most challenging owing to the range of skills required in order to perform it with any degree of competence. An in-depth understanding of health and safety and employment legislation is therefore required. Particularly pertinent is an appreciation of the requirements of the myriad of regulations covering both health and safety and disability, much of which results from the United Kingdom being part of the European Union. In 1992 six regulations under the Health and Safety at Work Act 1974 became law. These regulations are generally known as the 'six-pack'. A recurring theme is the need for both risk and health assessments. All employers are required to undertake a general risk assessment, supplemented with health surveillance, for people exposed to hazards that have an identifiable adverse effect on their health such as exposure to respiratory or skin sensitising agents. In addition to the need for a general risk assessment, further risk assessments are included within the 'six-pack' for workers who use computers or who manually handle loads or patients. OHNs are considered competent to undertake, or teach others to undertake, such risk assessments. They are able to contribute to the evaluation of control measures such as local exhaust ventilation extracting chemicals in work areas including laboratories or car spraying booths.

Many people work in industries that are intrinsically noisy. OHNs who practise in such industries are well placed to undertake a risk assessment to identify if employees are at risk, measure noise levels, comment on current exposure and suggest ways of reducing exposure by putting in place engineering or other controls. They are also able to comment on the suitability of personal protective equipment such as ear defenders including in-ear devices and ear muffs. They can interpret legislation covering noise in the workplace and decide which employees could be at risk of developing noise-induced hearing loss. Under such circumstances they undertake audiometry in order to detect its very early signs, enabling protective strategies to be instigated as a matter of urgency.

The educational domain of practice

The educational domain interlinks with the environmental domain previously discussed. It involves the OHN in teaching managers and workers on a range of issues as part of workplace health promotion. This is complementary to, but often different from, the health promotion interventions undertaken by nurses outside the OH setting. An example of such an activity is raising awareness of workplace hazards with managers and 'shop floor' staff and being involved in developing strategies and policies to prevent exposure. This may, for example, involve developing and presenting a health education package teaching people who work with hazardous chemicals how they can protect themselves from exposure. This may include highlighting safe and unsafe working practices during the storage, use and disposal of hazardous material and protective mechanisms including local exhaust ventilation and finally advising on the suitability of personal protective equipment. This is a health promotion activity but not as most nurses would recognise it.

Public health strategies

OHNs can influence the health of the community and as such they are public health nurses, and it is appropriate that those who hold a qualification in OH nursing are eligible to register as SCPHNs. Having discussed the domains of their practice, the contribution they are able to make to the Government's public health strategy will now be briefly explored. The end of the twentieth and start of the twenty-first century saw the publication of a number of public health documents including *Saving Lives: Our Healthier Nation* (DH 1999), *Revitalising Health and Safety* (Department of the Environment, Transport and the Regions 2000), and the Occupational Health Advisory Committee report on improving access to occupational health support (Health and Safety Commission 2000). These publications acknowledged the extent and costs of work-related ill health and recognised the potential for the workplace to become a platform to achieve the Government's overall aim of reducing accidents and improving the health of the population. They have influenced the practice of OHNs by engaging them in public health agendas and are essential if they are to meet the aims of the ILO and WHO already highlighted earlier in this chapter. The Department of Health in association with the RCN and Association of Occupational Health Nurse Practitioners has underlined the contribution of OHNs to public health in their document *Taking a Public Health Approach in the Workplace* (DH 2003). This guide states, 'Occupational health nurses are a key part of the public health workforce. Changing health needs, increasing public expectations and new government policies make this role more important than ever before'. It acknowledges the contribution that OHNs may make in reducing health inequalities and improving physical and mental health of the community through workplace interventions. Thornbory (2004) refers to the Health and Safety Commission's strategy for improving health and safety in Great Britain to 2010 and beyond whereby 'occupational health is acknowledged as a rising challenge now that "causes of safety failure" have been brought under some sort of control' (Health and Safety Commission 2004).

Specialist community public health nursing: Part 3 of the register maintained by the NMC

So what will the future hold for OH nursing? The year 2004 saw the NMC opening a new three-part register incorporating the 15-part register previously maintained by the United Kingdom Central Council for Nursing, Midwifery and Health Visiting (UKCC).

Incorporated within the register is one part specifically for SCPHNs. There is no direct access for those not already registered with the NMC. Health visitors along with those school and occupational health nurses holding appropriate qualifications are eligible to registration on this part of the register. The NMC have demonstrated their commitment to the public health agenda by supporting a new qualification for qualified nurses leading to additional registration on this part of the register. The NMC had debated whether the SCPHN qualification should be of a generic nature covering all aspects of specialist community public health nursing. This concept was rejected as it was quite rightly decided that it would be very difficult to ensure that graduates from such a programme would be 'fit for practice' across the whole field of public health nursing.

Previously, qualifications in OH nursing were recordable, but in contrast to the position with health visitors, such a qualification did not lead to registration of the holders on a special part of the register. The establishment of a part of the register for public health nurses, which includes OHNs, recognised their contribution to the public health agenda. In the view of many practitioners, a registrable qualification for OHNs is essential to ensure public protection. There may be implications for nurses who are practising in the OH setting without such a specialist practitioner qualification. However, validating a qualification leading to registration on a separate part of the nursing register was a significant move but not without controversy. There has been considerable debate regarding whether a separate part of the register for SCPHNs should continue, and the NMC are in the process of reviewing the structure, standards and proficiencies associated with this part of the register. Robust standards and the skill clusters required for effective and competent OHN practice and education within this review are paramount (Harriss 2011).

In conclusion, this chapter has presented to the reader an overview of the aim of OH services and the role of the OHN as a specialist practitioner within them. The context of their practice and historical perspective has been explored with particular reference to their contribution to public health initiatives. The OHN can directly influence the health, health and safety, and productivity of the workforce. They therefore make a contribution to promoting the health of the nation as a whole. It is an excellent career choice for nurses who enjoy a high degree of autonomy working with a predominantly well population.

References

Department for Work and Pensions (2008) *Working for a Healthier Tomorrow*, Stationery Office, London.

Department of Health (DH) (1998) *Report of the independent inquiry into the inequalities in health*, DH, London.

DH (1999) *Saving Lives: Our Healthier Nation*, DH, London.

DH (2003) *Taking a Public Health Approach in the Workplace*, DH, London.

Department of the Environment, Transport and the Regions (2000) *Revitalising Health and Safety: Strategy Statement*, The Stationery Office, London.

HM Government (2005) *Health, Work and Wellbeing – Caring for Our Future*, Department of Work and Pensions, London.

Harriss, A. (2011) Time to revamp degrees. *Occupational Health*, **63** (4), 18–20.

Health and Safety Commission (2000) *Occupational Health Advisory Committee: Report and Recommendation on Improving Access to Occupational Health Support*, The Stationery Office, London.

Health and Safety Commission (2004) *A strategy for Workplace Health and Safety in Great Britain to 2010 and Beyond*, The Stationery Office, London.

Health and Safety Executive (1995) *Good Health is Good Business: An Introduction to Managing Health Risks at Work*. HSE, London.

Health and Safety Executive (2005) *Hand-Arm Vibration: The Control of Vibration at Work Regulations 2005 Guidance on Regulations*, HSE Books, Norwich.

Health and Safety Executive (2011) *Health and Safety Executive Annual Statistics Report 2010/2011*. Available from http://www.hse.gov.uk/statistics/overall/hssh1011.pdf. Accessed on 14 June 2012.

Hillage, J., with others including Davidson, J., Irvine, I., Sainsbury, R. & Weston, K. (2012) *Evaluation of the fit for work service pilots: first year report – research report No. 792*. Department for Work and Pensions, London.

International Labour Organisation (ILO) (1959) *International Labour Organisation Occupational Services Recommendation No. 112*. International Labour Organisation, Geneva.

Lewis, J. & Thornbory, G. (2006) *Employment Law and Occupational Health a Practical Handbook*, Blackwell Publishing, Oxford.

Maltby, M. (2005) *Occupational Audiometry*, Butterworth-Heineman, Oxford.

Manos, J. & Silcox, S. (2007) Health, work and wellbeing: the occupational contribution. *Occupational Health Review*, **127** (May/June), 17–18.

Marmot, M. (2005) *Status Syndrome*, Bloomsbury Publishing, London.

Murugiah, S., Thornbory, G. & Harriss, A. (2002) Assessment of fitness. *Occupational Health*, 54 (4), 26–29.

Parliament (2012) *Health and Social Care Act, c.7.*, London.

Paton, N. (2012) OH is best fit for staff attendance. *Occupational Health*, 64 (1), 16–18.

Royal College of Nursing (2011) *Occupational Health Nursing: Career and Competence Development*, RCN, London.

Smedley, J., Dick, F. & Sadhra, S. (eds) (2007) *Oxford Handbook of Occupational Health*. Oxford Medical Publications, Oxford.

Thornbory, G. (2004) In with the new. *Occupational Health*, 56 (6), 20–21.

Waddell, G. & Burton, K. (2006) *Is Work Good for Your Health and Wellbeing?* The Stationery Office, Norwich.

Wilkinson, R. & Pickett, K. (2010) *The Spirit Level*, Penguin Books, London.

World Health Organization (WHO) (1973) *Environmental and health monitoring in occupational health. Report of a WHO Expert Committee. Technical Report Series 535*. World Health Organization, Geneva.

12

Caring for the Person with Mental Health Needs in the Community

Peter Sandy and Margaret Rioga

Faculty of Society and Health, Buckinghamshire New University, High Wycombe, UK

Introduction

It is fitting to commence this chapter with a brief discussion of the labels service users are ascribed and the impact of these on care provision. Terms such as depression, schizophrenia, psychosis and anxiety, frequently used in clinical practice, are the chains that fetter service users to mental health systems as well as sustain stigma and discrimination. These labels do not only serve as deterrent for developing better understanding of service users, but they may also distract healthcare professionals from providing individualised and compassionate care (Sandy & Shaw 2012). Added to this, they may make it difficult for service users to recover a place for themselves in society. In acknowledging this, the term 'mental distress' is used throughout this chapter to refer to service users who access mental health services. This is a less stigmatising term that takes into account experiences of human suffering or distress that may disrupt people's lives and subsequently bring them into contact with mental health services.

This chapter discusses community mental health nursing within a recovery framework. The authors used a case study to discuss the recovery 'journey' of a service user with a long history of mental distress. The notion of 'journey' is used here to illustrate the challenges the service user was confronted with and the changes achieved from the experience. It is an attempt to portray the fluidity of human existence and its associated

Community and Public Health Nursing, Fifth Edition. Edited by David Sines,
Sharon Aldridge-Bent, Agnes Fanning, Penny Farrelly, Kate Potter and Jane Wright.
© 2013 John Wiley & Sons, Ltd. Published 2013 by John Wiley & Sons, Ltd.

suffering and joy, alienation and connectedness, meaning and confusion people may experience. The chapter also focuses on the roles of CMHNs in facilitating the service user's recovery. To increase understanding of the service user's experience of the recovery process, key principles of a recovery approach to community mental health nursing are included in the discussion.

Background: Why bother with community mental health nursing?

The past six decades witnessed significant changes in the settings and manner in which service users with mental distress are cared for. Prior to the 1960s, most of the care offered to service users with mental distress in the United Kingdom and other parts of the world, such as Australia, the USA and the Netherlands, took place in institutional settings (Pols 2006). Service users' experiences of institutional care were generally negative. It is reported in the literature that care provision in institution may lead to apathy and passive dependence, which, additively, may hinder service users from resuming active roles in their communities (Ryan 2003). Such an impact has been noted with alarm by observers like Goffman (1987) and mental healthcare professionals in the United Kingdom who increasingly perceive institutional care damaging and unhelpful (Fletcher 2003). Recognition of the unhelpful nature of institutional care resulted in the introduction of care in the community policies in the 1980s, which subsequently triggered the closure of large psychiatric hospitals and their replacement with community-based services (Simmonds *et al.* 2001). This shift in focus of care was also a function of the view that people are more likely to receive quality care if they remained in the communities they are familiar with (Nolan 1992). It is therefore not surprising to note an increase in community services to support people with mental distress. In fact, most of the care of this user group now takes place in community settings, with community mental health nurses (CMHNs) being the main care providers (Healthcare Commission 2005).

Service users in the community have a wide range of needs, which may include social, vocational, educational, spiritual and residential. The primary goal of CMHNs is to enable service users to meet these diverse needs (Fletcher 2003). Working with service users to meet these needs requires diverse roles for CMHNs and a re-conceptualisation of how services should be organised and delivered. In relation to the latter, CMHNs are required today to adopt a recovery approach in mental health practice. In essence, this is an emphasis on the need for partnership and collaborative working between people with mental distress and CMHNs and for the former to be considered competent and capable persons who can live independently, maintain meaningful relationships, work and contribute to their communities.

Historically, community mental health nursing has been affected by negative media reports, which, in the main, relate to service users not being adequately supported. High-profile cases such as those of Christopher Clunis and Sharon Campbell have been used to highlight this (Coid 1994; HMSO 1994; Southill 1999). The negative publicity resulted in community mental health teams (CMHTs) placing more emphasis on risk assessment and management. CMHTs comprise social workers, occupational therapists, vocational workers, medical practitioners and CMHNs. CMHNs, generally described as 'gatekeepers', play an active role within CMHTs in ensuring the safety of the public as well as service users' prompt, timely assessments and access to appropriate therapeutic services. This 'gatekeeper' approach to care can contribute significantly to the support offered to service users, which might halt the development of severe mental distress and prevent hospitalisation.

Clinical profile: John

John is a 48-year-old man diagnosed with schizophrenia and substance dependence. He lives in the community in a 24-hour supervised hostel. He has lived in this accommodation for nearly 5 years. Recently, he asked his allocated care co-ordinator CMHN for a possible move to a bedsit. John has an extensive history of contact with mental health services, which started at the age of 16. Contact with his family is limited to frequent visits by his mother and occasional telephone calls from a childhood friend who lives many miles away from John's hostel. John is on antipsychotic oral medication, specifically olanzapine, but now on a weekly antipsychotic depot injection, fluphenazine decanoate, because of problems with medication adherence. The injection is usually administered every Wednesday morning by his care co-ordinator at a Community Mental Health Resource Centre (CMHRC). John hears voices, which he describes as tormenting. He also experiences periods of severe paranoia that include beliefs that people around him are planning to kill him. He thus spends most of his time alone in his hostel room, sometimes listening to music. He has expressed feelings of hopelessness and helplessness to his CMHN during some periods of severe experiences of paranoia, for example, in his words, 'my neighbours are aggressively following me, they want to kill me'. John has never worked and his personal hygiene is generally considered to be poor. John's CMHN and treatment team usually experience feelings of hopelessness as he continues to misuse substances and frequently fails to attend his therapeutic activities despite encouragement to do so. However, a change in treatment philosophy, adoption of a recovery-orientated approach by the CMHN and treatment team, have resulted in improvement in John's adherence to his therapeutic programme.

Recovery: Conceptual explanation

Recovery is one of the most commonly used terms in today's mental health services. It is acknowledged by service users and healthcare professionals to mean different things to different people. Watkins (2001) refers to recovery as an act of regaining self-confidence and control over one's life. Others consider it to be personal growth, a transition from lives devastated by chronic mental distress to gratifying and meaningful lives (Roe *et al.* 2004; Kelly & Gamble 2005). Although such transitions can be a lengthy and painful process, it is a journey that is recommended by service users of the authors' clinical settings because it enriches their connections with others and offers new meaning and purpose in life beyond their illness.

Noordsy *et al.* (2002) proffer a comprehensive definition of recovery. It is about being hopeful, taking personal responsibility and growing beyond the demands of their distress. Implicit in this definition is the view that recovery is not about 'cure' of mental distress, but it is about the reclaiming of personhood, roles and responsibilities, self-knowledge and people's acceptance of the limitations of their illness. Apparently, this is the case for many people as they live satisfying and contributing lives whilst still experiencing cognitive difficulties, hallucinations and other symptoms of their distress (Woodside *et al.* 2007). An 'expert by experience', Deegan (1993), supports this view:

Being in recovery means I know I have certain limitations and things I can't do. But rather than letting these limitations be an occasion for despair and giving up, I have learned that in knowing what I can't do, I also open up the possibilities of all I can do.

Anthony (1993), another 'expert by experience', offers a similar meaning of recovery:

It is a deeply personal, unique process of changing one's attitudes, values, feelings, goals, skills and roles. It is a way of living a satisfying, hopeful and contributing life, even with the limitations caused by illness.

The definitions thus far indicate that recovery is a complex personal process of discovery of new ways of living with mental distress that is unique to the individuals who embark on it. From a service user's perspective, the identification of new ways of living or recovery can be possible if individuals attribute personal meanings to their distress and explore ways of minimising the restrictions caused by these (Deegan 1993). In the authors' opinion, this can be achieved through an intrapersonal dialogue that is not based on pathology. Such an approach allows individuals to focus less on their distress and to think about constructive ways of giving their lives meaning. However, engaging in an intrapersonal dialogue requires courage, will and hopefulness, as people may recall challenges such as past abuses, and losses that may have negatively affected their lives (Noordsy *et al.* 2002). This intrapersonal nature of recovery suggests that it is a dynamic and ongoing process experienced by all human beings.

As humans, we all have embarked on a journey of recovery, for instance, from physical illnesses, losses, trauma and financial crisis to ultimate solutions to, or 'ways out of', these problems. The phrases 'solutions to' and 'ways out of' indicate 'stuckness', a critical stage of the recovery process (Woodside *et al.* 2007). In essence, 'stuckness' relates to stages in people's lived experiences when they are unable to grow or change because of their exposure to bewildering and overwhelming periods of distress. For Young and Ensing (1999), recovery starts with overcoming 'stuckness'. In other words, recovery is about empowering people to step out of 'stuckness' and face the opportunities and responsibilities of life. Thus, one of the focuses of recovery work is on enabling people to free themselves from the negative impact or trauma of their distress. Certainly, this requires some degree of planning. Arguably, recovery is an organising construct that can guide the planning and implementation of mental health services for people living with mental distress, including those in our communities. Responding to the needs and wants of service users in community settings requires CMHNs to adopt specific roles and responsibilities.

Development of therapeutic relationship

Mental health nursing is essentially an 'interactive activity' between service users and nurses with the ultimate aim of understanding and addressing the holistic needs of the latter. In essence, holistic needs include all aspects of a person, including his or her genetic make-up, lived experiences and social networks (Swinton 2001). It is critical to state that service users' experiences of mental distress and how they cope with it are influenced by the interplay between their holistic needs (Seedhouse 2000). These needs will often emerge within the framework of a therapeutic relationship, an important, if not the most important, aspect of working with people with mental distress.

A therapeutic relationship is a planned and goal-directed interactional process between a healthcare professional and a service user for the purpose of caring for the latter (Louise 2008). It is the needs of service users and nurses' commitment and willingness to work with the latter that form the basis of therapeutic relationships. One of the fundamental functions of CMHNs is to develop and maintain a therapeutic alliance or relationship with service users, which Louise (2008) claims should be underpinned by the principles of empowerment. In practice, this involves mental health nurses engaging with service users in a positive, respectful and collaborative manner, a view also acknowledged by some theorist in mental health nursing like Barker and Reynolds (1994) who state that

> The focus of mental health nursing is located in the careful examination of the whole lived experience of service users in care. This examination demands an active, collaborative relationship between nurses and service users.

It is evident from Barker and Reynolds (1994) assertion that caring for people with mental distress demands an intensified presence with a strong intention and commitment to be supportive and demonstrate understanding. Such a presence or 'involvedness' is particularly required in instances where service users experience difficulties with verbally expressing their needs. This case study illustrates how being present can enable service users to trust healthcare professionals and disclose issues they never talked about. The consistent and regular physical presence (visits) of the CMHN, which demonstrates willingness and readiness to listen and offer support, made John to talk about his desire to reunite with his son who he has not seen for over 7 years. Acknowledging this, it is safe to state that the presence of a professional who is able to express empathy and demonstrate acceptance and positive regard can mark a turning point for service users in their recovery journey. For John, the disclosure serves as personal power, which enhances his self-efficacy and led him to openly discuss his needs and difficulties in subsequent meetings with the CMHN. The disclosure helped the CMHN to gain some understanding of John's needs as well as strengthening the nurse–service user relationship. John's ability to engage in open discussions about his difficulties is a function of him feeling valued, respected, empowered and accepted as an individual by the CMHN. Schafer and Paternelj-Taylor (2003) agree with this by stating that seeing people as individuals with lives beyond their distress is imperative in making them feel accepted and empowered.

Empowerment is a significant factor for service users' recovery and the development of therapeutic relationships. Ahern and Fisher (2001) argue that the healing of mental distress is generally more effective in an empowerment culture than in the expert-centred culture of mental health systems. The question now arises, what is an empowerment culture? It is a therapeutic relationship that emphasises people's worth and capacity to live through distress and to learn and grow from their experiences (Adern & Fisher 2001). It is also perceived as a therapeutic relationship in which the subjective experience of the person seeking help is validated and where mutual respect and equality are fostered. Taking this into account, successful therapeutic relationships can only be established if service users and mental health professionals assume the role of team members or facilitators of the relationship rather than as leaders. The CMHN met with John on a number of occasions, and most of these meetings took place in cafes not too far from John's residence. The discussions during these meetings mainly centred on activities, such as listening to music, liked by both John and his CMHN. Participating in activities that do not make one person more dominant over the other, such as talking about mutual interest, can strengthen both therapeutic relationships and levels of equality shared between service users and CMHNs. In addition to this, being available to spend uninterrupted time with service users will make them open up and disclose personal issues that will enable mental health professionals to develop better understanding of service users' presentations and the meanings behind their narratives (Berg & Hallberg 2000). Arguably, a therapeutic relationship provides an essential interpersonal climate for nursing assessment.

Assessment of needs

All humans, particularly those with mental distress, have a wide range of unique and invisible personal experiences that are sometimes manifested through behavioural disturbances, such as aggression and isolation. Examples of these unique experiences, which are frequently consequences of mental distress, include traumas and losses. Mental health nurses cannot offer quality nursing care without effective assessment of service users' unique and invisible experiences. Thus, one of the core functions of mental health nurses is to work with service users to access and review their experiences and to enable them to adapt to their distress and problems associated with it. Nursing assessment is therefore not a unilateral process, but one that involves 'assessing with' rather than 'assessing the' service users. This collaborative approach to assessment is consistent with some of the key tenets of mental health recovery: the need to respect, value and accept people's individuality. Adopting these principles in the assessment process would enable service users to become responsible and resourceful individuals, able to influence the direction of their unfolding lives.

John actively participated in the assessment process. He led most of the discussions particularly those that relate to his experiences of traumas and loses. The CMHN perceived John as an expert of his experiences and was therefore encouraged to freely talk about his mental distress, including its associated meanings and impact. It is a well-established fact that repeated exposure to multiple traumas can have a devastating impact on the lives of people who experience them (LaFond 2002). For example, people may be left disconnected from themselves, others, their environment and purpose of life (McDonald 2005). For John, his distress, stigma and discrimination from people in his community caused him to feel disconnected from himself and society. John's feelings of disconnectedness were associated with a range of loses or needs, which were discussed concurrently with the roles of the CMHN and CMHT in healing the emotional wounds inflicted by his loss experiences.

Instilling hope

Loss of hope is a common feature of service users with mental distress (Noordsy *et al.* 2002). This is particularly the case where people are exposed to mental health services with little or no influence over the care they are offered. Service users with such exposure may, over a protracted period of time, acquire an attitude of learned helplessness that may involve doing nothing or doing something with no clear sense of direction or uncritically accepting requests or solutions suggested by others. Service users generally find the experiences of being and feeling controlled insulting and devaluing, and such feelings may lead to the giving up of hope (Sandy & Shaw 2012). Hopelessness and apathy can be seen as strategies service users employ to cope with the imbalance of power in mental health services. From experience, mental health services are very good at developing and reinforcing learned helplessness, usually associated with feelings of hopelessness, but they are generally poor at enhancing people's resourcefulness and self-efficacy. Thus, the task of CMHNs is to develop service users' self-efficacy, which, from a practical point view, can be achieved through setting realistic and achievable targets, focusing on strengths rather than weaknesses and maintaining a hopeful attitude.

John frequently expressed feelings of hopelessness, which were mainly centred on him not being able to gain employment despite numerous attempts to do so. Hope for people with mental distress usually comes from mental health professionals. However, Deegan (1996) warns that restoring hope for a person who has given up hope to protect himself or herself from potential additional experiences of trauma (like John) is a risky task to undertake. This is because individuals with these experiences may express anger and attempt to sabotage professionals' efforts to offer help. But because having a hopeful attitude would enable someone to believe in himself or herself, restoring hope is a task worth undertaking. This is because being hopeful serves as a 'secure base' from which people grow and discover new meaning and purpose in life (Bowlby 1988).

The CMHN discussed the issue of employment on a number of occasions both in person and on the telephone. It became apparent during the discussions that John would like to become a chef but lacked the necessary skills and knowledge for this responsibility. As a result, with the support of his CMHN, John decided to do a college course on catering, which he commenced, successfully completed and subsequently gained employment as a chef in an Italian restaurant. When persons with mental distress do find and keep employment, research indicates that they experience a decrease in symptoms, an increase in self-efficacy and self-esteem and improved integration into their communities (Kirsh 2000; Woodside *et al.* 2007). This was also the case for John, who on a number of occasions stated that he highly valued his work roles. Added to this, he claimed that his work role served as a distraction from the worries and anxieties about his son.

Promoting life beyond distress

Encouraging service users to engage in activities beyond their mental distress is a significant professional attitude for promoting recovery. Engagement in meaningful valued life roles, such as husband, father, mother, son, daughter and church member, is one of the activities considered by the authors to be critical for service users' recovery process. This is because service users with living mental distress are often assumed to be incapable of fulfilling these roles. Such assumptions, particularly when expressed by mental health professionals, frequently result in service users feeling devalued and pessimistic about their ability to perform these roles and to contribute meaningfully to their communities. It is evident in the literature that engagement in valued roles would enable people living with mental distress to perceive themselves as useful members of their communities (Noordsy *et al.* 2002), which in turn would protect them, at least temporarily, from the negative effects of their illness.

John frequently described deep feelings of frustration at not being able to have access to his son and made several requests for his CMHN to help in gaining visitation rights. The CMHN, with the help of other members of CMHT, collaborated with John to establish his capacity to parent. It was noted that John has a history of neglect and physical abuse towards his son when under the influence of cocaine and alcohol. John was aware that these substances, which were risk factors of physical abuse, would deter the prospect of him gaining access to his son. With his approval, John was referred to a drug and alcohol team for help with his substance misuse problem. Consequently, John ceased substance use and access to his son was arranged. The need for privacy was critical for John, especially during his son's visits. He frequently reiterated that this could be met if he was offered a suitable accommodation. For John, a bedsit would be suitable accommodation. Thus, his request to be moved to a bedsit was addressed by his CMHT to help him enhance relationship with his son and to connect with other family members.

Promoting connectedness

Finding the motivation to rebuild relationships or connections can be a difficult task for service users with mental distress who may also be taking psychotropic medication. Such difficulty is a function of disinterest and anhedonia (inability to express pleasure or emotions) caused by their distress and experiences of stigma and discrimination associated with the same (Davidson *et al.* 1998). Disconnectedness can therefore be seen as a strategy that service users employ to cope with these difficulties. It is a commonly held belief that encouraging people to deeply reflect on their life experiences will enable them to reveal meaning and purpose in their lives that may motivate them to engage in activities of their interest (Langdridge 2007). Arguably, motivation should not just be perceived as an outcome of the intrapersonal process, but it should also be considered as a product of interpersonal engagement (Miller & Rollnick 2002). Engagement in activities of interests can provide a stable foundation for re-establishing and/or building connections.

John liked listening to music and playing guitar. The CMHN expressed an interest in John's musical talent when he first saw him play his guitar. As a result, John played his guitar during every home visit and recorded tapes that were made available for members of the CMHT to listen to. The CMHN consistently acknowledged John's musical talent. The consistent praise offered eventually motivated John to share his experiences playing with professional musicians in his community. Connecting with professional musicians strengthened John's sense of self-worth, as the experience enabled him to perceive himself as a valuable and respected member of his community. The quality of his music improved with improvement in his mental state. Consequently, John realised the need to actively participate in his treatment programme.

Promoting personal responsibility

Taking personal responsibility for health and well-being may follow or precede service users' development of connectedness and engagement in meaningful and valued roles. From a clinical practice point of view, embracing responsibility for one's actions is usually associated with progress in service users' recovery journey, a view also acknowledged by Mead and Copeland (2000). Hence, a critical function of CMHNs is to enable service users to assume responsibility for their health and wellness. But it must be taken into account that service users may experience extreme difficulty with regaining autonomy and, in other words, take responsibility for their lives after many years of being entrapped in a dependent role. So, mental health professionals need to be easily accessible to offer support when allowing service users to exercise their judgement, determine their own priorities and meet their needs. They should also be optimistic about service users' capacity to grow and change. Adopting these approaches would enable service users to recognise and trust both their own inner strengths and resourcefulness. Podvoll (2003) considers such realisation as essential ingredients that would make people to stop leaning on others and begin to take responsibility for their health and wellness.

One of the key issues that was frequently discussed between John and his CMHN relates to medication adherence. John disclosed to his CMHN that he dislikes taking oral medication. As a result, he was not consistently taking his medication. He attributed his experiences of paranoia and auditory hallucinations to the difficulty with medication adherence. Deegan (1996) claims that acceptance for service users living with mental illness generally indicates their ability and need to find solutions to their difficulties. It is certainly an acknowledgment of their capacity to assume responsibility for their lives. On the basis of these assertions, the CMHT works collaboratively with John on the issue of medication adherence. To improve this, he suggested to his CMHN that his medication should be changed to a depot form, based on the belief that it would help alleviate both his hallucinatory and paranoid experiences, which in turn would enhance his connectedness and relationships with others and performance of valued roles.

Principles of community mental health nursing

CMHNs are the key professionals working with mental distress in the community. Thus, their roles and responsibilities for supporting services in their journey to recovery in these settings are critical. They have important roles to play in assisting service users to recover from the impact of multiple trauma and losses caused by mental distress. Following are a set of key principles that guide CMHNs in executing their supportive roles.

Examining experience with service users

Service users have a wide range of life experiences that are unique and constantly evolving. So, service users can be perceived as leading experts of their experiences that can be explored and understood. Because all experience is experience of something (Husserl 1970, 1982), mental health nursing is about trying to recognise and understand service users' 'whole experience' with the view of meeting their unique needs. This can be achieved if service users and nurses share their expertise. Thus, community mental health nursing is an 'inter-view-ing' or a 'learning together activity' that involves both service users and nurses examining the life experiences of the latter.

Linking experiences

People are inescapably social beings, as they always live in relation with others. This is what Heidegger (1962) accurately refers to as 'being-in-the-world-with-others'. This means that service users' experiences do not occur in isolation, but they always occur in relation to others. So, community mental health nursing is not just about examining service users' experiences (what is experienced) but also about developing and understanding of the mode of experiencing, in other words the manner in which something is experienced. This requires mental health nurses to explore the impact of service users' experiences on both themselves and others, including relatives and carers. Hence, the involvement of significant others in the care of service users should be an integral part of mental health nursing. They should be involved in the decision-making processes, which include planning, delivery and evaluation of care (DH 1999).

Acknowledging service users' wishes

The essence of the therapeutic relationship is referred to by Buber (1937, 1987) as the 'interhuman', which, as the term implies, is not owned by either the nurse or the service user, but exists between them. The underpinning assumption in Buber's philosophy of the interhuman is that to be human is to relate or interact with one another (Buber 1988; Slevin 1999). The practice of community mental health nursing is therefore located within the interhuman, and both service users and nurses have equal roles to play in this partnership. Community mental health nursing is therefore about co-partnership with service users to identify their needs, set specific goals, design and implement programmes to meet identified needs (DH 2006). To ensure effectiveness of this relationship, CMHNs need to respect service users' wishes.

Working together

Community mental health nursing recognises the diversity and breadth of the role of CMHNs who provide a proactive outreach service, which embraces a professional responsibility to seek out, challenge and influence public policy related to mental health. Whilst service users feel stigmatised and discriminated against by members of the public and even healthcare professionals, there is a growing belief that people with mental distress can be successfully integrated into the community if supported by community-based services (DH 2000). It must be stated that discrimination faced by service users with mental distress can be one of the most incapacitating aspects of their experiences. Therefore, challenging prejudicial attitudes should not only be an integral part of mental health promotion but should also be an activity for all healthcare professionals, including the Government, communities, service users and carers (DH 2001, 2006). Hence, the overall objective of CMHNs is to work with service users, their carers and communities to maximise overall mental health potential.

Therapeutic presence

Community mental health nursing in its uniqueness attributes precedence to the interpersonal, dynamic process of enabling individuals, families and nations to restore equilibrium between their internal and external worlds (Long & Chambers 1993). Communication, which is an important aspect of community mental health nursing, embraces the notions of giving and receiving, opening up, reflecting and responding. Working within a therapeutic encounter, communication also involves empathic being and having an ability to invite, 'stay with', contain and interpret service users' painful thoughts and emotions. Although these attributes would help service users to work through distressing experiences, nurses' unexplored and unresolved conflicts may render them unable to stay with and contain service users' painful thoughts and feelings. When this happens, a nurse's presence is no longer that of a catalyst for healing and recovery; rather, she/he becomes instead atherapeutic. Therefore, CMHNs require an understanding and awareness of their own therapeutic presence in order that they may be able to stay with and contain their service users' innermost thoughts, feelings and emotions. Otherwise, they may find it impossible to integrate their therapeutic presence into the nurse–service user relationship. Rogers (1961, p. 53) narrated:

> Recently I find that when I am closest to my inner intuitive self whatever I do seems to be full of healing, simply my presence is releasing and helpful.

Risk assessment and management

Risk is the chance of a target behaviour occurring, which, in the authors' views, can be influenced by the past. Thus, assessment of risk should be based on the past. This is not because of the relationship between the past and future behaviour but because the circumstances surrounding the past behaviour will provide useful insights to reduce the likelihood of its occurrence. Heidegger (1962), in his book, 'Being and Time', which focuses on individuals' experience of time, supports this assertion by stating that peoples' understanding of any event in the present always involves their past and projection of their future. Implicit in this statement is a call for all healthcare workers, irrespective of the settings they work in, to always engage in risk assessment with the view of predicting and preventing adverse events from occurring. Prevention is the key as neither practitioner nor service user wish to be on the giving or receiving end of serious harm. The role of CMHNs in this context is to safeguard the community and also identify and protect individuals 'at risk' from adverse events. It must be noted that it is extremely difficult, if not impossible, to eliminate all risks. As such, risk assessment aims mainly at minimising risk rather than eliminating it. Noting this, the concept itself is a misnomer, as it seems to suggest accurate prediction and risk elimination.

The area of prediction has garnered considerable empirical support over the years and is therefore considered to be essential to risk assessment. Because a person always lives with and influenced by others, an assessment of risk that the person may pose or expose to could lead to a range of possible outcomes. In summary, these may include inaccurate or accurate predictions. We therefore recommend risk assessment be continuous and routine throughout service users' care pathways. It is also critical to add that risk assessment is not about making accurate prediction, but it is about making informed, defensible decisions about behaviours. The management of risk, more accurately, its minimisation, should be influenced by these defensible decisions.

The most appropriate activity for risk minimisation is initiating and maintaining a safe and therapeutic relationship with the services that can be achieved, for example, through assertive outreach (Allen 1998; Morgan 1999). The provision of evidence-based psychosocial interventions together with collaborative approaches to medication management further enhances risk minimisation. Paradoxically, risk-taking is also an important part of risk assessment and management. Positive risk-taking means supporting service users to make and take decisions about their lives, to explore and test out their choices and to learn from the experience of 'failure' as this is what living is about. This suggests that CMHNs take positive risks when carrying out their role.

Conclusion

Mental health recovery has emerged as an important concept in the treatment of people living with mental distress in the community. This chapter has offered discussions of the role of CMHNs within a recovery framework using a case study. CMHNs are the main care providers in community-based services. They offer enormous support and care to communities, families and service users in their care. In doing so, they assume a wide range of roles to help them address the holistic of individuals and communities. Examples of these include developing therapeutic relationship, assessment of needs and promoting meaningful service user involvement. Some key issues that emerged from the CMHNs' roles are the need to empower service users and partnership working. Empowering service users not only promotes their recovery but also encourages their independence. So, the views and perceptions of service users are critical in community mental health nursing.

In addition to the roles of CMHNs, the chapter has discussed six important principles of community mental health nursing. Again, most of these principles emphasised the need for partnership with service users. In our view, it is the cornerstone of service users' recovery. CMHNs can learn a lot by working in partnership with service users. They can develop their skills and experiences whilst offering support to service users on their road to recovery. So, both service users and CMHNs can benefit from working together in partnership.

References

Ahern, I. & Fisher, D. (2001) Recovery at your own pace. *Journal of Psychosocial Nursing and Mental Health Services*, 39, 4.

Allen, D. (1998) *Mental Health and Nursing*. Sage, London.

Anthony, W.A. (1993) Recovery from mental illness: the guiding vision of the mental health system in the 1990s. *Psychosocial Rehabilitation Journal*, 16, 11–23.

Barker, P. & Reynolds, W. (1994) The proper focus of psychiatric nursing: a critique of Watson's caring ideology. *Journal of Psychosocial Nursing*, 22, 17–23.

Berg, A. & Hallberg, I.R. (2000) The psychiatric nurses lived experiences of working with inpatient care on a general team psychiatric ward. *Journal of Psychiatric and Mental Health Nursing*, 7, 323–333.

Bowlby, J. (1988) *A Secure Base; Clinical Application of Attachment Theory*. Tavistock/Routledge, London.

Buber, M. (1937) *I and Thou*. T & T Clark, Edinburgh.
Buber, M. (1987) *I and Thou*. Translated by Walter Kaufmann. Scribners, New York.
Buber, M. (1988) *Knowledge of Man: Selected Essays*. Humanities Press, Atlantic Highlands, New York.
Coid, J.W. (1994) The Christopher Clunis Enquiry. *Psychiatric Bulletin*, 18, 449–452.
Davidson, L., Stayner, D. & Haglund, K.E. (1998) Phenomenological perspectives on the social functioning of people with schizophrenia. In: *Handbook of Social Functioning in Schizophrenia* (eds K.T. Mueser & N. Tarrier). Allyn and Bacon, Boston.
Deegan, P.E. (1993) Recovering our sense of value after being labelled mentally ill. *Journal of Psychosocial Nursing*, 31, 7–11.
Deegan, P.E. (1996) Recovery as journey of the heart. *Psychiatric Rehabilitation Journal*, 19, 91–98.
Department of Health (DH) (1999) *National Service Framework for Mental Health: Modern Standards and Service Models*. DH, London.
DH (2000) *The NHS Plan: A Plan for Investment, a Plan for Reform*. DH, London.
DH (2001) *Making It Happen: A Guide to Delivering Mental Health Promotion*. DH, London.
DH (2006) *From Value to Action. The Chief Nursing Officer's Review of Mental Health Nursing*. DH, London.
Fletcher, F. (2003) *Mental Health Nursing*, 5th edn. Prentice Hall, Upper Saddle River, NJ.
Goffman, E. (1987) *Asylums: Essays on the Social Situation of Mental Patients and Other Inmates*. Penguin, London.
Healthcare Commission (2005) *Patient survey report 2004 – mental health*. Healthcare Commission, London.
Heidegger, M. (1962) *Being and Time*, Blackwell, Oxford.
HMSO (1994) *Report of the inquiry into the care and treatment of Christopher Clunis, presented to the Chairman of North East Thames and South East Thames Regional Health Authorities*. HMSO, London.
Husserl, E. (1970) *The Crisis of European Sciences and Transcendental Phenomenology*, Northwestern University, Evanston.
Husserl, E. (1982) *Ideas Pertaining to a Pure Phenomenology and to a Phenomenological Philosophy*. Kluwer, Dordrecht.
Kelly, M. & Gamble, C. (2005) Exploring the concept of recovery in schizophrenia. *Journal of Psychiatric and Mental Health Nursing*, 12, 245–251.
Kirsh, B. (2000) Work, workers and workplaces: a qualitative analysis of narratives of mental health consumers. *Journal of Rehabilitation*, 66, 24–30.
LaFond, V. (2002) *Grieving Mental Illness: A Guide for Patients and Their Caregivers*, 2nd edn. University of Toronto, Toronto.
Langdridge, D. (2007) *Phenomenological Psychology: Theory, Research and Method*. Pearson, England.
Long, A. & Chambers, M. (1993) Mental health in action. *Senior Nurse*, 13, 7–9.
Louise, R.S. (2008) *Basic Concepts of Psychiatric Mental Health Nursing*, 7th edn. Lippincott Williams and Wilkins, USA.
McDonald, A. (2005) *Milestone on My Recovery Road* (Online). Available from: http://www.scottishrecovery.net. Accessed on 20 November 2005.
Mead, S. & Copeland, M.E. (2000) What recovery means to us: consumer's perspectives. *Community Mental Health Journal*, 36, 315–328.
Miller, W.R. & Rollnick, S. (2002) *Motivational Interviewing: Preparing People for Change*, 2nd edn. Guildford, New York.
Morgan, S. (1999) *Assessing and Managing Risk*, Pavilion, London.
Nolan, P. (1992) *A History of Mental Health Nursing*, Stanley Thornes, Cheltenham.

Noordsy, D., Torrey, W., Mueser, K. & Mead, S. (2002) Recovery from severe mental illness: an intrapersonal functional outcome definition. *International Review of Psychiatry*, 14, 318–326.

Podvoll, E. (2003) *Recovery Sanity: A Compassionate Approach to Understanding and Treating Psychosis*. Shambhala Publications, Boston.

Pols, J. (2006) Washing the citizen: washing, cleanliness and citizenship in mental healthcare. *Culture Medicine and Psychiatry*, 30, 77–104.

Roe, D Chopra, M, Wagner, B., Katz, G. & Rudnick, A. (2004) The emerging self in conceptualisation and treating mental illness. *Journal of Psychosocial Nursing and Mental Health Services*, 42, 32–40.

Rogers, C. (1961) *On Becoming a Person*. Houghton Mifflin, Boston.

Ryan, D (2003) Community mental health care. In: *Psychiatric and Mental Health nursing: The Craft of Caring*. (ed. P. Barker), pp. 357–363. Arnold, London.

Sandy, P.T. & Shaw, D.G. (2012) Attitudes of mental health nurses to self-harm in secure forensic settings: a multi-method phenomenological investigation. *Journal of Medicine and Medical Science Research*, 1, 63–75.

Schafer, P. & Paternelj-Taylor, C. (2003) The therapeutic relationship and boundary maintenance: the perspectives of forensic patients enrolled in a treatment programme for violent offenders. *Issues in Mental Health Nursing*, 24, 605–625.

Seedhouse, D. (2000) *Practical Nursing Philosophy: The Universal Ethical Code*. Wiley, Chichester.

Simmonds, S., Coid, J. & Joseph, P. (2001) Community mental health team management in severe mental illness: a systematic review. *British Journal of Psychiatry*, 178, 497–502.

Slevin, O. (1999) The nurse-patient relationship. In: *Interaction for practice in community nursing*, (ed A. Long). Macmillan, London.

Southill, K. (1999) *Will They Do It Again? Risk Assessment and Management in Criminal Justice and Psychiatry*, Herschel Prins, London.

Swinton, J. (2001) *Spirituality and Mental Health Care*. Jessica Kingsley, London.

Watkins, P. (2001) *Mental Health Nursing: the Art of Compassionate Care*. Butterworth-Heinnemann, Oxford.

Woodside, H., Krupa, T. & Pocock, K. (2007) Early psychosis, activity performance and social participation: a conceptual model to guide rehabilitation and recovery. The Cleghorn Program, Ontario, Canada. *Psychiatric Rehabilitation*, **31**(Fall 2), 1215–1230.

Young, S.L. & Ensing, D.S. (1999) Exploring recovery from the perspective of people with psychiatric disabilities. *Psychiatric Rehabilitation Journal*, **22**(Winter 3), 219–232.

13

Caring for the Person with Learning Disabilities in the Community

Owen Barr

Faculty of Life Sciences, University of Ulster Magee, Londonderry, Northern Ireland, UK

Introduction

The chapter provides an introduction to the definition of specialist nursing practice before considering the definition of learning disabilities, an overview of the number of people with learning disabilities and their overall health status. This is followed by a review of the service principles within services for people with learning disabilities, and an outline of the role of community nurses for people with learning disabilities and their families is presented. Some key challenges related to providing an effective community nursing services for people with learning disabilities are then explored before considering the future direction for community nursing in services for people with learning disabilities.

Community nursing for people with learning disabilities has been present in the United Kingdom from the mid-1980s and initially was very much focused on supporting people with learning disabilities who were preparing to leave learning disability hospitals. However, as the service developed, it became clear that the role of the domiciliary community nurses for people with learning disabilities was a varied one and included a large element of working with people with learning disabilities (and their families) who had never lived in a learning disability hospital. The numbers, grades and qualifications of community learning disability nurses within the United Kingdom continue to be difficult to establish at a national level. It does appear as the health needs of people with learning disabilities have changed and services have reconfigured

Community and Public Health Nursing, Fifth Edition. Edited by David Sines, Sharon Aldridge-Bent, Agnes Fanning, Penny Farrelly, Kate Potter and Jane Wright.
© 2013 John Wiley & Sons, Ltd. Published 2013 by John Wiley & Sons, Ltd.

that there have been developments amongst the remits of learning disability nurses working in community settings, with changes such as acute liaison nurses, health facilitation, nurses within mental health services and nurses working in specific clinical areas such as epilepsy. It is unclear how much this has been a growth in posts or a redesignation of existing and former community learning disability nursing posts.

The qualification of community learning disability nursing has been a recorded specialist practice qualification since 1994. It was noted then and still applies now that 'there is a clear difference between practicing within a speciality and holding the recordable qualification of specialist practitioner'. A specialist practice qualification was defined as 'the exercising of *higher levels* (original emphasis from UKCC) of judgement, discretion and decision making in clinical care and their families' and having 'higher order responsibility in clinical care and that it is relevant, required and responsive to health needs'. It was envisaged that community nurses who held a specialist practice qualification 'would demonstrate higher levels of clinical decision making and so enable the monitoring and improving of standards of care through supervision of practice; clinical audit; development of practice through research; teaching and the support of professional colleagues and the provision of skilled professional leadership'. The same definition and standards for 'specialist practice' remain in place through the auspices of the Nursing and Midwifery Council. The need for the required 'higher level of clinical decision making is the foundation of specialist nursing practice and should be evident when observing or assessing the practice of a community learning disability nurse'. It is important that community learning disability nurses who hold a specialist practice qualification clearly demonstrate how they exercise the level of practice consistent with the definition of the recorded qualification.

People with learning disabilities

The term 'learning disability' is used within the United Kingdom in the context of service planning and provision. The definitions used in the current reviews in England, Scotland and Northern Ireland (SE 2000; DH 2001; DH, SSPS 2004) identified that learning disabilities are considered to have three components, namely:

- A significantly reduced ability to understand new or complex information and to learn new skills (impaired intelligence)
- A reduced ability to cope independently (impaired social functioning)
- Having started before adulthood (before the age of 18), with a lasting effect on development

Some clarification was provided within *Valuing People* (DH 2001) that 'the presence of a low intelligence quotient, for example an IQ below 70, is not, of itself, a sufficient reason for deciding whether an individual should be provided with additional health and social care support' (p. 15). The guidance went on to state that in determining the level of need, an assessment of social functioning and communication skills should also be undertaken. Furthermore, it was clarified that the definition of learning disability is not the same as the term 'learning difficulty', which has been defined more broadly within the corresponding legislation relating to education.

The position of adults with autistic spectrum disorders in relation to the definition of learning disabilities is not always clear. Within the definition used in *Valuing People*, it was further stated that the definition covers adults with autism who also have learning disabilities, but not those with a higher-level autistic spectrum disorder who may be of average or even above-average intelligence – such as some people with Asperger's syndrome (p. 22). Whilst the review undertaken in Northern Ireland does not include this caveat, a separate stream of work has been undertaken. In contrast within the policy review undertaken in Scotland (SE 2000), it was stated that the definition of learning disabilities was taken to include people with autistic spectrum disorders, for the purposes of that review (p. 116). The needs for services to respond effectively to the abilities and needs of people with autism and their families have now been strengthened with the passing of new legislation in England (Autism Act 2009) and Northern Ireland (Autism Act (NI) 2011). Key changes as a result of the legislation include changes to Disability Discrimination Act (DDA) definition of disability to now include people with autism and a corresponding increased access to services and benefits and the need for government departments responsible for health to act as the lead government agency in producing, reviewing and implementing a cross-department strategy, developing a data collection system to calculate current and future need for services for people with autism and their families for future planning including how the needs of families and carers will be met. (Further details are available at www.autismni.org/autism-act-(ni)-2011.html and www.autism.org.uk/Working-with/Autism-strategy/The-autism-strategy-an-overview/Autism-Act-2009.aspx.)

The earlier definitions of 'learning disabilities' and the legislation specific to people with autism, many of whom will also have learning disabilities, provide an overview of the criteria that may be applied by service planners and providers in determining who has learning disabilities, and it is accepted that the term may be viewed from differing perspectives and the detail of the interpretation of the nature of learning disabilities alters to some degree depending on the perspective it is being viewed. However, it is generally agreed that if services for people with learning disabilities are to be effective, they must be holistic in nature and provide an effectively coordinated interdisciplinary and interagency approach (DH 2007).

The number of people who have learning disabilities

The numbers of people in the United Kingdom who are considered to have learning disabilities are estimated based on the reported prevalence rates and are revised within major policy reviews or as a result of census findings. Within England, a prevalence rate of 3–4 people per 1000 of the population for people with severe and profound learning disabilities and 20–25 people per 1000 of the population has been used to estimate the numbers of people with mild and moderate learning disabilities. On the basis of these figures, it has been estimated that there are about 210 000 people with profound and severe learning disabilities in England, of which approximately 65 000 are children and young people, with 120 000 adults of working age and 25 000 older people. In using the prevalence rate of 25 people per 1000 for people with mild and moderate learning disabilities, it was estimated that there were 1.2 million people with this condition in England (DH 2001). A total figure of 120 000 has been given for the total estimated number of people with learning disabilities in Scotland, using a prevalence rate of 3–4 per 1000 for profound and severe learning disabilities and 20 people in every 1000 for people with mild/moderate learning disabilities. Increasingly, it was further estimated that only about a quarter of people with learning disabilities had regular contact with local authorities or the health service in Scotland. A survey to calculate the prevalence of people with learning disabilities in Northern Ireland reported the overall prevalence rate for all levels of learning disability as 9.7 persons per 1000 people in the population. In 2003, this is calculated to a population of 16 366 people with learning disabilities in Northern Ireland (McConkey *et al.* 2003). At present within the United Kingdom, there is no central robust database to provide details of the numbers, ages and abilities/needs of people with learning disabilities and their families on a national level of the type which exists in the Republic of Ireland and was set up to provide a demographic profile of people with learning disability in the Republic of Ireland, including their ages, gender and level of learning disability, and how have these changed over time. It is also able to provide details of the number of people with learning disability receiving specialised health services and what services do they receive and the number of people waiting for specialised health services, what service are they waiting for and when, in the next 5 years, do they need these services (www.hrb.ie/health-information-in-house-research/disability/nidd/).

The number of people with learning disabilities across the United Kingdom has been increasing since the 1960s with an estimated annual rate of increase of 1.2%. The life expectancy of people with learning disabilities has increased considerably in the past 50 years with many people living into their 60s, and although still lower, it is now approaching that of other members of the general population (Cooke 1997; Glover & Ayub 2010). At the other end of the age continuum, children with learning disabilities who may previously have died as young children now more frequently live into adulthood due to advances in and increased accessibility to treatment. At times, these children and young adults may have complex health needs, which can lead to an increased need for physical care and support, such as specialist seating equipment, intensive physiotherapy, the availability of suction equipment and enteral feeding.

Given the increasing success in children with profound and severe learning disabilities surviving into adulthood and the increasing life expectancy of adult people with learning disabilities, it is expected that the number of people with learning disabilities will continue to rise year on year. It has been projected that the rate of increase will be approximately 1%; this will primarily be seen amongst younger people with profound and severe learning disabilities and the growth in the number of older people with learning disabilities (SE 2000; DH 2001).

The majority of people with learning disabilities continue to live in community-based settings with almost all people under 20 years of age living in their family home, as do about three quarters of adults with learning disabilities (McConkey *et al.* 2003). Increasingly, people with learning disabilities who move out of their family home or from hospital settings into residential accommodation in the local community and a growing number are successfully living within supported living settings (Simons & Watson 1999; Sines *et al.* 2012). However, many adults with learning disabilities are living with older parents or other family carers; it has been reported that a quarter of people with learning disabilities live with a family carer over 65 years of age and 20% of people with learning disabilities have two carers aged 70 or over and 11% have only one aged 70 or over and can be forecast that these numbers will increase as life expectancy of people with learning disabilities and the general population increases (SE 2000). Some older parents and siblings are reluctant to see their son or daughter or sibling move into residential accommodation, and many have not developed clear agreed plans with other family members or service providers (Davys *et al.* 2010; Mansell & Wilson 2010). In some circumstances, the person with learning disabilities may become a 'carer' for a parent, and this adds another layer of complexity to the planning of future care for both the person with learning disabilities and their parent (www.learningdisabilities.org.uk/our-work/family-friends-community/mutual-caring/).

Service principles in learning disability services

An important dimension that needs to be considered is how devolution of power from the Westminster Government to alternative structures within the United Kingdom, including the Scottish Government, the Welsh Assembly and the Northern Ireland Assembly, has resulted in a number of policy documents within the United Kingdom. Community nurses should be up to date and have a working knowledge of the service principles and policy documents that apply in the jurisdiction they are working within as well as be aware of documents from other linked jurisdictions that they may have interactions with (Jukes & Aldridge 2007). Policy reviews were published in Scotland under the title of 'Same as You?' in 2000, and in England the first major review of learning disability policy in 30 years entitled 'Valuing People' was published in 2001. A new framework was presented in Wales during 2002 under the title of 'Fulfilling the Promises' (Welsh Office 2001), and the most recent review in Northern Ireland has been published under the title of 'Equal Lives' (DH, SSPS 2004). Across these policy reviews, a consistent emphasis on the rights of people with learning disabilities to be included as valued citizens in the countries they live can be seen in the principles identified to guide future services. The policy reviews within Scotland, England, Wales and Northern Ireland presented their future vision as a series of service principles (Box 13.1 and Box 13.2).

BOX 13.1   Principles identified in policy reviews in the Scotland, England and Northern Ireland since 2000

Scotland: *Same as You?* **(Scottish Executive 2000)**

- People with learning disabilities should be valued. They should be asked and encouraged to contribute to the community they live in. They should not be picked on or treated differently from others.
- People with learning disabilities are individual people.
- People with learning disabilities should be asked about the services they need and be involved in making choices about what they want.
- People with learning disabilities should be helped and supported to do everything they are able to.
- People with learning disabilities should be able to use the same local services as everyone else, wherever possible.
- People with learning disabilities should benefit from specialist social, health and educational services.
- People with learning disabilities should have services which take account of their age, abilities and other needs.

England: *Valuing People* **(DH 2001)**

Legal and civil rights: The Government is committed to enforceable civil rights for disabled people in order to eradicate discrimination in society. All services should treat people with learning disabilities as individuals with respect for their dignity and challenge discrimination on all grounds including disability. People with learning disabilities will also receive the full protection of the law when necessary.

Independence: The starting presumption should be one of independence, rather than dependence, with public services providing the support needed to maximise this. Independence in this context does not mean doing everything unaided.

Choice: This includes people with severe and profound disabilities who, with the right help and support, can make important choices and express preferences about their day-to-day lives.

Inclusion: Inclusion means enabling people with learning disabilities to do those ordinary things, make use of mainstream services and be fully included in the local community.

Northern Ireland: *Equal Lives* **(DH, SSPS 2004)**

Citizenship: People with learning disabilities are individuals first and foremost, and each has a right to be treated as an equal citizen.

Person centred: People with learning disabilities should be supported in ways that take account of their individual needs.

(continued)

BOX 13.1   (*Continued*)

> Participation: People with learning disabilities should be consulted about the services they want. They should be actively involved in making choices and decisions affecting their lives.
> Interdependence: People with learning disabilities should be valued and encouraged to contribute to the life of the community.
> Equality: People with learning disabilities should be able to use the same services and have the same entitlements as everyone else.

BOX 13.2   Principles that underpin the vision of future services for people with learning disabilities in Wales (Welsh Office 2001)

- Provide comprehensive and integrated services to achieve social inclusion.
- Be person centred.
- Improve empowerment and independence.
- Ensure effortless and effective movements between services and organisations at different times of life.
- Be holistic in approach and delivery taking fully into account an individual's preferences, hopes and lifestyle.
- Ensure that a range of appropriate advocacy services are available for people who wish to use them.
- Be accessible – in terms of both service users and their carers and families having full information.
- Have fully developed collaborative partnerships to deliver flexible services.
- Services should be developed on evidence of their effectiveness and transparency about their costs.
- Be delivered by a competent, well-informed, well-trained and effectively supported and supervised workforce.
- The early completion of the National Assembly's resettlement programmes to enable all people with learning disabilities to return to live in the community.

A report published 4 years after *Valuing People* presented the findings of a review of information from government departments and service providers. It concluded that after considering the responses received, there had been progress towards the implementation of the *Valuing People* policy including:

- People are being listened to more.
- Person-centred planning, done properly, makes a difference in people's lives.
- The Supporting People programme has helped many more people live independently.
- Direct Payments are helping to change people's lives.
- Organisations are working together better at a local level VPST (2005), p. 6.

However, it was also noted that change was not universal and in particular more work was needed to support people in ethnic minority communities. In responding to the report, the Department of Health noted that:

- There has been good progress in many areas but disappointing change in others.
- Getting some general healthcare services to be properly inclusive of people with learning disabilities has been difficult.
- Too many people and organisations have failed to deliver on the policy promises.
- Where change has happened, some people now feel it is getting difficult to move on to the next stage of change DH (2007), pp. 16–17.

Or put in the language of the original evaluation, 'Big change is only happening where people wanted it to happen and were willing to listen to why people with learning disabilities must be seen and treated as equal citizens. In some other places, little has changed. Put bluntly, too many people in public services see *Valuing People* as being 'optional' – something they can get away with not doing' (VPST 2005, p. 6). The report concluded that the major challenge to be overcome was to 'make sure that everyone takes the lives of people with learning disabilities a lot more seriously' (VPST 2005, p. 7).

Community nurses for people with learning disabilities have a role to play in the achievement of the objectives within the updated *Valuing People Now: The Delivery Plan (2010–2011)*. This has highlighted health, housing and employment as major aspects for service developments and listed the six key priorities for action for 2010–2011, which are:

- To have strong leadership and an effective Learning Disability Partnership Board operating in every local authority area
- To secure access to, and improvements in, healthcare, with strategic health authorities and primary care trusts responsible for and leading this work
- To increase the range of housing options for people with learning disabilities and their families, including the closure of NHS campuses
- To ensure that the Personalisation agenda is embedded within all local authority services and developments for people with learning disabilities and their family carers and is underpinned by person-centred planning
- To increase the number of people with learning disabilities in real paid jobs of 16 hours a week for all who can – including in the public sector
- To improve joint strategic planning, commissioning and service development across children's and adult services, so that people are supported to plan for future employment and a full life (DH 2010, p. 3).

However, despite the investment of time, education and service plans several high-profile independent investigative reports which highlighted the poor quality of care which had components of institutional abuse and promoting dependency in some services within newer models of services, including dispersed community housing, respite care, services for people who presented challenges to services and day activities (HCC/CSCI 2006; HCC 2007a, b; CQC 2011). These reports have criticised to the governance arrangements in place and the attention given to assessing, planning, implementing and evaluating care within services, and one challenged and criticised the actions of the body responsible for undertaking regulation and quality of services as not being effective.

The continued publication of such reports should be a reality check for people working in services for people with learning disabilities and impress on them the need for attention to person-centred care that focuses on the individual and does not become complacent about how much 'new' services have improved from the previous long-stay hospital services. There continues to be a need for community nurses for people with learning disabilities to pay attention to all stages of the nursing process from assessment to the evaluation of care, taking seriously their advocacy role in supporting people with learning disabilities and their professional accountability for actions and omissions as nurses, particularly in relation to escalating concerns about the quality of services (NMC 2010). The implications of failing to do so are clearly visible within these reports, which bear unsettling similarities to the reports which criticised the long-stay hospitals in the 1960s and 1970s such as Ely and Normansfield. The recent reports have clearly demonstrated that the belief that the removal of large hospitals and congregated living settings will resolve the problems of institutionalisation is not true. Institutionalisation and institutionalised abusive practice does not require a large hospital, if the essential ingredients of depersonalisation, 'block treatment' and failure to recognise the value of each person as a citizen are present in any service, including community teams that do not even have residential services (Barr & Fay 1993).

Moving forward

Despite the limitations highlighted in the previous reports referred to, much has been learnt about what characterises a 'good service'. The Healthcare Commission noted that it can be difficult to work in services for people with learning disabilities and that their review of 154 services (of which six were found to have safety concerns requiring immediate actions) that succeeded in providing a quality service as reported by people with learning disabilities had the following characteristics:

- Placed people with learning difficulties at the centre of care, particularly in relation to planning for their care and helping them to make choices
- Provided care in an attractive environment
- Had clear arrangements for safeguarding
- Provided access to independent advocacy services
- Were open to internal and external scrutiny, with the organisations' leaders playing an important role in this
- Had good practices in place for the training of staff (HCC 2007b, p. 5).

A central theme running across all policy reviews within the United Kingdom, including the most recent reports noted earlier, is the need to make the inclusion of people with learning disabilities as equal citizens in society a reality. Inclusion emphasises the rights to people with learning disabilities as citizens of their respective countries and as citizens of their entitlement to the same services as all other citizens. Inclusion challenges the need for people with learning disabilities to meet extra conditions/criteria to use community facilities, to make decisions about their lives or to receive the same services as other members of the local population. In developing and delivering an inclusive service, people with learning disabilities 'must be seen as valued citizens and must be fully included in the life of the community (e.g. education, employment and leisure, integration in living accommodation and the use of services and facilities not least in the field of health and personal social services)' (DH, SSPS 2004).

The respect of citizenship means that community nurses will have to further develop their knowledge and skills in the establishment of anti-discriminatory practice. This is a legal requirement, rather than an 'optional extra' (VPST 2005). Over the past few years, there have been implications from major changes in legislation such as the implementation of the DDA that covered access to areas such as goods, services and employment, together with the acceptance of the European Convention on Human Rights into UK law in 1997, and the corresponding Human Rights, Capacity/Incapacity and Autism-related legislation requires a considerable shift in emphasis in which the onus is on professionals, members of the public and local communities to make reasonable adjustments to accommodate people with learning disabilities, instead of the previous emphasis on people with learning disabilities having to 'fit in' to existing structures. Failure to make reasonable adjustments may be challenged as unlawful discrimination. The implementation of legislation such as the DDA, the Human Rights Act and Autism Act is being used to further support the move towards the development of inclusive services.

Another particular focus in policy reviews has been the need to deliver services in a person-centred manner and the need to promote choice for people with learning disabilities. The development of clearer policies in relation to consent to examination, treatment and care, as well as legislation covering capacity in Scotland and England, further reinforces the need to clear steps to be taken to include people with learning disabilities in all decisions that affect them to the degree to which this is possible, with each decision being treated separately, in so far as someone may be able to make a decision about day activities, but not surgery, and this should be accommodated. The starting point being the expectation that people will be involved, with the onus on services to make this a possibility and only when efforts taken and reasonable adjustments have been made that have not been successful should a best interests pathway be followed and the decision taking by others. Attention will also need to be given to the criteria for informed consent in order to ensure that the procedures involved in providing information to people with learning disabilities and including them in overall decision-making process are consistent with these guidelines. This is consistent with the expectations of citizenship, inclusion and a holistic model to services. A particular challenge in making active involvement in decision making a reality is access to information for people with learning disabilities. Whilst considerable progress has been made in increasing the amount of accessible information available, the lack of information, particularly about health care and health services, continues to be highlighted as a gap in services. Overcoming this will require a focus on the provision of information in a manner accessible to a person's individual abilities and needs. Community nurses should be aware of update to date accessible resources about healthcare such as 'Easyhealth' and be involved in using and developing these (www.easyhealth.org.uk/).

The health of people with learning disabilities

The need to improve the health and access to general healthcare of people with learning disabilities continues to be identified as a major challenge to future services (Michael 2008; Parliamentary and Health Services Ombudsman 2009; Mencap 2012). There is a body of evidence that has accumulated since the mid-1990s, which now conclusively shows that people with learning disabilities have a wide range of unmet health needs. Community nurses for people with learning disabilities have been identified as potentially having a significant role in promoting and maintaining the health of people with learning disabilities (DH 2001). However, in the past few years, further evidence about premature deaths amongst people with learning disabilities (Heslop *et al.* 2012) and concerns over the access to health care people with learning disabilities receive in particular the risk of diagnostic overshadowing with potentially fatal consequences, due to the lack of coordinated services between primary care, acute secondary care and learning disability services (Michael 2008; Parliamentary and Health Services Ombudsman 2009). It is worrying that community nurses for people with learning disabilities as collaborating partners with primary care and secondary care services, or advocates for people with learning disabilities and their families, are largely noticeable by their absence, rather than presence in these reports.

In order to benefit from increased longevity, people with learning disabilities need to be able to maintain a high level of overall health. Physical and mental health is crucial if people are to have a satisfactory quality of life and be able to avail of the developing opportunities for valued social inclusion. However, although the available evidence clearly shows an increasing life expectancy of people with learning disabilities, associated with this is the growing prevalence of physical and mental ill health. As for other members of the general population, the physical and mental health of people with learning disabilities is impacted upon by broad factors such as their living and working conditions, their behaviour and way of life and aspects within their wider environment including the degree of disadvantage or social exclusion they experience (DH, SSPS 2002). The influence of several of these factors may be stronger in the lives of people with learning disabilities; for instance, these may be a greater impact from disadvantage and social exclusion arising from higher rates of poverty, unemployment and low educational achievement (Northway 2001; Emerson 2003). Limited opportunities for involvement in local community activities arising from a number of factors including lack of awareness of these opportunities, dependence on others for transport (often older carers) and the costs involved can result in people with learning disabilities leading a more sedentary lifestyle. Furthermore, poor nutrition and the long-term use of a large number of medications (polypharmacy) have been identified as particular risk factors amongst people with learning disabilities (Beange 2002; Chapman *et al.* 2006).

In addition to the earlier factors, the health of people with learning disabilities may be further compromised by co-morbidity in which the presence of particular syndromes or conditions associated with their learning disabilities may increase their likelihood of having physical health problems (e.g. Down syndrome, epilepsy, associated physical disabilities) (Glover & Ayub 2010). The situation for people with learning disabilities may be future compounded by barriers in access to health care facilities and a resultant delay in the detection of their health needs and instigation of effective treatment (Michael 2008; Parliamentary and Health Services Ombudsman 2009).

Physical health

It is clear that the pattern of morbidity and mortality amongst people with learning disabilities is altering to become similar to that of the general population, with the increasing longevity of people with learning disabilities considered to be a major contributing factor to these reported changes. There has been an increase in deaths arising from cardiovascular disease and stroke and cancers; at the same time, there has been a reduction in the number of deaths arising from infections (Hatton *et al.* 2003). Respiratory disease is still the most common cause of death amongst people with learning disabilities at a rate twice that of general population, with cardiovascular disease the second most common but at a rate half that of the general population (Table 13.1). Recorded death from cancers and other growths amongst people with learning disabilities is still much lower than that reported in the general population (Glover & Ayub 2010).

Much debate has taken place in respect of whether the health of people with learning disabilities is comparatively less healthy than that of the general population. Two main strategies have been used to answer this question; the first approach has involved the inclusion of control or comparison groups within research projects investigating the health of people with learning disabilities. In the main these studies have focused on hearing and visual impairments, conditions of the nervous system, skin disorders and obesity. These conditions are more 'visible', and the data from observation and measurement can usually be collected to support the presence of these conditions without the need for most intrusive investigations that other conditions may need to

Table 13.1   Top ten causes of death amongst people with learning disabilities in comparison to general population[a]

Cause of death	People with learning disabilities (%)	General population (%)
Respiratory disorders	52.0	28.9
Circulatory diseases	12.1	25.6
Infectious disease	6.2	4.4
Nervous system disease	5.3	1.3
Other signs and symptoms	4.5	6.9
Congenital conditions	4.0	—
Cancers and other growths	3.8	22.0
Injury poisoning	2.6	2.7
Digestive system disease	2.6	4.0
Mental health/behaviour	—	1.0

[a]Glover and Ayub (2010).

confirm their presence. In undertaking a review of comparative studies on the health problems of people with learning disabilities, Jansen *et al.* (2004) located eight studies that they considered robust and included control groups undertaken since 1995. The evidence from these studies indicates that people with learning disabilities have increased prevalence rates for epilepsy, diseases of the skin, sensory loss and increased risk of fractures.

A second approach for conditions that require more intrusive investigation or have a lower frequency has been the comparison between the reported rates of particular conditions and illness amongst people with learning disabilities and the national prevalence rates for that condition. The most comprehensive review in this area has been undertaken in relation to cancer amongst people with learning disabilities. The authors concluded that although the overall prevalence rates of cancer amongst people with learning disabilities are similar to that of the general population, there is evidence of an increased prevalence of particular types of cancer amongst people with learning disabilities (Hogg *et al.* 2000). Cancers of the stomach and oesophagus, as well as testicular cancer, have been reported at rates higher than those present in the general population. Conversely, people with learning disabilities appear to have lower rates for lung, breast, urinary tract and prostate cancers (Cooke 1997; Duff *et al.* 2001; Patja *et al.* 2001).

Irrespective of whether the overall rates for the earlier conditions are higher amongst people with learning disabilities, there is growing evidence of unmet health needs amongst people with learning disabilities in a number of areas (Table 13.2).

Mental health

A review of available studies found reported that the prevalence rates of mental health problems (excluding challenging behaviour) amongst adults with learning disabilities range from 25% to 40% (Emerson *et al.* 2001). This compares with the rates of 15–25% for adults without learning disabilities. A population-based study reported

Table 13.2   Overview of the findings of health screening projects within the other areas of the United Kingdom and internationally for people with learning disabilities in Northern Ireland[a]

Area of health screen	Examples of conditions detected
Optical/visual impairments	Reduced vision, need for prescription glasses, cataracts, eye infections
Ear, nose and throat	Hearing loss, ear wax
Dermatology	Eczema, psoriasis, dry skin
Mobility problems	Arthritis, obesity, foot problems
Dental health	Problems with teeth, gums and mouth ulcers
Sexual health	Menstrual problems, testicular and breast anomalies
Cardiovascular	Obesity, hypertension
Endocrine	Diabetes, thyroid problems
Gastrointestinal	Pain and discomfort, reflux problems, peptic ulcers, constipation
Continence problems	Reduced continence, urinary tract infections, pain and discomfort

[a]Turner and Moss (1996); Horwitz *et al*. (2000); Hunt *et al*. (2001); Cassidy *et al*. (2002); and Hatton *et al*. (2003).

prevalence rates of mental health problems amongst children with learning disabilities as 39% compared to a rate of 8.1% for children who did not have learning disabilities (Emerson 2003).

A consistent finding across studies investigating the mental health of people with learning disabilities is that a wide range of mental health problems, similar to that found amongst the general population, can be present. In addition, on occasions, the presentation of the mental health problems amongst people with learning disabilities may be atypical due to their level of verbal and cognitive abilities. Furthermore, some mental health problems may be over-prevalent amongst people with learning disabilities, including affective disorders, phobic states and dementia (Hassiotis *et al*. 2003). In children, similar rates have been reported for depressive disorders, eating disorders and psychosis, with higher rates reported for conduct disorders, anxiety disorders, hyperkinesis and pervasive developmental disorders (Emerson 2003). Whilst any attempt to provide definitive prevalence rates of mental illness amongst people with learning disabilities comes up against a number of difficulties, it appears that children and adults with learning disabilities are diagnosed with mental health problems and at a higher rate than members of the general population (FPLD 2002; Fraser & Kerr 2003).

Action to promote and maintain the health of people with learning disabilities is likely to become an increasing area of work for community nurses, in relation to both the direct care they provide and the need for more effective collaboration with staff in primary care, acute general hospitals and mental health services. Research on the role of community nurses demonstrates that they have already taken steps to improve the health status of people with learning disabilities, amongst a range of other roles they fulfil in the present services. However, despite this process, many mental health services available to other members of the general public continue to present barriers for people with learning disabilities wishing to access services and do not seem to have made the process towards inclusive services that has been achieved within primary care and general acute services (FPLD 2002; DH, SSPS 2004; Hardy 2006).

What community nurses for people with learning disabilities do?

The first research papers on the role of the CNLD appeared in the late 1980s (Mackay 1989), with several others published since that time. The findings emerging from these studies show that community nurses for people with learning disabilities report that they have a reasonably consistent range of reasons for visiting people with learning disabilities. These include support in responding to the presence of challenging behaviour, mental health problems, physical disability, epilepsy and sensory disability (Mackay 1989; Jenkins & Johnson 1991). More recently, the degree of community nurse support for issues relating to physical care needs and issues associated with people with learning disabilities growing older and sexuality appears to become more prevalent (Parahoo & Barr 1996). It is also noted that although the majority of people with learning disabilities visited by community nurses are adults, community nurses are also actively involved with people with learning disabilities across a wide age range from young children to people with learning disabilities who are over 60 years of age.

Mobbs *et al.* (2002) used postal questionnaires, this time to managers of CNLD services across 170 NHS Trusts in England, and obtained responses from 136 NHS Trusts (81%). The findings of this study showed that 99% of NHS Trusts responding employed one or more CNLDs. However, it is clear from the information provided on clinical grades, which range from A to I, that this survey sought information on all nurses working in community learning disability services. It was reported that 44% of NHS Trusts employed support staff at B grade, whilst staff at clinical grades D, E, F, G and H were employed by 12, 57, 30, 97 and 43% of NHS Trusts, respectively, but no information was provided on the numbers of staff employed at each grade or grade mixture within individual services. Mobbs *et al.* (2002) outlined the increasing range of specific posts within community nursing services for people with learning disabilities and reported the presence of dedicated clinical posts in the following percentage of NHS Trusts surveyed: challenging behaviour (27%), child health (25%), epilepsy (20%) and forensic (18%). However, despite these developments, this study also reported that CNLDs were not employed to work with children less than 5 years of age or between 6 and 19 years of age in 27% and 21% of NHS Trusts, respectively. They also reported that 18% of NHS Trusts provided an out-of-hours or on-call service.

The top ten areas of clinical practice as identified by the managers on the basis of the time they felt allocated by nurses were:

- Assessment
- Advice and support
- Health monitoring (ongoing)
- Nursing care
- Counselling
- Health promotion
- Clinical procedures

- Health screening (assessment)
- Crisis intervention
- Client reviews

Whilst this study provides an overview from the perspective of managers, it does not provide information on the composition of services or the function of nurses within individual services. The authors also acknowledge that the views of managers may not reflect the views of individual community nurses in practice settings. It also appears that all nurses working with community services for people with learning disabilities have been considered as a homogenous group, despite the range of specific posts identified, which will impact on the activities the individual nurses will undertake.

In a qualitative study into the role of community nurses for people with learning disabilities, Boarder (2001) interviewed 20 experienced CNLDs (>5 years of experience as a CNLD) in Wales about the key aims and features of their role. Participants reported caseloads of between 15 and 35 clients, 3 working with children and 17 with adults. In the analysis of the interview data, a number of main themes were identified pertaining to the role of community nurses. Participants highlighted the increasing health focus on the community nurses and the continuing development of dedicated clinical posts, such as those reported by Mobbs *et al.* (2002).

They reported an emphasis on interdisciplinary teamwork, and a wide range of tasks undertaken by community nurses were identified. These highlighted the role of community nurses in working with people with learning disabilities in relation to health maintenance and responding to specific physical and mental health difficulties they may experience. Community nurses also had key roles in respect of assessment, advocacy, assisting to maintain people with learning disabilities in a range of community settings and supporting people who present with behaviours that challenge behaviour, skills development and personal relationships. Unfortunately, the findings of this study may be confounded by the fact that two nurses were not RNMH qualified and four nurses (20% of sample) although working in community did not work as part of community learning disability nursing teams but rather in two residential settings, one in a challenging behaviour service and one within a case management team (Boarder 2002).

The views that other professionals within community learning disability teams had of community nurses for people with learning disabilities were explored by Mansell and Harris (1998). They used postal questionnaires to collect information from a range of 96 professionals (including 32 nurses) working in community learning disability teams in South Wales and achieved a response rate of 83%. Respondents identified the top five skills of nurses to be:

- Client-based interventions
- Coordination and planning of care
- Training
- Care management
- Health promotion

The authors reported that the majority of respondents (74 of the 96) indicated that if the registered nurse learning disability was not a team member, another professional could not undertake their role.

Powell *et al.* (2004) reported similar support of the role of community nurses by other health and social services staff community based within residential services. In a questionnaire-based survey of 40 staff, the top five areas reported as part of the role of community nurses were consultancy, assessment, treatment, training and promoting access to services, care planning and health promotion. The need to improve communication with other services and the need to take further action to promote the health of people with learning disabilities were identified as two areas that the services provided by community nurses could be further improved upon. Overall, the respondents rated the community nursing service as effective and valued the broad and varied role that community nurses undertook.

These developments in the role of community nurses are further evidenced in the published papers on individual service developments that provide a detail of similar developments (Barr *et al.* 1999; Hunt *et al.* 2001; Cassidy *et al.* 2002; Martin 2003). Overall, the emerging research knowledge on the role of community nurses for people with learning disabilities demonstrates a continued wide-ranging role of community nurses for people with learning disabilities but also the increasing focus on health orientated and an increasing number of people appointed into dedicated clinical posts. These studies also provide a growing body of evidence as to the value attached to the role of community nurses by other health and social care professionals. In particular the importance attached to the comprehensive knowledge and package of skills community nurses have to work with people with learning disabilities across a wide range of tasks (Mansell & Harris 1998; Stewart & Todd 2002).

Whilst the earlier research findings do show considerable progress in the development of the role of community nurses for people with learning disabilities, four challenges that need to be considered in developing future services were also reported. Firstly, the emphasis on trying to justify the role of the CNLD by reducing it into tasks undertaken risks missing the key value of a CNLD, which is not the individual tasks they undertake or skills they possess that is crucial. Individually, each of the discrete skills can be found in other professionals in the community and amongst other carers, but the fact that it is combination of knowledge, skills and expertise that they bring which is the contribution that CNLDs bring to services. Secondly, there appears to have been a reduction in the number of community nurses who work with children with learning disabilities, as it has been reported that up to a quarter of community nurses for people with learning disabilities in England do not work with children under 5 years of age and one fifth do not work with children under the age of 16 years old (Mobbs *et al.* 2002). Thirdly, there continues to be a lack of recognition and understanding by staff in mainstream services as to the role of the community nurses for people with learning disabilities and the need for greater role clarity within learning disability services. Finally, there is a need to develop strong links with the development of dedicated clinical posts in areas such as metal health, epilepsy and liaison posts and care management/coordination type of posts as distinct from engaging in direct caseload work with individuals whilst keeping under review the potential impact that the changes may have on the fragmentation of services and the effect this has on continuing role of the specialist practice of the domiciliary community nurse for people with learning disabilities.

The future role of community nursing services for people with learning disabilities

A major report entitled 'Strengthening the Commitment – the report of the Modernising Learning Disability Nursing Review was published in April 2012 (Scottish Government 2012). This major report was supported by the four chief nursing officers in the United Kingdom and highlighted both their recognition of the value of learning disability nursing and their commitment to its development. The report focused on the development in four main areas, namely, strengthening capacity, capability, quality and the profession. The report provides clear examples of innovative practice amongst community nurses for people with learning disabilities and makes recommendations for the development of the profession and some with particular relevance to community nurses.

Building on the reports discussed earlier in this chapter, the direction of the future role of CNLD services will continue to evolve to be within a more health-orientated framework, incorporating the need to work effectively with children and older people with complex physical and mental health needs and to have a greater role in facilitating access to general primary, secondary and tertiary care services, including the need for active involvement in public health activities. At the same time, it is essential that community nurses demonstrate positive outcomes for people with learning disabilities and their families through a refocusing on the role and contribution of the 'nursing' component of the community nursing role and an increased 'throughput' in caseloads with more effective admission and discharge procedures and measurement against agreed outcomes and recognised matrixes.

Existing services in many areas continue to be characterised by either perceived 'medical' or 'social' models of care. At times, these models are unfortunately portrayed as having irreconcilable differences and that the medical model is less acceptable in developing services for people with learning disabilities. It has been highlighted that both models have their strengths and limitations, and it is important that a medical model is not mistaken as representing all healthcare provisions (Scottish Government 2012; Thomas and Woods 2003). Evidence has clearly shown the high level of unmet health need amongst people with learning disabilities, and action must be taken to address this (Michael 2008; Parliamentary and Health Services Ombudsman 2009). Future services will be required to become more holistic and accommodate a broader 'health' perspective, including the need to become actively involved in the developments in public health activities and delivering these to people with learning disabilities. Health is holistic in nature as it encompasses physical, psychological and social aspects as well as primary, secondary and tertiary aspects. The emphasis should be on comprehensive holistic assessment of an individual's abilities and needs whilst giving due recognition to their social circumstances (Jukes & Aldridge 2007). A holistic model of health such as that proposed by Seedhouse (1986) who defined health as 'the set of conditions which fulfil or enable a person to work to fulfil his or her realistic chosen and biological potentials' (p. 61) is consistent with the service principles identified as guiding future services for people with learning disabilities and is in keeping with the need for increase interdisciplinary and interagency collaboration. There is a need to become directly involved in addressing the growing complexity of health needs of children and older people. This can be achieved through the provision of family support, early intervention and skills teaching, and community nurses need to develop links with children's nurses and public health nurses in order that they work closely together to maximise the potential of children and older people with complex health needs and reduce the development of longer-term health issues (Scottish Government 2012). There is a need for community nurses for people with learning disabilities to also ensure they have current knowledge and skills to support people with complex health needs and support other staff in making reasonable adjustments to support effective access to services (Michael 2008). Within the development of public health, community nurses for people with learning disabilities should become actively involved in local and national public health activities, for instance, in the areas of cancer prevention (Hanna *et al.* 2011), alcohol misuse and the update of vaccinations.

All community nurses, in particular those who hold specialist practice qualifications, have a valuable role to contribute in the completion of comprehensive assessments. The assessment of health requires interdisciplinary collaboration; a key rationale for a comprehensive assessment is bringing together the thoughts of the main people involved. Each professional inputs into their assessment either with a specific assessment instrument or in the process of joint assessments with other people. Nursing assessments can provide important information on which future decisions will be based, and it is essential that nursing assessments are grounded in nursing frameworks. Community nurses must be careful to match the nursing assessment instrument/strategy they choose to the abilities and needs of the person with learning disabilities. Following the completion of a nursing assessment, nurses will be able to contribute to a comprehensive assessment. Failure to complete a 'nursing' assessment and instead relying only on limited information obtained in a more restricted assessment or a broader ranging but more superficial assessments considerably weakens the nursing contribution to a comprehensive assessment (Barr & Devine 2006).

As more people with learning disabilities have their health needs met within primary care and other general healthcare services, community nurses for people with learning disabilities will increasingly become a secondary specialist service working with people with more complex needs than can be meet within general healthcare services alone. This will involve the continued need for frequent visits to people with learning disabilities and their families together with close liaison with other support services that are being provided. Community nurses will need to develop closer links with colleagues in other health to support the transition between services such as community children's services and staff in dedicated clinical posts such as behaviour support, epilepsy services, mental health and child and adolescent psychiatry services, primary care, general hospitals and palliative care services (McLaughlin *et al.* 2009). Collaborative working in which some joint visits, as well as the exchange of knowledge and skills will need to be further developed to move beyond the separateness of some of these services, which now often work in comparative isolation from each other with differing priorities, aims and objectives.

Whilst this does not necessarily require community nurses to be physically based within primary and general healthcare, at the very least, it requires the development of more formal links between nurses and other professionals in learning disability and primary care services. For instance, community nurses for people with learning disabilities could attend local community nurse meetings within their trust and forge links with nursing colleagues or be nominally attached to general practitioner practices and develop effective liaison with local acute general hospitals. Actively promoting these links will increase the opportunities for CNLDs to make positive contributions in collaboration with other community nursing services to the lives of people with learning disabilities and their families. In relation to adults with learning disabilities, such links will assist in overcoming barriers to accessing primary and acute care services for the increasing number of people with learning disabilities who need to access such services. In contrast, the continued 'isolation' of community nurses within separate learning disability and social work networks will do little to inform other nursing colleagues of their role and possible contributions.

Whilst it is important that more people become aware of the possible contribution of CNLD services, the admission to the people to caseloads should be more effectively managed and prioritised (Caffery & Todd 2002; Barr & Devine 2006). Only on the completion of a nursing assessment and consideration by the CNLD of the contribution they can make in relation to specific nursing objectives should an individual be admitted to a CNLD caseload. This is not to argue against the need for person-centred planning approaches, and it is strongly believed that nursing assessments should contribute to person-centred planning discussions; however, it is not acceptable professionally that nurses should become involved in nursing care that is not based on a nursing assessment. Nor is it acceptable to deliver nursing care to people and not record this intervention, for instance, in case of the nurses who have direct involvement with people not on their nursing caseload. Whilst it is recognised that nurses may be asked for advice and support, it is recommended that a note (not necessarily a complete file) be kept of this interaction. Such changes as outlined earlier are likely to require a revision of nursing assessments to ensure these reflect current approaches to nursing assessment and are suitable to CNLD services. More specific nursing assessment and determination of nursing needs will also go some way to removing the vagueness and uncertainties around the role of the CNLD (Boarder 2001). Community nurses for people with learning disabilities also need to be able to clearly demonstrate the impact in outcome terms what they have achieved for people who have been working with, and there is a growing need to consider the more targeted and formal use of outcome measures to improve safety, productivity and effectiveness alongside traditional person-centred approaches. Examples may include improvements in health status, increasing access to general health services, promoting independence and social functioning, improving nutrition, enhancing psychological and emotional well-being or reducing frequency of seizures (Scottish Government 2012).

When a nursing assessment identifies no nursing need (defined as a need identified within a structured nursing assessment undertaken by a registered nurse), then this should be communicated to the referring professional, and alternative services can then be sought by them. It should not fall to the CNLD to fill the gap in existing services by responding to non-nursing needs; rather, this should be identified as an unmet need and dealt with by the person making the referral through local arrangements for responding to such needs. A more focused approach to nursing assessment will contribute to smoother admission processes and to more effective discharge procedures. It follows that if an individual is admitted to a nursing caseload with specific identified objectives, then once these objectives are achieved, the person could be potentially discharged. However, in order for this to happen, there is a need for comprehensive discharge policies that clearly provide procedures to staff as evidence exists that without such policies that address staff concerns, they will not discharge clients (Caffery & Todd 2002; Walker *et al.* 2003). CNLDs should start this process by reviewing the nursing needs of all people they have infrequent contact with (more than once a month) and determine what the current nursing needs are that justify retaining these people on a CNLD caseload. If the need identified is primarily one of monitoring health (physical or mental), then steps should be taken to work collaboratively with primary care services towards a situation when they undertake this monitoring as they would for other members of the community with ongoing health needs.

Conclusion

Community nurses continue to work with people who have a wide range of abilities and needs; however, there are strong indications that a particular emphasis on their future role will be with people who have increasingly complex physical and mental health needs. However, CNLDs must remain cognisant of the core values within policy reviews and the limitations of services highlighted within independent reviews (HCC/CSCI 2006; HCC 2007a, b) and take seriously their role to support people with learning disabilities and their families through the provision of high-quality, person-focused and coordinated services.

The continued development of CNLD services requires the commitment of community nurses, their immediate managers and those managers within the services responsible for agreeing service structures and policies. Service planners need to consider how the comprehensive package of skills that a community nurse for people with learning disabilities brings to community services can be most effectively used within services that seek to take forward services for people with learning disabilities in line with revised principles that should underpin future services. Equally, there is also a need for CNLDs to recognise that although the role they have performed for many years has been valued, it also will need to evolve further if it is to continue to be of value to people with learning disabilities and their families.

References

Barr, O. & Devine, M. (2006) Care planning in community learning disability nursing. In: Care planning and delivery in Intellectual Disability Nursing, (ed B. Gates), pp. 212–238. Blackwell Science, London.

Barr, O. & Fay, M. (1993) Learning disabilities. Community homes: institutions in waiting? *Nursing Standard*, 6 (41), 34–37.

Barr, O., Gilgunn, J., Kane, T. & Moore, G. (1999) Health screening for people with learning disabilities by a community nursing service in Northern Ireland. *Journal of Advanced Nursing*, 29, 1482–1491.

Beange, H. (2002) Epidemiological issues. In: *Physical health of adults with intellectual disabilities*, (eds V.P. Prasher & M. Janicki), Blackwell Publishing/IASSID, London.

Boarder, J.H. (2002) The perceptions of experienced community learning disability nurses of their roles and ways of working: an exploratory study. *Journal of Learning Disabilities*, 6 (3), 281–296.

Boarder, J. (2001) *Perceptions of experienced community learning disability nurses of their roles and ways of working: an exploratory study*. Report for Welsh National Board Training Research Fellowship, Cardiff.

Caffery, A. & Todd, M. (2002) Community learning disability teams: the need for objective methods of prioritisation and discharge planning. *Health Services Management Research*, 15 (4), 223–231.

Care Quality Commission (CQC) (2011) *Review of Compliance: Castlebeck Teeside Ltd*, CQC, London.

Cassidy, G., Martin, D.M., Martin, G.H.B. & Roy, A. (2002) Health checks for people with learning disabilities: community learning disability teams working with general practitioners and primary care teams. *Journal of Learning Disabilities*, 6 (2), 123–136.

Chapman, M., Gledhill, P., Jones, P., Burton, M. & Soni, S. (2006) The use of psychotropic medication with adults with learning disabilities: survey findings and implications for services. *British Journal of Learning Disabilities*, 34 (1), 28–35.

Cooke, L.B. (1997) Cancer and learning disability. *Journal of Intellectual Disability Research*, 41 (4), 312–316.

Davys, D., Mitchell, D. & Haigh, C. (2010) Futures planning, parental expectations and siblings concerns for people who have a learning disability. *Journal of Intellectual Disabilities*, 14 (3), 167–184.

Department of Health (DH) (1998) *Signpost for Success*, HMSO, London.

DH (2001) *Valuing People. A new strategy for learning disability for 21st century*, DH, London.

DH (2007) *Valuing People Now. From Progress to Transformation*, DH, London.

DH (2010) *Valuing People Now: The Delivery Plan 2010–11*, DH, London.

DH, Social Services and Public Safety (DH, SSPS) (2002) *Investing in Health*, DH, SSPS, Belfast.

DH, SSPS (2004) *Equal Lives: Draft Report of Learning Disability Committee*, DH, SSPS, Belfast.

Duff, M., Hoghton, M., Scheepers, M., Cooper, M. & Baddeley, P. (2001) *Helicobacter pylori*: has the filler escaped from the institution? A possible cause of increased stomach cancer in a population with intellectual disability. *Journal of Intellectual Disability Research*, 45 (3), 219–225.

Emerson, E. (2003) Prevalence of psychiatric disorders in children and adolescents with and without intellectual disability. *Journal of Intellectual Disability Research*, 47 (1), 51–58.

Emerson, E., Hatton, C., Felce, D. & Murphy, G. (2001) *The Fundamental Facts*, Foundation for People with Learning Disabilities, London.

Foundation for People with Learning Disabilities (FPLD) (2002) *Count us in: the report of the Committee of Inquiry into meeting the mental health needs of young people with learning disabilities*, FPLD, London.

Fraser, W. & Kerr, M. (eds.) (2003) *Seminars in the Psychiatry of Learning Disabilities*, 2nd edn. Gaskell Press, London.

Glover, G. & Ayub, M. (2010) *How people with learning disabilities die*, DH, London.

Hanna, L.M, Taggart, L. & Cousins, W. (2011) Cancer prevention and health promotion for people with intellectual disabilities: an exploratory study of staff knowledge. *Journal of Intellectual Disability Research*, **55** (3): 281 291.

Hardy, S. (2006) *Mental Health Nursing of Adults with Learning Disabilities*. Royal College of Nursing, London.

Hassiotis, A., Tyrer, P. & Oliver, P. (2003) Psychiatric assertive outreach and learning disability services. *Advances in Psychiatric Treatment*, 9, 368–373.

Hatton, C., Elliot, J. & Emerson, E. (2003) *Key highlights of research evidence on the health of people with learning disabilities*. Available from http://www.doh.gov.uk/vpst/latestnews. htm#newdocs).

Healthcare Commission (HCC) (2007a) *Investigation into the service for people with learning disabilities provided by Sutton and Merton Primary Care Trust*. HCC, London.

HCC (2007b) *A life like no other: a national audit of specialist inpatient healthcare services for people with learning difficulties in England*. HCC, London.

Healthcare Commission/Commission for Social Care Inspection (HCC/CSCI) (2006) *Joint investigation into the provision of services for people with learning disabilities at Cornwall Partnership NHS Trust*, HCC, London.

Heslop, P., Blair, P., Fleming, P., Hoghton, P., Marriott, A. & Russ, L. (2012) *Confidential Inquiry into premature deaths of people with learning disabilities. Interim Report 2*. Norah Fry Research Centre, University of Bristol, Bristol. Available from www.bris.ac.uk/cipold/. Accessed on 2 December 2012.

Hogg, J., Northfield, J. & Turnbull, J. (2000) *Cancer and People with Learning Disabilities*, British Institute of Learning Disabilities, Kidderminster.

Horwitz, S., Kerler, B.D., Owens, P. & Zigler, E. (2000) *The health status and needs of individuals with mental retardation*, Yale University, New Haven, CT.

Hunt, C., Wakefield, S. & Hunt, G. (2001) Community Nurse Learning Disabilities – a case study of the use of an evidence-based health screening tool to identify and meet health needs of people with learning disabilities. *Journal of Learning Disabilities*, 5 (1), 9–18.

Jansen, D., Krol, B., Groothoof, J. & Post, D. (2004) People with intellectual disabilities and their health problems: a review of comparative studies. *Journal of Intellectual Disability Research*, 48 (2), 93–102.

Jenkins, J. & Johnson, B. (1991) Community nursing learning disability survey. In: *The Community Mental Handicap Nurse-Specialist Practitioner in the 1990's. (ed. P. Kelly)*, pp. 39–54. Mental Handicap Nurses Association, Penarth.

Jukes, M. & Aldridge, J. (eds.) (2007) *Person Centered Practices: A Therapeutic Perspective*. Quay Books, Michigan.

McConkey, R. Spollen, M. & Jamison, J. (2003) *Administrative Prevalence of Learning Disability in Northern Ireland. A Report to the Department of Health, Social Services and Public Safety.* DH, SSPS, Belfast.

McLaughlin, D., Barr, O. & McIlfatrick, S. (2009) Delivering palliative care to those with learning disabilities. *European Journal of Palliative Care*, 16 (6), 302–305.

Mackay, T. (1989) A community nursing service analysis. *Nursing Standard*, 4 (2), 32–35.

Mansell, I. & Wilson, C. (2010) 'It terrifies me, the thought of the future': listening to the current concerns of informal carers of people with a learning disability. *Journal of Intellectual Disabilities*, 14 (1), 21–32.

Mansell, I. & Harris, P. (1998) Role of the registered nurse learning disability within community support teams for people with learning disabilities. *Journal of Learning Disabilities for Nursing, Health and Social Care*, 2 (4), 190–195.

Martin, G. (2003) Annual health reviews for patients with severe learning disabilities: five years of a combined GP/CLDN Clinic. *Journal of Learning Disabilities*, 7 (1), 9–22.

Meehan, S., Moore, G. & Barr, O. (1995) Specialist services for people with learning disabilities. *Nursing Times*, 91 (13), 33–35.

Mencap. (2012) *Death by Indifference: 74 Deaths and Counting.* Mencap, London.

Michael, J. (2008) *Healthcare for all: report of the independent inquiry into access to healthcare for people with learning disabilities*, The Stationary Office, London.

Mobbs, C., Hadley, S., Wittering, R. & Bailey, N.M. (2002) An exploration of the role of the community nurse, learning disability, in England. *British Journal of Learning Disabilities*, 30, 13–18.

Northway, R. (2001) Poverty as a practice issue for learning disability nurses. *British Journal of Nursing*, 10 (18), 1186–1192.

Nursing and Midwifery Council (NMC). (2010) *Raising and Escalating Concerns. Guidance for Nurses and Midwives.* NMC, London.

Parliamentary and Health Services Ombudsman (2009) *Six Lives: the provision of public services to people with learning disabilities: overview and summary investigation reports HC 203-I*, The Stationery Office, London.

Patja, K., Eero, P. & Iivanainen, M. (2001) Cancer incidence among people with intellectual disabilities. *Journal of Intellectual Disability Research*, 45 (4), 300–307.

Parahoo, K. & Barr, O. (1996) Community mental handicap nursing services in Northern Ireland: a profile of clients and selected working practices. *Journal of Clinical Nursing*, 5, 211–228.

Powell, H., Murray, G. & McKenize, K. (2004) Staff perceptions of community learning disability nurses' role. *Nursing Times*, 100 (19), 40–42.

Scottish Executive (2000) *The Same as You? A Review of the Services for People with Learning Disabilities*, SE, Edinburgh.

Scottish Government (2012) *Strengthening the Commitment – the report of the Modernising Learning Disability Nursing Review*, Scottish Government, Edinburgh.

Seedhouse, D. (1986) *Health: Foundations for Achievement*, Wiley, Bristol.

Simons, K. & Watson, D. (1999) *The view from Arthur's Seat: Review of services for people with learning disabilities – a literature review of housing and support options beyond Scotland*, Scottish Executive Central Research Unit, Edinburgh.

Sines, D., Hogard, E. & Ellis, R. (2012) Evaluating quality of life in adults with profound learning difficulties resettled from hospital to supported living in the community. *Journal of Intellectual Disabilities*, 16 (4), 247–264.

Stewart, D. & Todd, M. (2002) Role and contribution of nurses for people with learning disabilities: a local study in a county of the Oxford-Anglia region. *British Journal of Learning Disabilities*, 29, 145–150.

Thompson, J. & Pickering, S. (eds.) (2002) *Meeting the Needs of People with Learning Disabilities*, Bailliere Tindall, London.

Thomas, D. & Woods, H. (2003) *Working with People with Learning Disabilities: Theory and Practice*, Jessica Kingsley Publishers, London.

Turner, S. & Moss, S. (1996) The health needs of adults with learning disabilities and the Health of the Nation strategy. *Journal of Intellectual Disability Research*, 40, 438–450.

Valuing People Support Team (VPST) (2005) *Valuing People: The Story so Far*, VPST, London.

Walker, T., Stead, J. & Read, S.G. (2003) Caseload management in community learning disability teams; influences on decision-making. *Journal of Learning Disabilities*, 7 (4), 297–321.

Welsh Office (2001) *Fulfilling the Promises*, Welsh Assembly, Cardiff.

14

Leadership: Measuring the Effectiveness of Care Delivery

Agnes Fanning

Leadership, Management and Measuring the Effectiveness of Delivery, Faculty of Society and Health, Buckinghamshire New University, High Wycombe, UK

Introduction

Working in the community setting requires leadership skills and styles that recognise the uniqueness of the service that is being delivered. To care for a person in their own home, requires skills of diplomacy, tact, sensitivity, yet at the same time possession of the knowledge that is needed for their particular care to be carried out effectively.

The purpose of this chapter is to address the various approaches to leadership that are deployed within the community and considers how these can impact on the effectiveness of the delivery of care. Leheney (2008, p. 14) suggests that there are five commitments to being a leader; these are commitments to **self, people, the organisation, the truth and to leadership itself**, and these will be intertwined throughout this chapter. This is an interesting concept as Leheney (2008) is suggesting that if a person is not committed to actually leading, then potentially they may not be able to drive change. It is therefore crucial for a leader to have self-belief. To take the lead in a community setting can be a lonely experience as securing the immediate support of other managers and colleagues may not be possible. A leader working in the community must be confident and comfortable with their accountability and their decision-making, which is why belief in self is so important.

Community and Public Health Nursing, Fifth Edition. Edited by David Sines,
Sharon Aldridge-Bent, Agnes Fanning, Penny Farrelly, Kate Potter and Jane Wright.
© 2013 John Wiley & Sons, Ltd. Published 2013 by John Wiley & Sons, Ltd.

In recognising Leheney's (2008) position, consideration must be given to the various layers of leadership that occur within organisations. Leadership is not only a top-down approach, but it also involves a number of people within an organisation to help drive forward the many changes that are occurring; this is particularly applicable to the National Health Service (NHS) today. After all, there are a number of subgroups, such as those that are provided by voluntary and charitable organisations within the community that also require support and direction. The complexities of leading in the community demand front-line staff and their managers to apply flexible styles of leadership that are not reliant on the previously dominant 'command and control approach' and in their place should be alternative systems that seek to coordinate multi-agency working and teamwork.

Influences on leadership

It is often claimed that people are born with inherited traits, such as those particularly suited to leadership, reinforcing the view also that leaders are 'born and not made'. Yet reviewing descriptors such as those presented next by Stogdill (1974; Table 14.1) suggests that these views could be challenged as Taffinder (2006, p. 3) claims that anyone can learn leadership skills and can be successful in leading others.

In 1939, Kurt Lewin carried out research to identify the different kinds of leadership styles that people used, and he focused on three particular styles: authoritarian (autocratic), participative (democratic) and delegative (laissez faire). In different situations, one style may be more dominant than another, but a good leader will use all three styles, depending on what forces are involved between the followers, the leader and the situation (http://www.nwlink.com/-donclark/index.html). Therefore, emotional intelligence is required for effective leadership, and individuals leading, at whatever level, must have an awareness of their own knowledge and that of their colleagues and those of the patient or client if the move of direction is to be successful.

Table 14.1   Stogdill's leadership descriptors

Traits	Skills
Adaptable to situations	Clever (intelligent)
Alert to social environment	Conceptually skilled
Ambitious and achievement orientated	Creative
Assertive	Diplomatic and tactful
Cooperative	Fluent in speaking
Decisive	Knowledgeable about group tasks
Dependable	Organised (administrative ability)
Dominant (desire to influence others)	Persuasive
Energetic (high activity level)	Socially skilled
Persistent	
Self-confident	
Tolerant of stress	
Willing to assume responsibility	

The community setting is a complex area within which to work as decisions are often made about an individual in their own private home, and such decisions cannot be made without the involvement of the patient or client and, where relevant, their carers. On these occasions a symbolic or emotional language of leadership may be required (Rowe 2006). Over the years user involvement has been encouraged, but this has not always been acted upon. The Government is now insisting that the involvement of service users is essential if services are to be focused on the needs of patients and clients. *The Guidance on Involving Adult NHS Service Users and Carers* (NHS 2010) stresses the importance of involving service users and carers to ensure a service is planned that will meet the needs of the wider public following constructive input from people who are actually using the service. Service users are also going to be asked about the effectiveness of their care, and as such users will be playing an important part in evaluating service delivery. Such involvement will require leadership and the provision of support and guidance to assist the service users to develop the relevant skills required to contribute as co-agents of change. Service user engagement will require the use of a range of diplomatic skills when addressing the needs of patients and clients, and it must be made clear that there is a difference between a 'need' and a 'want'. So often a patient is misguided because they want something, for example, a specific chair. Yet, having had a physiotherapy assessment the chair they want would actually cause them increased mobility problems. Such occasions will require the practitioner to have researched evidence to support their decision and to assist them to formulate a clear explanation for the patient/client to understand the reasons why this decision has been taken. This is leadership at a local level, and it is often such informal leadership actions that are remembered by patients and clients.

Those who have worked in the NHS are familiar with change, but at this particular time the NHS is at a crossroad in terms of its commissioning and delivery structure, with the introduction of Health Education England (HEE), Public Health England (PHE), NHS Commissioning Boards, Local Education and Training Boards (LETBs) and Clinical Commissioning Groups (CCGs), with associated changes in the locus and focus of power across the whole organisation. What is important though is the realisation that the operation of these combined forces will bring about profound change across the entire social welfare system (Senge 1997, p. 122). In order to accommodate such inevitable challenges, the NHS, social enterprises, charities and voluntary organisations will be required to develop a clear and compelling statement of strategic direction and intent.

All organisations need to have a clear strategy, and in order to deliver their services, they will require possession of a series of requisites for effective delivery. A key element to effective leadership is for the whole workforce to be aware of the vision and philosophy of the organisation, ensuring that there are clear and open communication channels to enable free-flowing communication in both directions. This will require knowledge of the health needs of local specific communities and an understanding of the deployment of relevant resources necessary to deliver local health care. Various modes of communication will be needed to support the dissemination of the service vision and philosophy to penetrate through the numerous layers of organisational management structure. There are many debates about what is the difference between a manager and a leader, and a frequently quoted statement is: 'Managers do things right, but leaders do the right things' (Bennis & Nanus 1997). It is imperative that managers and leaders work together sending the same message to organisations, teams, patients and clients. A potential difficulty of leading in a community setting is the diversity of populations that might reside within any one particular CCG. Nevertheless, there will also be the need to develop a strategy for an overall population. Creative styles of leadership and management will be required if such multifarious local demands are to be met.

The key leadership quality referred to in this chapter is about people having a vision and giving direction to others in their organisation to take this vision forward. Revisiting Leheney's (2008) thoughts, the leader must have belief in themselves if there is any chance of taking others with them on the journey of change. This view is also held by Ferguson-Pare (2011) who claims that leadership should emanate from every nurse and should 'come from within yourself' (Ferguson-Pare 2011, p. 393).

To build on the concept of 'self', reference will be made to Lombardi, who in 1959 made the famous statement that 'Leaders are born and not made'. Looking inwards towards ourselves as individuals, is it possible to recognise the leadership qualities that each of us possess? At some stage every person reading this chapter will have taken the lead in some activity throughout their life. This role may have taken place during school days, the workplace or in family or social life. Teachers in primary school are often heard to make statements such as 'that child will be a leader someday'. What are the qualities that have been recognised in this child? Whether self-belief stems from early childhood and people see potential in the individual, or whether it is a skill that has been developed over the years due to life experience, belief in oneself is necessary if the organisation, department, team, patient or client is going to put their trust in you. As will be discussed throughout this chapter, a leader will not possess expertise in all areas, but they will have conviction, which Owen (2005) suggests is the emotional bedrock of leadership. Individual leaders will possess and display a variety of characteristics that might range from introversion to extrovert tendencies. Neither tendency can be judged to be either right or wrong, the relevance here is for a leader to recognise the style that best conveys their message effectively to their teams, patients and clients to subsequently influence and embed change.

Leadership in the community setting will be directed and determined strategically by a number of key sources:

- Department of Health/NHS Commissioning Board/HEE/PHE
- LETBs
- Health and well-being boards
- CCGs
- Local authorities

- Service providers
- Local stakeholders
- Local communities
- Patient/client

This list is not exhaustive as many other agency influences such as local authorities, charities, the independent sector and/or voluntary organisations may also form part of the overall local strategic vision.

Government policies

The NHS Plan (DH 2000) set out a 10-year strategy to build an infrastructure fit for the twenty-first century and to improve the quality of care for patients, with improved access to health care. Shortly after this, Wanless (2002) suggested that there should be more clearly defined performance outcomes that would assist in measuring and monitoring the effectiveness of existing services so as to assist them to plan for service improvement, informed by reported outcomes. Thirteen years on, the Government is looking at restructuring the NHS once again by removing primary care trusts and replacing these with CCGs. With the abolition of primary care trusts and the introduction of CCGs, a new shape of service provision, commissioning and configuration is emerging. Micromanagement is to disappear and resources will be released increasingly to the front-line clinicians (Lansley 2011). Such initiatives will increase autonomy to those commissioning the care for people who require community services, whilst new, flexible and dynamic leaders will emerge at all levels of the service, from board to the front line of community service delivery. The new NHS Commissioning Board is expected to 'liberate' those delivering the services (Nicholson 2013). This is welcome news at a time when the NHS is facing a series of challenges from the media. It would be fair to say that since the inception of the NHS in 1948, there has never been so much negative publicity about leadership within the NHS. Recent reports such as the Francis Report (2013) and the Winterbourne Report (2012) have claimed that inadequate leadership has been to blame for poor and unacceptable practice within the NHS service. Leonard and Frankel (2012) reiterate the importance of creating an environment where no one is frightened to voice a concern, applying this principle to both professionals and caregivers. Health Secretary Jeremy Hunt has implied that he would like to see the NHS adopt the airline industry's standard of zero tolerance of error, stating that senior managers should be dismissed from post if an NHS organisation fails to meet quality and safety standards (Hunt 2013). In March 2013, new legislation has been introduced breaking the 'gagging law' that prevented so many people from reporting poor practice that jeopardised the delivery of safe and effective patient care. If people are free to whistle blow and report bad practice, this will enable prompt action to be taken that will impact on the overall measurement and standard of care delivery.

In 2011, the King's Fund set up a commission on leadership and management in the NHS, and one of the suggestions resulting from their work was to 'move beyond the outdated model of heroic leadership'. This can only be regarded as a positive move as leaders will now be scrutinised far more than ever, suggesting that some people may shy away from undertaking leadership roles because they will be publicly accountable. The changing structure of the NHS will now ensure that all commissioning decisions will be scrutinised through board decisions and there will be improved monitoring of budgets and quality of care.

The Secretary of State for Health in 2012 advised that the Government is committed to putting the right people in charge. Ministers have stated that they will remove obstacles and provide clear guidelines to support people who are in leadership positions in order to promote the delivery of excellent, harm-free care. Leaders will therefore need to be clear about their duties and responsibilities, and their ambitions should be matched with reality, ignoring the divergent tendencies that are often found in community settings. Bernstein *et al.* (2010) also say that there needs to be a more innovative mechanism to identify the roles of different government departments. With this in place and with leadership being high on the Government agenda, it might just be possible that the key message from the Government to promote integrated care and to increase patient choice will be feasible, as coordinated action will be promoted across service delivery lines.

Lansley (2011) stated that effective leadership should be promoted at all levels and suggested that leaders should be prominent in every professional clinical role, this being the only way that fully integrated care can be realised. Recognising that the demands to lead services are at their peak, people with knowledge of long-term conditions, specialist care, end of life care and other complex care will be required to be more creative in their thinking and to engage in new forms of service delivery (DH 2009). Whilst the 'Big Society' supports creative ways of working and promotes social entrepreneurship within the National Health System, this is still spasmodic, only happening in some areas across the United Kingdom. Some (Rickman 2011) have even said that the 'Big Society' was already occurring prior to the Coalition Government presenting this concept in 2010. The Government's ideal of realising a more participative and entrepreneurial society provides a great opportunity for health and care ventures to be explored (Wyatt & Loder 2010, p. 18). Unfortunately, the system at present is not designed to exploit such an approach, but if the Government is true to its word, then managerial bureaucracy will be removed and common sense will prevail. Managers will be free to enable clinicians to lead their teams without fear of being reprimanded because a 'box has not been ticked' or a 'target has not been met'. It is the lack of commitment to creativity from leaders within the NHS that is preventing innovative practitioners being able to improve patient care. Opportunities may arise to introduce innovation into the health and social care settings following the Government's desire to promote a clinically led health service, where providers of health-care services will be in competition with each other (competing on price, service quality and creativity of service delivery). Any qualified provider (AQP), which can include non-NHS providers, will drive competition within provision, giving patients the opportunity to choose from at least three locally selected providers of community services (NHS 2012).

The Care Quality Commission (2013) produced a report stating that the number of people being cared for in their own homes is increasing, resulting in an increase in demand for home care services. In 2011–2012, there was a sixteen per cent rise in home care services, and in the first 6 months of 2012–2013, this increased again by a further 6%. Whilst many of these services are delivered outside of the NHS, it is necessary for NHS staff to be aware of this. Those agencies delivering home care will need to work with the professionals who are also delivering specialist clinical skills to many of the same patients. The lead in these organisations has a responsibility to ensure that staff who are working in home care have the relevant communication skills, competencies and core values of caring and empathy. This will promote positive interagency working in the community and effective leadership skills to coordinate this care.

For many years the Government has been promoting the transfer of care closer to home and transforming community services (DH 2010), but not enough thought has been invested into underpinning this change of direction. It is not just a matter of moving services from the acute setting to a community setting. It requires a complete change of attitude and a profound change of mindset. You cannot simply transpose a structure from an acute setting to a home setting. Take the example of name bands for patients in an acute setting or insisting that patients are bathed before a visit. How ethical would it be to bring such a practice to an individual's private home? These are some of the challenges that staff are confronting. Service managers should recognise that to successfully lead in the community, there must be an acknowledgement that practitioners are visiting patients and clients in their own homes and they cannot dictate to them. It is a cliché, but all practitioners visiting patients and clients in their homes are guests and therefore must respect and be sensitive to the rights and needs of the vulnerable and unwell people they work with. The Queen's Nursing Institute in 2010 suggested that:

> It is time to recognise the significant difference between nursing in clinics, surgeries and other clinical premises in primary care; and nursing in patients' homes (QNI 2010, p. 5).

This highlights that even within community settings there must be recognition of the different requirements for those patients that are housebound. Leaders driving the community services must understand this and be able to work with the diverse and complex requirements of our multicultural and multi-pathological society.

Front-line staff

Many of the changes recommended as care moves closer to home can only take place if responsibility for leadership can be given to the clinicians who are at the front line of care, offering more control to those who understand the patient best

(Lansley 2011). Yet clinicians have been seen and not heard for too long (Ferguson-Pare 2011), but Lansley's vision is now giving permission for front-line staff to make a difference by being encouraged to influence change. The NHS is delivering a service that is free at the point of delivery and need. These core values must continue if the NHS is to remain as a major public organisation with patient safety and quality care at the centre of their philosophy. *High Quality Care For All* (Darzi 2008) advocated quality being at the centre of patient care, supporting the view that leaders who are skilled at working across systems and boundaries are more likely to deliver transformation (DH 2009). Even though leadership may be seen to be directed by a singular clinician, this is not the true picture. If leadership is to be effective and the patient's needs are at the forefront of all care, then there should be leaders at all professional levels, enabling and promoting truly integrated care, embracing people with different skills and backgrounds (DH 2009). Leading is not about one person but about groups of individuals who are mandated to lead with a common purpose, promoting good health and care for those that are unwell and vulnerable. This can be achieved by improving the patient experience, increasing the quality of care and reducing morbidity.

As alluded to at the beginning of the chapter, leading and managing services in the community setting can be very complex, and the Department of Health in 2009 (DH 2009) recognised this, claiming that if leaders and workforce itself are not representative of the communities they serve, it will be a struggle to deliver locally driven services that are responsive to the needs of individual patients. CCGs will be expected to encourage patients to be involved in their own care, and the Health and Social Care Act (2012b) states that it is the duty of the service providers to involve patients in decisions about the provision of services generally, supporting them to make informed choices about their own health care. This will mean that CCGs will be required to offer a range of services and treatments from more than one provider in order to provide patient choice (DH 2012b). This potentially may lead to a fragmentation of services, but if this information is shared with patients and clients, then they will feel empowered to make an informed decision based on the information they have (Leheney 2008). If the information shows that providers have not met the commissioning for innovation (CQUIN) targets, their funding will be withheld. It is therefore in the best interest for all if leaders can work with their teams to promote innovation and demonstrate a positive leadership approach from the onset. A successful trait of a good leader is the ability to listen to the needs of others and to respond, thus maintaining their motivation. At times they may have to work with uncertainty, but their skill set should equip them with the ability to be responsive to needs at the same time as having a strategic overview and knowledge of commissioning and policy developments (Frost 2011).

Covey (1999) discusses the various approaches to influencing people. As a leader, influencing is an approach often used by people in a position of power to gain support from their teams and staff. Influence is used across the spectrum of management layers that are evident in the range of community settings. To achieve the most positive

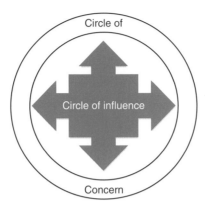

Figure 14.1   Circle of influence. (Covey 1999)

outcome from staff, the adoption of a proactive focus can be an encouraging way to deal with staff and patients to get things done. The positive energy of the leader encourages this attitude in others, and therefore, their circle of influence is increased (Fig. 14.1). For this type of leader, the more their circle of influence increases, the circle of concern reduces. This will build an environment where the positive attitude will make all things seem possible, thus increasing empowerment for staff, patients and clients.

For influence to be beneficial and accepted, it is anticipated that the leader will have the trust and respect of their followers. Many leaders in the community will be leading a multidisciplinary team, and this will bring challenges in gaining acceptance from those colleagues outside of their own profession, so belief in their leader will be essential if team members are going to be successful in working together. The leader will be required to have an overall understanding of the different professions that fall under their management structure. This will bring challenges as they work towards gaining an acceptance from the team and also whilst they cross service and agency boundaries in addressing service needs. Recognising that it is acceptable to be an expert in one professional area, but not in all aspects, will gain respect from their team. This style of leadership will also empower all of the professions to have a voice when decisions are made about the provision of their service. An essential part of leading such a team will be to build a sense of team belonging across a diverse range of people (Frost 2011, p. 2). To be effective they must have the ability to be fluid and flexible (Frost 2011, p. 3). It is important for any form of leadership to respect the opinions and actions of others, this being extremely relevant when dealing with multi-professionals from different agencies since this approach is a prerequisite to creating mutually satisfying solutions and responses to the requirements of the service provision.

The underpinning success of any teamwork is communication, and the concept of emotional intelligence as a predictor of success highlights two essential

BOX 14.1   Excercise 1

You are a health visitor lead with a team of health visitors, school nurses, district nurses, community staff nurses, nursery nurses, speech and language therapists, podiatrists, physiotherapists and occupational therapists.

Scenario 1: You have been asked to look at how services in the community are being delivered to patients who have diabetes. You ask all members of your team to give you a breakdown of what input they are giving to these patients, asking them to identify the multi-pathology of the patients and tell them that you must have these statistics by the end of the month with no excuses for delay.

Scenario 2: You ask your team to gather information about patients with diabetes where they are inputting services. You explain that some of the patients will have a number of other medical conditions that may have been predisposed by diabetes. In gathering all of this data, you will be able to look at what health promotion and preventative care can be planned for future patients. You say that this data is being collected from all of the teams in your region and will be sent to the clinical commissioning boards within the next 2 months, with a view to reviewing the provision of services for diabetic patients and potentially other diabetic-related conditions. You ask the team if they have any other questions in relation to this task.

BOX 14.2   Excercise 2

You are a district nurse visiting a patient (Mr. James) who is a new patient, not known to you. The patient is housebound and you are assessing a wound that has developed into a venous leg ulcer.

Scenario 3: You ring and arrange a time to visit Mr. James. When you arrive you assess the wound and tell Mr. James that the wound has been aggravated by wearing tight socks and you are very firm in stating that he must not wear these socks if he wants his leg ulcer to heal. When you visit the next day, you are cross to see that Mr. James has continued wearing the socks. You say in a very firm voice 'this wound will never heal if you don't do as I say'. You look angry and sound angry. Mr. James is upset at your tone and attitude and makes a decision that once you have left his home, he will put his socks back on.

Scenario 4: You ring and arrange a time to visit Mr. James. When you arrive to assess the wound, you notice that the socks he has been wearing are very tight and they have constricted the blood flow, causing extra pressure on the wound and therefore making the area around the wound very inflamed. You explain to Mr. James that this will delay the healing process and ask him if he has any other socks he could wear. He allows you to look at his other socks and you find a pair that are not tight fitting and will not hinder the wound. When you visit the next day, the inflammation around the leg ulcer has reduced, and Mr. James does not seem so anxious and does not have any pain.

qualities: empathy and sincerity. Borg (2010) purports the view that interpersonal intelligence and intrapersonal intelligence go hand in hand with empathy and sincerity and claims that as communication is transmitted through our attitude, it is not enough just to be competent in these areas but that it also requires empathy and sincerity, which in turn leads to persuasion. When working with teams, patients and clients, a great deal of persuasion can be effected by the way communication and interpersonal skills are used. As a leader in any context if positive interpersonal skills are used, such as smiling and positive body language, then there is a greater chance that this will influence the outcome. Owen (2005) makes an interesting statement in saying that if a message is portrayed in a positive way with the use of positive interpersonal skills, then the receiver of the message will remember who delivered the message more than the message itself, claiming that 'you' are the message.

Take a look at the exercises in Box 14.1 and Box 14.2 and identify the learning that can be taken from all four scenarios.

Spend some time looking at these four scenarios

Scenario 1 and scenario 2 are possibly recognised as being similar to many requests received by team leaders and service directors. Some may not see anything wrong with either approach. In looking at scenario 1, a particular leadership style has been used (autocratic). In scenario 2 another approach has been used (democratic), evidencing clarity about why this information is needed.

Reading these scenarios may make some readers feel patronised and enable them to recognise that scenario 3 is a common occurrence in district nursing practice, requiring patients to comply with instructions. Others will look at scenario 4 and recognise that the power of influence can be used at all levels of communication, realising that it can make a difference to compliance and the well-being for patients.

Only you will recognise the type of leader you are in relation to the earlier four scenarios. Spend some time and contemplate on what you can do to give those you work with the best quality experience they can receive from you. Radcliffe (2009) encourages people to actively look for opportunities to engage people, stressing that it is not only having the ability to getting a task done, but it is the act of gaining commitment from people that will demonstrate true leadership qualities.

Working within organisations it is common to be confronted with such characteristics as seen in Fig. 14.2. Resistance is difficult because resistors cannot see the relevance or do not want to see the relevance in what you are trying to achieve. Resistance at least consists of an emotion that can be challenged, whereas Radcliffe (2009) claims that apathy is the most difficult state of mind to work with as it is difficult to get people to move or shift from this mindset. The root cause of the apathy should be addressed as excuses for the appalling care reported in the Francis Report (2013) suggests that this was allowed to continue because nurses and staff were apathetic due to being

The Future I Want

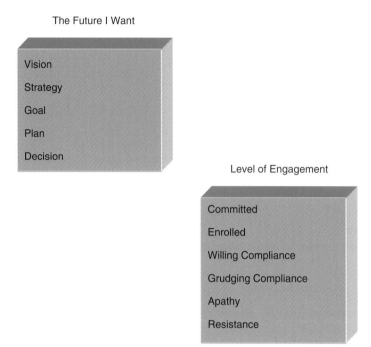

Figure 14.2   My preferred future

demoralised and working in an under-resourced environment (Donnelly 2013). The quality of the leadership in Staffordshire has been challenged following this damming report and represents an extreme case of apathy that had disastrous consequences. Grudging compliance will require some effort on behalf of the leader to get people with this attitude on side. Often tokenism is applied as a means of just going along with an idea. Where willing compliance is seen, there is an audience willing to travel with you and your vision. Once people are enrolled, they are on board, but they can become distracted, so they will need to be monitored. When a person becomes committed, they bring their enthusiasm and desire to work with you, and they are fully engaged and really do want to work with you. Whether a leader or a member of a team, it is worth contemplating whether you display any of the earlier traits, and if so, why and how can you change this? As a leader it will be difficult to take people with you and lead them if you are working out of a sense of compliance yourself (Leheney 2008). Where there are high levels of engagement, it is possible to get things done and motivation is increased. This is not only noticeable within the workforce, but patients and clients will be able to read the signals where there is either contentment or discontent. Therefore, as professionals, no matter how poorly motivated a team or an organisation may be, it is imperative that positive messages and confidence are portrayed to patients, clients and carers.

Effective leaders also have a responsibility to address disruptive or disrespectful behaviour, and they must be consistent in holding people accountable for any such behaviour (Leonard & Frankel 2012). A report produced by Hartley and Bennington (2011) has shown that leadership in the NHS is being viewed in a far more critical way than previously, referring to the 'dark side' that can be destructive as well as constructive.

Measuring the effectiveness of delivery

Leadership in the community setting has been discussed at length earlier, and the focus now moves to address how leadership and management can play a part in measuring the effectiveness of service delivery. In order to answer this question, which aspect of delivery being investigated needs to be known. The one area that automatically comes to mind is to look at the quality of care being given to patients and clients. Measuring the effectiveness of quality is bigger than only measuring the quality of care; according to the NHS Institute for Innovation and Improvement (2010), it involves:
  Patient and staff experience and satisfaction

- Patient safety
- Quality of care
- Clinical outcomes
- Prevention
- Population health
- Staff productivity

On the other hand, the National Nursing Research Unit (Maben and Griffiths 2008) carried out a survey to look at what is meant by good-quality nursing care, and the following was identified:

1. A holistic approach to physical, mental and emotional needs, patient-centred and continuous care
2. Efficiency and effectiveness combines with humanity and compassion
3. Professional, high-quality evidence-based practice
4. Safe, effective and prompt nursing interventions
5. Patient empowerment, support and advocacy
6. Seamless care through effective teamwork with other professions

No one would disagree with the six points earlier, but how can these six factors be measured? Bernstein *et al.* (2010) in their independent report on enabling effective delivery of health and well-being have recommended that there should be better data on cost-effectiveness and return on investment, reinforcing a number of previous views mentioned, that there needs to be clarity of high-level goals across the various systems, claiming that this can all be done without added expense. Changes within the

NHS introducing the Friends and Family Test (Cain 2013) are a means of measuring the quality of care delivered to patients in the acute setting and A & E, and it will just be a matter of time before such a framework will be set up to measure the quality of care for patients in the community.

To measure effectiveness there must be clarity around what is being measured, and all those involved are required to have an understanding of the value and benefits of gaining this information. There may be apathy and resistance to gathering information, and this is often due to not having all of the information to hand in an intelligible and reliable format. The leader has a responsibility to inform their teams, patients and clients as to why this information is required and, more importantly, what will be done with this information. They also have a responsibility to feedback on outcome measurement and on the interpretation or meaning attributed to the collected information (Neath 2010). If an outcome measurement tool is used, then greater acceptance will be shown as there is visible concrete evidence of performance and client/patient need. One such system that is being used in a number of community health-care settings is the RIO system. This is an electronic health-care record that enables shared information about patients to be communicated across the multidisciplinary team. It brings together the key elements of an electronic patient record that provides a single source of information about patients, providing improved levels of care. These records are a tool that demonstrates the care plan and care-related activities that are provided to patients and provides a means to measure the effectiveness of patient care.

A key message that has emerged from further research conducted by the King's Fund has stressed the importance of early intervention for all patients, irrespective of their presenting condition or care pathway. Integration and coordination of care for people with chronic diseases and complex needs was highlighted by the Department of Health in 2007 as an area for priority investment and has remained ever since at the heart of the planned care agenda. The provision of care closer to home will become a key area of activity and investment for all providers of integrated health and social care, resulting in more effective and responsive care delivery and enhanced service user satisfaction.

Conclusion

When leading teams, organisations, communities, patients or clients, it is essential to recognise what has been an enabling factor in successfully driving forward an initiative or vision. It is also necessary to address the inhibitors that have restricted service improvement or innovation. Evaluation should be common practice to ensure all avenues have been explored so that new ways of leading can be exercised. The influence of leadership on the overall shape and design of local services and their impact on the quality of service delivery must be acknowledged, and where good practice is witnessed, this should be held as an accolade for other areas. Sharing of good practice is something that is not an automatic occurrence, and this should be encouraged. It is one way of celebrating success and can be liberating for all those involved. A successful leader will not let disappointments prevent them from pursuing their goal. They will acknowledge that their leadership style should match the development needs of their team or their patient/client. If effective delivery is to be a priority in primary care, then health and social care leaders must aim to promote a society where both physical and psychological health and well-being are a requisite for the well-being of the community.

References

Bennis, W. & Nanus, B. (1997) *Leaders – Strategies for Taking Charge*, (2nd edn). Harper Business, New York.

Bernstein, H., Cosford, P. & Williams, A. (2010) *Enabling Effective Delivery of Health and Wellbeing*. Crown, London.

Borg, J. (2010) *Persuasion: The Art of Influencing People*. Pearson, Harlow.

Cain, J. (2013) The NHS Friends and Family Test: Publication Guidance, 7 February 2013. Department of Health, Leeds.

Care Quality Commission (CQC) (2013) *Care Update*, CQC, Newcastle.

Covey, R. (1999) *The 7 Habits of Highly Effective People*. Simon & Schuster, New York.

Darzi, A. (2008) *High Quality Care for all; NHS Next Stage Review*. Department of Health, London.

Department of Health (DH) (2000) *The NHS Five Year Plan 2000–2005*. DH, London.

DH (2009) *Inspiring Leaders: Leadership for Quality*. Workforce Directorate, DH, London.

DH (2010) *Transforming Community Services: Overview*. DH, London.

DH (2012a) *Department of Health Review; Interim Report Winterbourne View*, DH, London.

DH (2012b) *Transforming Health and Social Care: The Social Enterprise Investment Fund*, HMSO, London.

Donnelly, H. (2013) Apathy stops many of us from exposing poor care. *Nursing Standard*, 27 (25) 27–30.

Easton, J. (2010) *Measurement for Quality and Cost (2010)*, NHS Institute for Innovation and Improvement, London.

Ferguson-Pare, M. (2011) Perspectives on leadership: moving out of the corner of our room. *Nursing Science Quarterly*, 24 (4), 393–396.

Francis, R. (2013) *Independent Inquiry into care provided by Mid Staffordshire NHS Foundation Trust January 2005–2009*, vol. 1. The Mid Staffordshire NHS Foundation Trust Inquiry Stationery Office, London.

Frost, N. (2011) *Guide to leading multi-disciplinary teams*. Leeds Metropolitan University Blog. Available from http://www.ccinform.co.uk/articles/article.aspx?IiArticleID=5706&Prin. Accessed on 19 February 2013.

Hartley, J. & Benington, J. (2011) *Recent Trends in Leadership*. King's Fund, London.

Hunt, J. (2013) Hospital deaths are as bad as air crashes, *The Times*, 17 March 2013, p. 22.

Lansley, A. (2011) *2011 Modernisation Speech*, King's Fund Leadership Conference, May 18. DH, London.

Leheney, M. (2008) *The Five Commitments of a Leader*. Management Concepts, Vienna.

Leonard, M. & Frankel, A. (2012) *How Can Leaders Influence a Safety Culture?* The Health Foundation, London.

Lewin, K. (1939) Available from http://www.nwlink.com/-donclark/index.html. Accessed on 15 February 2013.

Lombardi, V. (1959) *1959 Green Bay Packers Season*. Available from http://www/en.wikipedia.org/wiki/1959_Green_Bay_Packers_season#cite_ref-1. Accessed on 16 March 2013.

Maben, J. & Griffiths, P. (2008) *Nurses in Society: Starting the Debate*. National Nursing Research Unit at Kings College, London.

Neath, A. (2010) *Report from WebEx, 16th April 2010*. NHS Institute for Innovation and Improvement, Warwick.

National Health Service (NHS) (2000) *The NHS Plan: A Plan for Investment, a Plan for Reform*. NHS, London.

National Health Service (2010) *Guidance on Involving Adult NHS Service Users and Carers*. National Leadership and Innovation Agency for Healthcare, Wales.

National Health Service (2012) *NHS Confederation Annual Conference and Exhibition 2012*. Available from www.nhs.confed.org/2012. Accessed on 16 March 2013.

Nicholson, D. (2007) *What Matters to our Patients, Public and Staff*. DH, London.

Nicholson, D. (2013) *Equity and Excellence: Liberating the NHS*. DH, London.

Owen, J. (2005) *How to Lead*. Pearson, Harlow.

Queen's Nursing Institute (2010) *2020 Vision – Focusing on the Future of District Nursing*. QNI, London.

Radcliffe, S. (2009) *Future, Engage, Deliver*. Troubadour Publishing, Leicester.

Randall, S. (2013) *Leading Networks in healthcare*. The Health Foundation, London.

Rickman, D. (2011) *The Big Society – Anarchy with a Middle Class Twist?* Huffington Post Politics, UK.

Rowe, J. (2006) Non-defining leadership. *Kybernetes*, 35 (10), 1528–1537.

Senge, P. (1997) Through the eye of the needle. In: *Rethinking the Future* (ed. R. Gibson, pp. 122–146. Nicholas Brealey, London.

Stogdill, R. (1974) *Handbook of Leadership: A Survey of Theory and Research*. Free Press, New York.

Taffinder, P. (2006) *The Leadership Crash Course: How to Create a Personal Leadership Value*, 2nd edn. KoganPage, London.

Wanless, D. (2002) *Securing our future health: taking a long-term view – the Wanless Report*. DH, London.

Wyatt, S. & Loder, J. (2010) How big society ideas can break new ground. *Health Service Journal*: 18–19.

15

Social Innovation and Enterprise

Agnes Fanning

Faculty of Society and Health, Buckinghamshire New University,
High Wycombe, UK

Introduction

Over the past decade, we have witnessed a drive to deliver care closer to home (DH 2010a), and with the decline in staff numbers and the merging of organisations, staff are being encouraged to be creative in their practice yet remain within the boundaries of their professionalism. There is limited evidence, however, to determine how community practitioners are prepared for such changing roles and their associated impact as new demands will require practitioners to address the Government's drive to bring care closer to home (DH 2010a) through demonstration of innovative practice. To enable government initiatives to be implemented, community practitioners will have to confront existing professional boundaries, work with limited resources and work more cost-effectively without compromising care quality. Community practitioners of the future are going to have to be ambitious to enable them to find ways to improve community healthcare services.

The Department of Health (DH) in 2006 stated that they would 'bring health into the local community'; this can only be done effectively if practitioners can listen to the needs of their patients/clients and introduce new initiatives, which will involve the local communities. There has to be an element of entrepreneurial spirit if a practitioner is going to work outside of the normal parameters and social innovation in the community setting will attract community practitioners who are ambitious to find ways to improve community health services. This chapter will address some of the ways that innovation can be captured to best serve the health and social needs of the communities.

Community and Public Health Nursing, Fifth Edition. Edited by David Sines,
Sharon Aldridge-Bent, Agnes Fanning, Penny Farrelly, Kate Potter and Jane Wright.
© 2013 John Wiley & Sons, Ltd. Published 2013 by John Wiley & Sons, Ltd.

What is social innovation?

The term social innovation entered the vocabulary in the aftermath of the French revolution and has been used since the seventeenth century, being used regularly in the 1860s and ensuing decades (Social Innovation 2012). Social innovation as an activity was often regarded negatively and was frequently considered to lead to risks with uncontrollable consequences. Social innovation is about individuals who propel social change through transformative forces, and it also refers to new strategies, concepts, ideas and organisations that meet social needs (Oxford Dictionary 2011). It is not a new concept, it has been in existence since the beginning of the seventeenth century, but it is relatively new in the health field (McSherry & Douglas 2011). A resurgence of social innovation occurred, however, in the second half of the twenty-first century with a number of social entrepreneurs emerging who are already waiting and ready to be discovered and nurtured into positive action (Clark 2009).

The terms social enterprise and social innovation are often used interchangeably, but it should be understood that social enterprise refers to organisational change, whilst social innovation refers to the individual who presents with innovative ideas and who can influence and improve society (in the case of the health service, such persons would normally be part of a social enterprise but could also be a member of a National Health Service (NHS) Community Trust). In the United Kingdom, there are currently 68,000 social enterprises, and health-related social enterprises make up a small percentage of these, with an increase in activity expected in the health and social care field.

The overarching theme of social innovation is to identify new ways of working and participating with the local community. It is not meant to be a replacement for services already in place, but should be seen as a support by introducing innovation within existing services. It encourages participation and working with individuals and communities to promote well-being not only *for* them but also *with* them (Hubert 2010). An intuitive social innovator will have identified a need to experiment and introduce new ways of working to provide an effective alternative to bring about this social change. Social innovation relies on schemes, suggesting that it goes hand in hand with subversion and revolution, leaving no system unchallenged (Bornstein 2007, p. 13), providing a means for transforming society.

The philosophy of social innovation encourages the joining together of individuals with an innovative concept. Practitioners are encouraged to work within this concept with individuals from the community to enable innovative 'ideas' to become a reality. Practitioners will need to develop these skills to make this happen whilst recognising that transforming a new concept from the planning stage into reality suggests that an element of risk must be evident. However, such changes will not just happen passively – they will need to be developed actively, and on occasions, change may cause disharmony and disagreement amongst team members and managers. However, social innovation can serve to demonstrate positive connectivity between the perceived innovation and government and local public policies, and when this occurs, opportunities exist for service redesign and the creation of service improvement. It is for this reason that community practitioners must be vocal in their attempt to promote this new way of working. They must be able to plan, develop and put their ideas into practice (Bornstein 2007, p. 22). In doing so, policymakers become aware of the benefits of working with social innovators, thus breaking down many of the barriers that exist today between public sector organisations and social enterprises.

Social innovators provide challenges and activities that will stretch their teams to work beyond their comfort zone in crossing boundaries to achieve a desired outcome. Social innovators will require knowledge in areas such as budgeting, project management, finance, pitching for investment and business planning. If a community practitioner does not innately have these skills, they will invariably find ways to obtain these skills – it may mean attending study days on budgeting and working with a finance department for a short time, or, in many cases, the innovation they wish to pursue may present with a sense of immediacy, therefore requiring advice and support from experts to assist in the development of the innovation. Social innovators possess vision and an inner drive and passion to improve quality of care for their patient/client. Such qualities should be recognised as central tenets of any social change model (Bornstein 2007, p. 27).

Fundamental to professional practice are the linkage of theory and practice and the acquisition of knowledge to blend in within the practice setting, encouraging imaginative and innovative solutions (Raelin 2000). Knowledge is learnt for work, through work and in work (Rounce & Workman 2005). However, successful innovation also demands that practitioners are confident and skilled in the art of promoting change and service transformation in order to secure and deliver real benefits for their patient/client groups. They will also need to work with commissioners, accountants and chief executives to execute their vision and ensure active engagement with their colleagues and other agencies.

Research on social innovation

There is limited evidence to determine how community health professionals are prepared for the role and impact of innovative practice. However, a number of global research studies have been conducted on social innovation (Gardner *et al.* 2007; Goldenberg *et al.* 2009; Goldsmith 2010; Murray *et al.* 2010) that have no direct relevance to community health in the United Kingdom. However, there are lessons to be learnt such as the inner drive and passion that each social innovator appears to hold. Ross *et al.*'s (2011) study, however, did look at the professional and personal features and mechanisms on innovation and outcomes in nursing, which claimed that the link between a supporting organisation and personal characteristics is influential in the context of transacting the innovation. A further study by Redfern and Harris (2011) claims that innovation in nursing requires managerial support and that nurses need to be skilled in driving innovation forward. Frequently, nurses are directed towards management courses to further their leadership skills, and many of these focus on how best to motivate staff and how to work effectively in teams (Frankel 2008). However, many of these leadership and management programmes do not tackle the issue of innovation in any depth and may therefore limit skills acquisition on how best to make a noticeable impact on innovative practice. Despite the existence of a paucity of primary research in this area, a wealth of literature does exist beyond the United Kingdom (Maddock *et al.* 2006; Welch *et al.* 2008; Suhonen & Paasivaara 2011). A number of agencies are also promoting innovative practice, and organisations such as the Florence Nightingale Institute, the Royal College of Nursing, The Queen's Nursing Institute and The Young Foundation are all engaged in the support of individual nurses who display potential as aspiring social innovators. The Young Foundation is another pioneer in the field of social innovation, having always had their roots in the community and encouraging service transformation and service improvement.

Within the NHS, the issue of social enterprise and social innovation has grown in importance since the DH (2010c) carried out an evaluation of 26 social enterprises across the health and social care sector. This evaluation demonstrated that social enterprise was a catalyst for delivering services in an innovative way. The DH (DH 2009, p. 43) has claimed that they will 'align its entire work programme to support NHS organizations to meet the challenges ahead'. However, the importance of supportive management cannot be emphasised enough if this is to happen.

Characteristics of a social innovator

The traditional caricature of social innovation is that the innovator may be regarded a little eccentric, often a loner, but committed to making changes within society. Bird and Roddick (1991), who founded *The Big Issue* as a means of offering homeless people the opportunity to earn a legitimate income, are an example of such innovators. Their way of achieving this passion was to observe people and learn from them and to have the ability to visualise a better life for homeless people. This innovation has gone on to improve the lives of many homeless people, which has eased a social problem and is still going strong 20 years on. This innovation was successful because Bird and Roddick believed that they could make a difference to society. Community practitioners wishing to introduce innovation into their practice will be expected to be committed to making this happen and to ensure that such changes impact positively on the services that they deliver to their client group. The NHS, however, are not always ready to take on the challenges presented by proactive practitioners or by individuals with maverick tendencies (Prentis 2011). Nevertheless, whilst the manager may not be the innovator, their role is to support those practitioners who do have innovative vision. Often the innovation may require the need to change systems, attitudes, expectations and behaviours (Bornstein 2007, p. 47). Someone who did just that was Florence Nightingale, who when she was faced with the high mortality rate of soldiers in Scutari set about looking at the public health issues, which were impacting on the loss of lives. She reorganised the military hospital, introduced laundry rooms, ensured soldiers ate with sterilised cutlery and requested that all clothes were laundered in boiled water. This was no easy feat for a woman in the nineteenth century, but her resilience and determination and her knowledge of medical commissions and medical reports and statistics (Bornstein 2007, p. 43) enabled her to use her innovative approach, power and unwavering belief in the rightness of her ideas (Bornstein 2007, p. 47) to introduce a new approach to nursing.

Florence Nightingale displayed characteristics such as those listed in the succeeding text, and these same characteristics are required of social innovators in 2013. Social innovators will be required to:

- Challenge existing practice
- Listen to people's views
- Get involved in public consultation and influence change and policy
- Work with local people and Clinical Commissioning Groups (CCGs) to indentify local needs
- Become involved with shaping future services
- Work with restructuring of services
- Understand white board economics
- Demonstrate resilience
- Be flexible
- Be able to survive adversity
- Demonstrate visionary leadership
- Utilise technical support effectively
- Be involved with risk-taking activities
- Work within the systems and processes to create and sustain their vision.
- Embrace failure and learn from the experience.

Social innovation and community health

There is recognition amongst politicians, policymakers and the healthcare community that more healthcare provision needs to be delivered through primary and community-based care, underpinned by public involvement in health improvement in order to enable a shift away from over-reliance on acute sector care. Such policy imperatives assist the healthcare service to evolve to meet the increasing challenges presented by an ageing population and by an increased demand for case management of those with long-term, complex conditions, in a way that allows patients to retain and regain an active role in society.

The NHS reviews of the last decade (Wanless 2002, 2004), the Darzi Report (DH 2010a), the World Health Organisation (2000), the Prime Minister's Commission on the Future of Nursing and Midwifery in England (DH 2010a) and the Royal College of Nursing (2010) have all recognised the need to upgrade the role of community nursing in order to respond to government policy. The 2012 coalition government also recognised the need for greater emphasis to be placed on the delivery of innovative, public health-oriented healthcare in the community, with social enterprise being seen as central to the delivery of improved health outcomes (DH 2010d). Empowered community health practitioners can play a significant part in designing and delivering the neighbourhood-based, joined-up approach that the Government envisions in its new public health service. Government policies offer a real opportunity to empower community health providers to develop and deliver innovative new health services that save money and improve quality of life.

Primary care is where the majority of services are being delivered to patients/clients, thus requiring that traditional practices must be challenged to make way for innovative approaches to care (Sines *et al*. 2009). The NHS Institute for Innovation and the Improvement and National Innovation Centre (NHS 2011) claim that most innovation actually comes from staff who operate at the interface of primary care and who are working close to the patient and not, as may be suggested, by more remote policymakers and senior physicians. The Darzi Report (DH 2010a) recommends the provision of care closer to home. Increased patient choice places community practitioners in a central position to drive the innovation that will create an NHS where more of service is focused on prevention and provided increasingly in the community and in people's homes. More innovation should come from the front line of nursing and other allied health professionals who 'put the patient first', challenging the top-down, target-driven culture that underlies the low morale found in so many parts of the NHS. Community health professionals face serious challenges ahead and will require new knowledge and resilience to be able to respond effectively if they are to meet the needs, and wishes, of service users within the context of a new NHS, which supports Lansley's (2012) view that the NHS 'requires healthy competition, which potentially will result in innovation'.

The NHS Institute for Innovation and Improvement has been recognising and awarding innovation through their NHS Innovation Challenge, and the DH (DH 2009) has also stated that they will respond to the challenges ahead and will support and empower clinicians who want to drive improvements. One example of positive practice, 'The Right to Provide' (DH 2011), is a delivery model championed by the Government (Prentis 2011). For positive practice to be effective, health professionals need to have belief in the innovative changes that they want to introduce, and they need to have confidence that this innovation will enhance the quality of care to patients/clients in their homes, at the same time as being cost effective to the organisation. These views do appear to be shared by the Government (DH 2011), but it does not solve the dilemma that many of the staff working in the NHS do not currently possess such prerequisite entrepreneurial skills.

Government policy provides huge opportunity for innovation, and the 'Health and Social Care White Paper' (DH 2010c) promotes innovation and supports The Big Society agenda in two ways: first, by challenging the bureaucratic and hierarchical management model of the NHS and devolving power to local organisations in order to design the best responses to public health issues and, second, by putting the patient at the heart of the process with clinicians, nurses and allied health professionals playing an essential mediation role in working with patients, communities, GPs and local authorities to deliver improved health and public health outcomes through innovative practice. Examples of successful innovation have been recognised by the NHS Innovation Challenge. The introduction of these awards in 2011 recognises innovation in organisations and teams and looks particularly at how organisations are working towards finding solutions and not focusing solely on the problem. Topics such as reducing avoidable GP/primary care attendances, innovative approaches to controlling infection and community engagement projects for the early detection of cancer are just a few of the innovations that have been recognised over the past few years. However, there are a number of other community innovations that are being implemented across the country, ranging from community developments that will lead to increased community activity to the generation of support networks that enable local community residents to take greater control of their lives. Other examples relate to the deployment of 24-hour coverage specialist nurses undertaking integrated care/multi-professional assessments, carried out in one location for children with complex health and social care needs. Such services reduce the anxiety and stress faced by families who so often report of the need to retell their story over and over again to various professionals in different locations. Other innovations such as setting up a lymphoedema service for non-cancerous patients have improved the lives of people who would normally not be offered such a service and who may often have been inappropriately treated in leg ulcer clinics. Such a provision is addressing social inequalities of care provision. Similarly, the formulation of a proactive caseload management tool for District Nurses aims to prevent the number of hospital admissions. The setting up of an integrated service between mental health services and the functions performed by diabetes specialist teams provide further evidence of health improvement and service innovation.

The Organisation for Economic Co-operation and Development (2011) suggests that social innovations such as those illustrated in this section can be seen as dealing with the welfare of individuals and communities, both as consumers and producers, confirming that these combined elements enhance both quality of life and activity levels.

Commissioning

The role of commissioning has taken on a major role in the procurement of care and has become increasingly important to the health system in England (DH 2012a). CCGs will be controlling the commissioning budgets from April 2013, and the NHS Commissioning Boards will be commissioning primary care and community services. At this time of change within the NHS, social innovators will also have the opportunity to market their services. In selling their service to CCGs, they will need to demonstrate that their service is delivering a safe, quality service that is also cost effective. The commissioners will need to be persuaded that the innovative practitioner has piloted their idea and that it has proven to be beneficial to client and the organisation. One of the key functions of the NHS Commissioning Board is to improve quality and outcomes and demonstrate value for money (NHS 2012).

The NHS commissioning for quality and innovation (CQUIN) standard framework provides an ideal platform within which social innovators are able to demonstrate the effectiveness and productivity of their schemes and innovative practice. The CQUIN payment framework gives commissioners the power to reward excellence, by linking a proportion of English healthcare providers' income to the achievement of local quality improvement goals (DH 2012b). In 2012, for example, Yorkshire and Humber were awarded £150,000 for three innovative community projects. It is likely that these services will continue to be commissioned in the longer term as they are recognised as adding value to both patients and the organisations that procure them.

Approaches to social innovation

Often an innovation is an idea that occurs and it does not necessarily have any specific boundaries. An idea comes about that makes a practitioner think 'this could be done so much better and could be more cost effective if transacted differently'. Such ways of thinking often result in a change in relationships within local delivery teams or within the organisations that support them. Innovation though needs careful planning and demands the creative blending of ideas from a variety of sources (Murray *et al.* 2010, p. 8), with most people trying to innovate being aware of only a fraction of the methods they could be using (Murray *et al.* 2010, p. 2). Innovation is a combination of ideas, actions, environmental conditions, structural systems and resources applied to a range of social and health conditions. Combining these provides an effective recipe for a social innovation. The Centre for Social Innovation (2012) suggests that the introduction of diversity into any given situation will provoke discovery and that by balancing these characteristics a dynamic approach will be stimulated that enables new ideas to germinate and blossom.

Innovation therefore has a vital role to play if the NHS is to continue to improve outcomes for patients and deliver value for money (DH 2012a). The NHS has recognised this and has promoted and encouraged such innovation through their NHS innovation challenges whereby practitioners are invited to design and support the creation of a culture of innovation in the NHS. The DH sees this as an essential part of the NHS leadership role.

Community health practitioners are in an influential position by being able to contribute to local needs assessment and mapping. These views are endorsed by The Queen's Nursing Institute (QNI 2009) which claims that 'Community Nurses in England are at the centre of one of the most significant developments in the health service since its origin in 1948'. Innovation is also recognised through organisations such as the Royal College of Nursing Frontline First Innovation Awards that expose excellent practice and encourage wider dissemination of service transformation initiatives that are at the cutting edge of thinking (McLellan 2012). Bornstein (2007, p. 121) claims that social innovators do not immediately make themselves or their idea known, but they just do things naturally. It is almost as if it is second nature to them, but they can sometimes become frustrated at the bureaucracy that often accompanies the implementation phase of a new idea. One such example is that of The Open Door Project (www.opendoorcare.co.uk), which was set up by a Health Visitor who had been working in one of the most deprived areas in England. It was recognised that there were a high number of homeless people (more than 1000) in the area; many were asylum seekers and drug users and were not registered with a GP. It took some time for this to be acknowledged by the local team and for funding to be arranged to support this group of people. The project eventually came together with the result that the majority of emergent new services are being delivered by Specialist Nursing Teams and community support workers. The overall philosophy of The Open Door Project is to work with the public health agenda to promote screening alongside the provision of housing and benefit advice. The impact such an innovation has had on the population of this deprived area has had life-changing consequences for a number of the service users who have accessed the service. A project such as this could not have been carried out in isolation but was successful due to collaborative working practices between health and social care and voluntary agencies. Another example of a successful collaborative project is the Newquay Pathfinder pilot project, which seeks to provide an inter-agency approach between health and social care and the voluntary sector that aims to reduce the risk of inappropriate hospital admissions for older people. The project co-ordinates and navigates the most appropriate volunteer service to the individual, helping to manage the demand for health-related services by mainstreaming prevention at a local level so that older people receive better and more appropriate care closer to home. The DH (DH 2009) promotes the concept of collaborative working, giving examples of integrated teams and health and social care organisations working together. As mentioned earlier, there are currently 68 000 social enterprises in the United Kingdom (a selection of these being in the health field). This does prove the point that individuals are taking ownership of their ideas and are taking charge of their 'vision' by translating innovation into practice.

Social innovation as a concept

Innovation is very personal to each individual and individual area, and as such, each innovation must be judged against the impact that the proposed service change will have on the local community.

Imagine a conversation between the District Nurse team leader and the Chief Executive of the organisation:

DN   'I would like to discuss a new service that I wish to develop'.
CEO   'What is wrong with the service we are currently delivering?'

Case study no. 1

You have recently joined a District Nursing team working in an inner-city team where you will be the team leader. Your team consists of 2 District Nurses (1 full time (you) and 1 × part time 0.5), 1 staff nurse (full time) and 3 × band 4 healthcare practitioners (1 × full time and 2 × 0.5). No 24-hour service exists for patients/clients on your caseload, but this is something that you would like to implement. You see this as a means of improving the quality of service for patients/clients.

What are you hoping to gain from introducing this service?
What is the problem you are seeking to solve and what your intended solution?
What steps will you have to take to begin the process?
Who will you need to discuss this with?
Will you require additional funding?
How will you calculate the additional funding?
How will you begin the process of implementing this plan?
What time limit have you set for implementation of this plan?
How will you evaluate the success of your planned interventions?

DN 'Patients are not getting 24 hour care in their homes'.

CEO 'Why do they need to have 24 hour care?'

DN 'Patients are calling emergency services unnecessarily at night'.

CEO 'How do you know this, are you making an assumption?'

DN 'I have the 'stats' here – DN produces the stats for the past 3 months showing the number of call outs that have been requested from patients on the DN caseload'.

CEO 'Just because these patients have been seen at night either by a duty doctor or taken to the emergency department does not show that this would have been prevented by the provision of a 24 hour service'.

DN 'The stats show that patients were seen in the emergency department and were sent home again with either a change in their treatment or to be told to visit their GP the next day. A number of these patients have been seen three times in 3 months in A & E. The District Nursing team would know their patients and would have been able to assess the situation and if appropriate would have been able to prescribe requisite medicines. Overall the patient would have had a much better experience and would have been able to remain in their own home at no extra cost to the organization'.

CEO 'There would have been a cost though for the provision of your service'.

DN 'Having looked at the skills within the team, 24 hour cover could be arranged by increasing the staff with a 0.5 DN and a 0.5 staff nurse. This would cost the organization approximately £30000.00 in extra salary support. However if only 10 patients were admitted over a 12 month period you would break even. A 6 month pilot study could be arranged to prove these facts'.

CEO   'Carry out the pilot and I would like to see a monthly breakdown of the A & E stats and the number of times that the 24 hour DN service has been called upon'.

DN   'Thank you, I know this will be beneficial to both patients and the organization'.

This innovation was recognised as being a project that could potentially save the organisation a substantial amount of money. This project may not have been considered if the District Nurse had not been prepared to present an evidence-based solution to the problem. It is not enough to identify a problem; the answer is in having a sensible, realistic solution. In this situation, the District Nurse had calculated how much each visit to the A & E Department was costing, which was approximately £70.00 per visit for each individual patient seen (nationally it is shown that 41% of all A & E patients were discharged with no follow-up required; DH 2011), and then if the patient was admitted to hospital, on average, this was costing £3000 per patient stay in hospital. The cost of staff salary had been calculated enabling the District Nurse to show the cost benefit to the organisation.

Later two further case studies are presented, work through the process of solving the problem and creating a solution to the problem identified.

Case study no. 2

You are working as a Health Visitor in a rural village. Your team consists of one full-time Health Visitor (you), one staff nurse (children's nurse) and one nursery nurse. All staff are full time. You have had a number of requests from mothers to deliver a sleep clinic as there are a number of mothers who are challenged by not being able implement effective sleep patterns for their children with the consequence that they were missing out on sleep themselves.

You would like to set up a clinic where mothers can attend to receive specific advice on sleep patterns and sleep behaviour. The key questions to ask are:

What is the solution to this problem?
Can a service be delivered with the current resources?
What will the benefit be of such a programme?
Who would be involved in the service?
How will you know whether the service is successful?
What will the overall value of your solution be?
What measures will be used to calculate the value of this provision?

Case study no. 3

You are working as a Community Learning Disability Nurse and you have identified that patients who have a learning disability are not being followed up for conditions such as cardiac obstructive pulmonary disease (COPD). You would like to set up a clinic to invite patients with learning disability to attend so that you can assess their long-term conditions and arrange their longer-term management plans. The key questions you need to consider are:

What is the problem?
What is the solution?
How are you going to access the names of patients that fit this category?
Will you require extra resources?
Who do you need to discuss this plan with?
Where will these assessments take place?
Who will be involved?
How will consent be obtained?
How frequent will the clinics be held?
Have you considered which referral system you will use?
Is there a time plan for the implementation of this project?

This is a group of patients/clients living in the community who often are 'the forgotten ones'. As a learning disability nurse, you will be used to being an advocate for your patients/clients, but at the same time you are promoting their independence and autonomy. Consider this when addressing the earlier points.

On occasions, it is important to recognise that requests from patients/clients will not always yield an answer to their problem. However, on working through the earlier questions, you will be able to identify whether it is worth pursuing a project.

Conclusion

In conclusion, this is the right time for innovation in community healthcare to be recognised. There are four primary reasons for this:

1. Shift of power: The NHS White Paper (DH 2010b) has recognised that there needs to be a shift of power over health budgets to patients and GPs. This shift in policy towards patient choice has the potential to drive and reward innovation provided by community health services as they seek more cost-effective and better ways to deliver patient care.
2. New types of providers: In line with 'The Big Society' healthcare reforms now promote the delivery of public services by social enterprises. This will enable staff to take control of public services and run them as public sector cooperatives.

3. NHS budget reforms: The NHS White Paper promises a real-term increase in spending on the NHS, with an increased demand on service delivery; there is a need to realise £20 billion in efficiency savings by 2014. These savings will include a 45% reduction in spend on NHS management, thus affording front-line workers the opportunity to develop their innovative and entrepreneurial skills.
4. Opportunities for innovation: There is a shift away from a target-driven culture to one focusing on a limited number of key outcomes. Healthcare providers will have more opportunities to be innovative in their provision of services and will have greater encouragement to test new ideas for service provision.

Community healthcare is changing rapidly, and practitioners will be required to be flexible, responsive and be able to deliver quality, cost-effective care with limited resources. Innovation provides an opportunity for many community health practitioners to demonstrate what their 'idea' can do for their community. Now is an exciting time for all community practitioners to grasp clinical challenges by creating innovative solutions, which can be implemented to drive their innovation forward. The current climate in the NHS is encouraging creative, innovative, safe and cost-effective practice. Community practitioners should embrace these opportunities with confidence and courage.

Eagles Flourish when they are free to fly (Blanchard 2003, p. 74).

References

Blanchard, K. (2003) *The Heart of a Leader*, Lighthouse Books, Boulder, CO.
Bird, J. & Roddick, G. (1991) Available from www.bigissue. Accessed on 20 August 2012.
Bornstein, D. (2007) *How to Change the World: Social Entrepreneurs and the Power of New Ideas*, Oxford University Press, Oxford.
Centre for Social Innovation (2012) *Where Change Happens*, CSI, Toronto.
Clark, M. (2009) *Social Business*, DH, London.
Department of Health (DH) (2006) *Our Health Our Care Our Say*, Crown, London.
DH (2009) *Working to Put People First: The Strategy for the Adult Social Care Workforce in England*, DH, London.
DH (2010a) *Front Line Care. Report by the Prime minister's Commission on the Future of Nursing and Midwifery in England.* Crown, London.
DH (2010b) *High quality care for all, next stage review*, Darzi Report, DH, London.
DH (2010c) *Equity and Excellence: Liberating the NHS (White Paper)*, Crown, London.
DH (2010d) *Leading the way through social enterprise: the Social Enterprise Pathfinder Programme evaluation.* Crown, London.
DH (2011) *A Guide to the Right to Provide*, Crown, London.
DH (2012a) *Using the Commissioning for Quality and Innovation (CQUIN) payment framework.* Crown, London.
DH (2012b) *Public health, adult social care, and the NHS, Innovation.* Crown, London.
Frankel, A. (2008) What leadership styles should senior nurses develop? *Nursing Times, 104* (35), 23–24.

Gardner, C., Acharya, T. & Yach, D. (2007) Technological and social innovation: a unifying new paradigm for global health. *Health Affairs, 26* (4), 1052–1061.

Goldsmith, S. (2010) *The Power of Social Innovation: How Civic Entrepreneurs Ignite Community Networks for Good*, Jossey Bass, Philadelphia, PA.

Goldenberg, M., Kamoji, W., Orton, L. & Williamson, M. (2009) *Social Innovation in Canada: An Update*, Canadian Policy Research Networks, Ontario.

Hubert, A. (2010) *Empowering people, driving change: social innovation in the European Union, innovations in primary care, 2005*. IPC, Hampshire.

Lansley, A. (13 February 2012) *The Guardian*, London.

Maddock, A., Kralik, D. & Smith, J. (2006) Clinical Governance improvement initiatives in community nursing. *Clinical Governance: An International Journal, 11* (3), 198–212.

McLellan, A. (2012) HSJ Awards 2012-cutting-edge thinkers triumph. *Health Service Journal, 21*: 1–36.

McSherry, R. & Douglas, M. (2011) Innovation in nursing practice: a means to tackling the global challenges facing nurses, midwives and nurse leaders and managers in the future. *Journal of Nursing Management, 19* (2), 165–169.

Murray, R., Caulier-Grice, J. & Mulgan, G. (2010) *The Open Book of Social Innovation*, The Young Foundation & the National Endowment for Science, Technology and the Arts, London.

National Health Service (NHS) (2011) The NHS Institute for Innovation and the Improvement and National Innovation Centre, London.

NHS (2012) *Developing the NHS Commissioning Board*, NHS, London.

Open Doors Project Available from www.opendoorcare.co.uk. Accessed on 12 September 2012.

Organisation for Economic Co-Operation and Development (2011) *Fostering innovation to address social challenges*. www.oecd.org/science/innovationinsciencetechnologyandindustry/47863.

Oxford Dictionary (2011) *The Oxford Mini English Dictionary*, Oxford University Press, Oxford.

Prentis, D. (2011) In: *Social Enterprises and the NHS: Changing Patterns of Ownership and Accountability* (eds L. Marks & D. Hunter). pp. 2, Foreword. Centre for Public Policy and Health, Durham, NC.

Raelin, J. (2000) *Work-Based Learning: The New Frontier of Management Development*, Prentice Hall, Upper Saddle River, NJ.

Redfern, S. & Harris, R. (2011) The impact of nursing innovations in the context of governance and incentives. *Journal of Research in Nursing, 16* (3), 274–294.

Ross, F., Redfern, S. Harris, R., & Christian, S. (2011) The impact of nursing innovations in the context of governance and incentives. *Journal of Research in Nnursing*, May Vol. 16, (no. 3), 274–294.

Royal College of Nursing (RCN) (2010) *Pillars of the community: the RCN's policy position on the development of the registered workforce in the community*, RCN, London.

Rounce, K. & Workman, B. (2005) Introduction to work-based learning in health and social care. In: *Work-Based Learning in Health Care: Applications and Innovations* (eds. Rounce, K & Workman, B.). pp. 145–160. Kingsham Press, Chichester.

Sines, D., Saunders, M. & Forbes-Burford, J. (2009) *Community Health Care Nursing*, 4th edn. Wiley-Blackwell, Oxford.

Suhonen, M. & Paasivaara, L. (2011) Nurse Managers' challenges in project management. *Journal of Nursing Management, 19*, 1028–1036.

The Queen's Nursing Institute (2009) *2020 Vision: Focusing on the Future of District Nursing*, QNI, London.

Wanless, D. (2002) *Securing Our Future Health: Taking a Long-Term View*, DH, London.

Wanless, D. (2004) *Wanless report: health spending and public health*. DH, London.

Welch, R., Mooney, J., Shindul, J., *et al.* (2008) The university/community partnership: transdisciplinary course development. *Journal of Interdisciplinary Care, 22* (5), 461–474.

World health Organisation (WHO) (2000) *The World Health Report 2000 – Health Systems: improving performance*. WHO, Switzerland.

16

Adult Vulnerability in the Community

Jason Schaub

Faculty of Society and Health, Buckinghamshire New University,
High Wycombe, UK

Introduction

When examining the adult safeguarding literature for community health-care nurses, there are a number of areas of note that arise including mental health, disabilities, domestic abuse and alcohol/substance misuse. The first two of these groups are well represented in the literature, but the latter two less comprehensively (Peckover & Chidlaw 2007). Given their prevalence and impact upon communities, it seems reasonable to explore them more fully. As a result, this chapter will describe the shifting framework for adult safeguarding and then explore domestic abuse and alcohol/substance misuse.

Adult safeguarding

Beginning in the 1970s, adult abuse first entered the public sense with 'granny battering' (Baker 1975). Since then, adult safeguarding has had a slow and inconsistent development to our current provision of safeguarding guidance and legislation.

Safeguarding adults as an area of work has been described as having unclear boundaries, and in 'England it is recognised only piecemeal in legislation' (Mandelstam 2009, p. 22). It is not as enshrined in legislation, or public concern, as child protection (DH 2009). However, it appears that the implementation of local safeguarding adult boards

Community and Public Health Nursing, Fifth Edition. Edited by David Sines,
Sharon Aldridge-Bent, Agnes Fanning, Penny Farrelly, Kate Potter and Jane Wright.
© 2013 John Wiley & Sons, Ltd. Published 2013 by John Wiley & Sons, Ltd.

will soon be required to be statutory (Spencer-Lane 2011). In the past several years, there have been a number of safeguarding adults policies, consultations and inspectorate reports published (DH 2009, 2010; Law Commission 2010, 2011; NHSLA 2010; Mandelstam 2011). With this recently produced array of guidance, it may be helpful to describe some definitions of adult safeguarding and the basic legislative guidance as they currently exist.

Definitions of abuse of adults

The Department of Health guidance *No Secrets* defines a vulnerable adult as a person 'who is or may be in need of community care services by reason of mental or other disability, age or illness; and who is or may be unable to take care of him or herself, or unable to protect him or herself against significant harm or exploitation' (DH 2000, pp. 8–9). The updated legal framework published by SCIE, in collaboration with Department of Health (DH) defines more clearly and delineates the different areas of abuse as harm that is 'physical, sexual, psychological, financial or material, neglect and acts of omission, discriminatory or institutional' (Mandelstam 2011, p. 2). The Law Commission report, *Adult Social Care*, identifies harm as:

- Ill treatment (including sexual abuse, exploitation and forms of ill treatment that are not physical);
- The impairment of health (physical or mental) or development (physical, intellectual, emotional, social or behavioural);
- Self-harm and neglect;
- Unlawful conduct, which adversely affects property, rights or interests (e.g. financial abuse). (Spencer-Lane 2011, p. 277).

This framework has importantly added self-neglect to the considerations for adult abuse for England and Wales. The term 'adult at risk' has supplanted vulnerable adult in the Government language, and adult safeguarding has superseded adult protection. The Government's framework for safeguarding adults contains three concepts: protection, justice and empowerment (Minister of State 2010). With these changes in definition, it can appear that the situation is in flux for the sector, which can cause confusion about process and procedural implementation for practitioners. What can be helpful however is to note that the definitions appear to becoming more expansive and definitive as we begin to scrutinise the abuse of adults with some of the vigour that has only previously been applied to child abuse. A noted concern within the safeguarding adult's literature, for example, is the financial abuse of older people and the abuse of adults by those closest to them, whether they be family members or paid carers.

The prevalence of abuse of adults is difficult to accurately determine, and studies claiming veracity often have a number of qualifiers, which restrict their scope. One of the most comprehensive recent projects is the O'Keefe *et al.*'s (2007) UK *Study of*

Abuse and Neglect of Older People: Prevalence Survey Report, which suggested that 2.6% of the population is likely to have suffered abuse or neglect over the past year, approximately 227 000 older people per year. Importantly, this study did not include abuse or neglect of older people by nonfamily members or institutions and only focused upon the abuse of those over 66 years of age. These exclusions are likely to cause expectations that adult abuse might be less prevalent than it actually is and compounded by the specific issues for adults to feel able to self-report abuse. Some nurses have also advised that they do not regard themselves to be skilled in detecting or responding to adult protection incidents (Ramsay 2009).

Given this lack of clarity, the flow chart for referring and responding to adult abuse concerns is replicated in this chapter from *Clinical Governance and Adult Safeguarding* (DH 2010) (Fig. 16.1).

This flow chart shows how concerns for abuse should be progressed and the stages of the process. What is important in this process is that 'the person discovering/witnessing the event' is to report his or her concern to the Local Safeguarding Team (DH 2010, p. 8). These reports are to be reviewed within 24 hours in local arrangements between health- and social care agencies. These arrangements seek to foster better communication

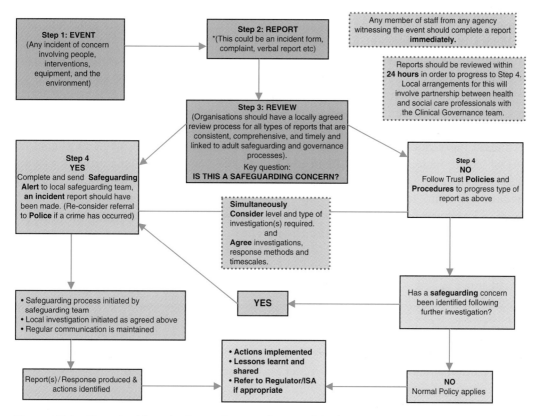

Figure 16.1   Flow chart for referring and responding to adult abuse concerns

and inter-agency working in these complex situations, which often occur across a number of different settings and require a high degree of co-operation between sectors.

Legal framework of adult safeguarding

As described earlier, the legal structures that underpin adult safeguarding are poorly defined and very recent in comparison to child protection. In the United Kingdom, the inception was with the implementation of the practice guidelines *No Longer Afraid: The Safeguard of Older People in Domestic Settings* (DH 1993), which suggested that 'elder abuse' was an issue that required attention of services. These guidelines were revised in *No Secrets* (DH & Home Office 2000)[1], which provides guidance for service providers, primarily local authorities. It set out a framework that placed local authorities at the helm of investigations and responses to the abuse of vulnerable adults. In comparison to other guidance, it is much less prescriptive, for it does not require the establishment of adult protection committees but only recommends that they be convened. Importantly, this document is only statutory for local authorities and remains advisory only for other agencies, including the NHS. This delineation confirms that the status of adult safeguarding has not had the same level of penetration in the sector compared to child protection legislation and guidance. The *No Secrets* guidance (DH & Home Office 2000) identifies institutional abuse as one of its areas of concern, noting that adults at risk of harm are particularly prone to institutional forms of discrimination and abuse.

More general obligations are prescribed for NHS trusts and their employees under the NHS Act 2006, but there are no specific acts that cover adult safeguarding. As a result, we must examine guidance and frameworks from further afield. The Association of Directors of Social Services (ADSS) published a national framework of standards (ADSS 2005), which described the need for clear joint working and planning of a number of service organisations, including police and probation, NHS and voluntary organisations (who provide a remarkable amount of service provision for adults that might be at risk of harm). This framework was also advisory but proposed improvements to inter-agency team working with the effectiveness of health- and social care responses to adult safeguarding.

Mental Capacity Act 2005

The Mental Capacity Act 2005 has some far-reaching effects on service provision because it attempts to both protect and empower individuals at the same time (Mandelstam 2009). Included in its tenets is the right to 'make an unwise or eccentric

---

[1] This is for England only; Wales had similar guidance adopted in the same year (National Assembly of Wales, 2000).

decision' (Manthorpe *et al.* 2009). The Act suggests that persons should be thought to have capacity until assessed as not, which appears to be a departure from some normative practice, particularly with older people. A further core principle represented in the Act is that people may lack capacity for one decision but have the capacity to make a decision in another area; so each decision must be contextually assessed for capacity. It makes other provisions for specific circumstances, such as the Deprivation of Liberty Safeguards (DoLS) and Best Interest Assessments (BIA), which are applied in specific settings.

Recent adult safeguarding guidance

A review into the *No Secrets* guidance undertaken by the DH (2009) suggested that the NHS struggled to 'own' adult safeguarding and that implementation of the 2000 guidance was 'slow, patchy and inconsistent and...that much more needs to be done' (DH 2009 p. 37). This review also recommended an increased engagement in adult safeguarding as an area of note, with particular reference to the potential abuse adults might experience within institutional settings. This call for increased scrutiny within the NHS is likely to increase with the potential statutory setting for local safeguarding adult boards.

In addition to the review into *No Secrets*, there have been other changes occurring within the legal framework for adult safeguarding. The Law Commission was commissioned in 2008 to consult on the 'complex and confusing patchwork of legislation' for adult social care (Spencer-Lane 2011, p. 275), with a completed final report being published in 2011. This Commission consulted widely, and its report suggests that individual well-being must be the basis for all decisions made and actions carried out under the statute. It also takes into effect some of the principles of the Mental Capacity Act 2005 but suggesting that people are the best judge of their own needs, unless their capacity is compromised. Importantly for nurses in the community, another recommendation is for each local authority be given the responsibility to investigate concerns of abuse or neglect but that these investigations can be delegated to health services. Of equal importance was a recommendation that carers should be assessed without the need for them to make a formal request for an assessment and to remove the requirement for them to be providing a 'substantial amount of care on a regular basis' (Law Commission 2011, p. 69). This recommendation recognises the significant expectations placed upon carers by our society and the growing need for support for them. Lastly, a further recommendation for local safeguarding adult boards to become a statutory requirement seems to provide evidence of the need to provide a more robust structure for the protection of adults, akin to those provided for child protection.

This increased emphasis placed upon adult safeguarding is not enough, and further work needs to be undertaken, as research into practitioner responses to adult abuse suggests that a 'discrepancy ... often exists between the response outlined in policy documents and the views of staff about their own response' (Jenkins & Davies 2006, p. 37; see also Northway *et al.* 2004). This discrepancy was also highlighted by the previously mentioned DH review into *No Secrets* (2009). This gap might suggest that practitioners are potentially less clear about how and when to act upon potential abuse of adults in comparison with the more robust and embedded guidance that they refer to for child protection. This suggests that there might be a need for a higher level of scrutiny within the NHS to better observe and refer concerns of abuse or neglect of adults.

One of the confounding factors confronting community practice relates to the inter-professional nature of practice interventions. Safeguarding adults requires robust inter-agency working because of the demands and challenges that relate to information sharing and decision making (McKeough 2009; Reeves *et al.* 2011; Williams 2011). Such inter-agency working can be problematic for those working at the interface between health- and social care organisations or when service users are facing a change in their circumstance (for instance, when moving from home to a managed care setting).

Moving on from the policy and legislative setting for adult safeguarding, the next two sections discuss specific issues about the support of adults in the community: domestic violence and alcohol/substance misuse.

Domestic violence

Domestic violence is an issue requiring the consistent attention of community health-care nurses, health visitors, midwives and for those nurses in acute care settings (as well as other professionals, including social workers). Its impacts are widely researched and there are various programmes and support services that focus upon the provision of support to those people (the vast majority of whom are women and their children) that are experiencing abuse from their partners and ex-partners. This section does not aspire to provide an exhaustive delineation of the situation but rather to provide a description of key issues that influence community health-care nursing practice.

For context, the Home Office defines domestic violence as:

Any incident or pattern of incidents of controlling[2], coercive or threatening behaviour, violence or abuse between those aged 16 or over who are or have been intimate partners or family members regardless of gender or sexuality. This can encompass, but is not limited to, the following types of abuse:

- psychological
- physical
- sexual
- financial
- emotional (Home Office 2012)

---

[2] The Home Office defines controlling behaviour as 'a range of acts designed to make a person subordinate and/or dependent by isolating them from sources of support, exploiting their resources and capacities for personal gain, depriving them of the means needed for independence, resistance and escape and regulating their everyday behaviour. Coercive behaviour is: an act or a pattern of acts of assault, threats, humiliation and intimidation or other abuse that is used to harm, punish, or frighten their victim' (Home Office, 2012).

This definition suggests that there are various facets of abuse that may not be easily identifiable to those outside the relationship itself (such as psychological or sexual abuse). The controlling aspects of domestic violence can wreak havoc on individuals' life choices and significantly restrict their ability to engage meaningfully and confidently with the rest of society.

The prevalence of domestic violence in the United Kingdom

Every week two women are murdered by a current or former partner (DH 2005), and 54% of rapes in the United Kingdom were committed by a current or former partner (Walby *et al.* 2004). One out of every four women, or 4.8 million, between the ages of 16 and 59 has been affected by domestic violence (Home Office 2010). These statistics should suggest that the problem is not an isolated concern for certain groups or sectors but is actually a pervasive issue throughout our communities. Of note is the fact that more than 90% of domestic abuse is committed by men against women, even though there are other forms of domestic violence (such as violence from women against men or same-sex domestic violence) with less sweeping presentation (DH 2005).

Of interest for when domestic violence begins and occurs is that research into the health of mothers and children showed that 30% of domestic abuse began during pregnancy (The Confidential Maternal and Child Health Enquiry in England and Wales, cited by Humphreys & Houghton 2008). This study highlights the need for professionals to be aware that there are points in women's lives that are associated with higher risks of domestic abuse and that these periods require more scrutiny in order to elicit new experiences of domestic violence.

Effects of domestic violence

Some of the effects of domestic violence are not easy to define or detect, since they occur within the almost sacrosanct boundaries of people's homes. These effects, though, are significant and result in a range of concerning presentations for health-care professionals. A meta-analysis of a North American research, for example, showed that domestic violence is the cause of most mental health problems in women (Campbell 2002), with a stronger correlation found between domestic abuse and depression and post-traumatic stress disorder (PTSD) than any correlation associated with childhood sexual abuse. This same meta-analysis suggests that 'economic and educational resources might not protect women from being abused, but makes it easier for them to relatively quickly escape or end the violence, thus rendering them less likely to be currently abused' (Campbell 2002, p. 1331). This stronger correlation between domestic violence and mental health problems conflicts with our current societal construction of childhood sexual abuse being one of the most difficult experiences to suffer and suggests that the recovery from the former may be more difficult than that of the latter issue. Also, women with the requisite economic resources at their disposal may be able to escape violence more easily, but are not necessarily any less likely to experience the violence itself.

This ability to escape bears noting for situations where health professionals are engaging with families from different social classes. What must be remembered for these women, though, is that when they are able to escape a violent setting, the losses 'are concrete and immediate: loss of home, money, neighbours, pets and perhaps even children. The gains are vague and long term: freedom and independence. It takes great courage to make that move' (Thomas 2008). In addition, trauma resulting from abuse often remains unrecognised, and blaming the victim is not uncommon amongst health-care professionals (Humphreys & Thiara 2003). What is also helpful to consider is that the health burden of domestic violence is significantly greater than smoking and obesity or indeed any other risk factor (Humphreys *et al.* 2008). This burden can create stresses upon services, particularly those in the community, and needs further exploration so as to more adequately explain.

Whilst not pertinent to all cases, the effects of domestic violence on children in these homes are as worrying as those effects on their mothers. Children that live in families with domestic violence are more likely to suffer significant harm (Cleaver *et al.* 2011; see also Peralta *et al.* 2010), as defined by the Children Act 1989. Of particular concern is that in a national study of serious case reviews into child deaths (or severe maltreatment), nearly 'three quarters of the children [...] had been living with past or current domestic violence and or parental mental ill health and or substance misuse – often in combination' (Brandon *et al.* 2010, p. 112). This toxic combination is often impenetrable for services and may require significant inter-agency working in order to address and alleviate the consequences of such complex presentations.

Contextual issues

Whilst the prevalence and effects of domestic violence are of importance when examining this issue, contextual issues need to be also explored. Research exists to suggest that poverty, and community context, has an impact upon rates of domestic violence (Pearlman *et al.* 2003; Benson *et al.* 2004; Cleaver *et al.* 2011). These reports suggest, however, that the picture is not clear and much more research is needed to explain the contextual nature of domestic violence. This community context may be of issue when health-care professionals are tasked to engage within particular community groups, since it might appear that the presentation and effects of domestic violence can differ depending upon the community within which practitioners operate.

Research has also shown that the process of disclosing domestic abuse may require the support of a series of encounters with professionals, given the number of barriers that women have to overcome to seek assistance (Hester *et al.* 2007; Bourassa *et al.* 2008). This extended disclosure process is often frustrating to professionals, when processes request a linear, chronological and logical disclosure description. These disclosures require the use of risk assessments. Such risk assessment tools have a traditional place within services in the community and are used by both nurses and social workers. Their ability of such tools to predict risk accurately is often disputed, and as such research recommends that they are used with caution (Hoyle 2008). As such community health-care nurses need always to continue to be open to the potentiality of abuse occurring within the home.

Lastly, the RCN advises that in some areas of nursing (community nursing, health visiting, midwifery, A & E, mental health services, etc.), all patients should be screened for domestic abuse issues (Royal College of Nursing 2000, p. 7). This guidance recognises that the widespread prevalence and staggering impacts of domestic violence require that nurses should be ever mindful of the societal and health impacts of domestic violence and of their key role in identifying and addressing it.

What is important to note as a contextual issue is the different cultural presentations of domestic violence (Farrant 2003; Parmar *et al.* 2005). Whilst there is no significant difference in domestic violence rates between ethnic groups, women from Black and Minority Ethnic (BME) groups are much less likely to access statutory services (Batsleer *et al.* 2002). This difference in engagement requires that practitioners make specific efforts to support women from BME groups to access services and to encourage them to seek help. In particular, issues of language, mistrust of services and immigration issues all have impacts upon women's reporting of domestic violence, not to mention concerns that Children's Social Care services will remove their children (Rose *et al.* 2011). There are some cultural settings where the community pressure to avoid shame and dishonour are more pressing than in others, with a resulting array of forces that intersect differently. It is important that community nurses are mindful of these different presentations and needs.

Substance and alcohol misuse

In addition to the impacts of domestic violence, the related but discrete concerns for substance and alcohol misuse should also be considered (Plant *et al.* 2002). In fact, those sectors of society that have previously been thought to be immune to substance misuse are showing significant increases in abuse, older people being among them (Beynon 2009; Moy *et al.* 2011). Alcohol abuse amongst older people has been a noted issue for some time (Reid & Anderson 1997), with growing concern about the impact of this for older people (O'Connell 2003). This increased understanding suggests that there is yet more to learn about this burgeoning issue. What is interesting is that some research suggests that a third of older people begin misusing alcohol later in life (Resnick *et al.* 2003) and that up to 30% of men and 15% of women are drinking more alcohol than is recommended (Gossop & Moos 2008).

A further issue relates to the rise of substance misuse issues amongst older people. There are now likely to be twice as many older people needing treatment for a substance misuse issue between 2001 and 2020 (Gossop & Moos 2008). There are two factors that are affecting this rise: the first is the widely noted size of the 'baby-boom' generation (accepted as being born between 1946 and 1964) and, secondly, the comparatively higher incidence of substance use within this generation. The current societal construction of the substance misuser as a relatively younger, disengaged person may need some significant examining in order to shift the focus of services for the older, more established person with substance issues. These changes are already beginning to increase the financial burden upon service providers, because of the recent introduction of this previously missing service user profile. The issues of cost are important for the NHS, for alcohol alone has an estimated annual cost to the NHS of £2.7 billion (The NHS Information Centre, Lifestyles Statistics 2011a). The costs for substance misuse are less definitive, because of the relatively more hidden nature of the issue, but the range of figures given are between £3.7 and £6.8 billion to the NHS, criminal justice system and state benefits (BBC News 2002).

Similarly to the aforementioned concern for the differing presentation for domestic violence in communities, there is a noted regional variation to both substance and alcohol abuse (The NHS Information Centre, Lifestyles Statistics 2011a, b). This issue is of concern throughout the United Kingdom, with significant resources used to support people suffering from addictions. There may be less of an issue for substance misuse than for alcohol abuse, depending upon the region, but the effects and the need for targeted services for people with these issues are clear and relevant throughout the United Kingdom.

A concerning fact for working with these individuals is their complexity of their presenting needs. There are, for example, issues relating to dual diagnosis of substance misuse and mental health problems (Phillips & Johnson 2003), with 75% of users of substance misuse services reporting mental health problems (Weaver *et al.* 2002 cited in Cleaver *et al.* 2011). With this potential constellation of issues, providing community-based health care can be complicated. These concurrently presenting difficulties can create a web-like system of apparent impenetrability, making engagement with patients in these circumstances thorny and challenging.

Of note for community health nurses is that they are integral to the continued decrease of substance and alcohol issues (Owens *et al.* 2000; Keleher *et al.* 2009) but often feel that medical issues are given primacy of attention over health-promoting tasks (Wilhelmsson & Lindberg, 2009). Research has also found community nurses to be 'ill-prepared for working with substance misusers' (Peckover & Chidlaw 2007, p. 243). Peckover and Chidlaw (2007) have suggested that the discourse of care for these patients is absent within the district nursing literature. They found a reductionist provision of care to substance misusers, in marked contrast to the holistic care suggested as integral to community nursing. Some writers posit that this could be a result of increased risk when visiting substance misusers' homes (Peckover & Chidlaw 2007; Nursing Standard 2012), an issue not faced by nurses within acute care contexts. Conversely specialist nurses can assist with working with patients with alcohol misuse issues in the community (Fernandez 2009). Importantly, school nurses are being seen as increasingly important in educating young people about substance use, both alcohol and illegal substances (Stead & Stradling 2010), in the hope of increasing our societal engagement with this issue from an earlier age.

Conclusion

Whilst this chapter has explored some far-ranging issues for community nursing practice, there is a need to see them as being integral to the current work of community practitioners. The rapidly changing (and poorly defined) framework for adult safeguarding is an issue that requires attention by those practitioners within the community (which also includes social workers and other practitioners). What is known is that the changes in this arena are not likely to discontinue for the foreseeable future, and it is imperative that practitioners that engage with adults are aware of the changing nature of the context in which they practise. It is clear from the review of *No Secrets* (DH 2009) that there is further work to be undertaken in this area, which the Law Commission highlights in its call for further clarity and statutory foundations for the safeguarding of adults.

It might seem a large leap to look at the experience, impact and prevalence of domestic violence in the United Kingdom, but given its apparent presence in all areas of our society, it can be seen as one of the primary issues of vulnerability for adults. The place of community nurses within the homes of those that are vulnerable makes them key practitioners to identify and respond to new concerns about domestic violence and requires them to make these issues known to other agencies (particularly to the police and social services).

Lastly, the changing context of alcohol and substance misuse within the United Kingdom is likely to impact increasingly upon those practitioners in the community because of their relationship to local families and communities. They are very well placed, but appear to struggle, to identify and support those individuals with substance issues. It is important to also recognise that the demographic profile of substance abuse is shifting, given the effects of the baby-boom generation and their less conservative views of substance use than their parents' generation.

These issues, when taken in conjunction, suggest that whilst the setting for community health nursing practice is shifting, community nurses are well placed to engage with these issues. Further consideration needs to be given to these topics in both the literature and research in order to more adequately inform the profession and to assist in the enhancement improved service responses to clients and families.

References

Association of Directors of Social Services (ADSS) (2005) *Safeguarding Adults: A National Framework of Standards for Good Practice and Outcomes in Adult Protection Work*. ADSS, London.

Baker, A.A. (1975) Granny battering. *Modern Geriatrics*, **5** (8), 20–24.

Batsleer, J., Burman, E., Chantler, K., *et al.* (2002) *Domestic Violence and Minoritisation: Supporting Women to Independence*. Manchester Metropolitan University, Women's Studies Research Centre, Manchester.

BBC News (2002) *Drugs cost society £18.8bn* 2 2002. British Broadcasting Corporation, London.

Benson, M.L., Wooldredge, J., Thistlethwaite, A.B. & Fox, G.L. (2004) The correlation between race and domestic violence is confounded with community context. *Social Problems*, **51** (3), 326–342.

Beynon, C.M. (2009) Drug use and ageing: older people do take drugs! *Age and Ageing*, **38** (1), 8–10.

Bourassa, C., Lavergne, C., Damant, D., Lessard, G. & Turcotte, P. (2008) Child welfare workers' practice in cases involving domestic violence. *Child Abuse Review*, **17** (3), 174–190.

Brandon, M., Bailey, S. & Belderson, P. (2010) *Building on the Learning from Serious Case Reviews: A Two-Year Analysis of Child Protection Database Notifications 2007–2009 – Research Brief.* Department for Education, London.

Campbell, J.C. (2002) Health consequences of intimate partner violence. *Lancet*, **359** (9314), 1331–1336.

Cleaver, H., Aldgate, J., Unell, I. & Great Britain. Department of Education and Science (2011) *Children's Needs – Parenting Capacity: Child Abuse, Parental Mental Illness, Learning Disability, Substance Misuse, and Domestic Violence*, The Stationery Office, London.

Department of Health (DH) (1993) *No Longer Afraid: The Safeguard of Older People in Domestic Settings.* HMSO, London.

DH (2005) *Responding to Domestic Abuse: A Handbook for Health Professionals.* The Stationary Office, London.

DH (2009) *Safeguarding Adults – Report on the Consultation on the Review of 'No Secrets': Guidance on Developing and Implementing Multi-Agency Policies and Procedures to Protect Vulnerable Adults from Abuse*, The Stationary Office, London.

DH (2010) *Clinical Governance and Adult Safeguarding: An Integrated Process*, The Stationary Office, London.

DH & Home Office (2000) *No Secrets: Guidance on Developing and Implementing Multi-Agency Policies and Procedures to Protect Vulnerable Adults from Abuse.* DH, London.

Farrant, A. (2003) Fighting back. *Nursing Standard*, **17** (51), 20–21.

Fernandez, J. (2009) Nurse-led detox in primary care. *Journal of Community Nursing*, **23** (8), 18–23.

Gossop, M. & Moos, R. (2008) Substance misuse among older adults: a neglected but treatable problem. *Addiction*, **103** (3), 347–348.

Hester, M., Pearson, C., Harwin, N. & Abrahams, H. (2007) *Making an Impact: Children and Domestic Violence: a Reader.* 2nd edn. Jessica Kingsley Publishers, London.

Office, H. (2010) *Crime in England and Wales 2009/10: Findings from the British Crime Survey and Police Recorded Crime*, Home Office Research, Development and Statistics Directorate, London.

Home Office (2012) *Domestic Violence.* Available from http://www.homeoffice.gov.uk/crime/violence-against-women-girls/domestic-violence/. Accessed on 25 September 2012.

HoyleC. (2008) Will she be safe? A critical analysis of risk assessment in domestic violence cases. *Children and Youth Services Review*, **30** (3), 323–337.

Humphreys, C. & Houghton, C. (2008) The research evidence on children and young people experiencing domestic abuse. In: *Literature Review: Better Outcomes for Children and Young People Experiencing Domestic Abuse: Directions for Good Practice*, pp. 14–28. Scottish Government, Edinburgh.

Humphreys, C. & Thiara, R. (2003) Mental health and domestic violence: 'I Call it Symptoms of Abuse'. *British Journal of Social Work*, **33** (2), 209–226.

Humphreys, C., Houghton, C. & Ellis, J. (2008) *Literature Review: Better Outcomes for Children and Young People Experiencing Domestic Abuse: Directions for Good Practice.* Scottish Government, Edinburgh.

Jenkins, R. & Davies, R. (2006) Neglect of people with intellectual disabilities A failure to act?. *Journal of Intellectual Disabilities*, **10** (1), 35–45.

Keleher, H., Parker, R., Abdulwadud, O. & Francis, K. (2009) Systematic review of the effectiveness of primary care nursing. *International Journal of Nursing Practice*, **15** (1), 16–24.

Law Commission (2010) *Adult Social Care: A Consultation Paper.* Consultation Paper No 192. The Law Commission, London.

Law Commission (2011) *Adult Social Care.* The Stationary Office, London.

Mandelstam, M. (2011) *Safeguarding Adults at Risk of Harm: A Legal Guide for Practitioners.* Social Care Institute for Excellence, London.

Mandelstam, M. (2009) *Safeguarding Vulnerable Adults and the Law.* Jessica Kingsley Publishers, London.

Manthorpe, J. Rapaport, J. & Stanley, N. (2009) Realising the potential of the Mental capacity Act 2005: early reports from adult safeguarding staff. *Journal of Adult Protection*, **11** (2), 13–24.

McKeough, C. (2009) Reflections and learning from adult protection policy development in Kent and Medway. *The Journal of Adult Protection*, **11** (1), 6–12.

Minister of State (2010) *Government Response to the Consultation on Safeguarding Adults; The Review of the No Secrets Guidance.* Ministerial Statement by Minister of State, Phil Hope regarding safeguarding vulnerable adults. DH, London.

Moy, I, Crome, P., Crome, I. & Fisher, M. (2011) Systematic and narrative review of treatment for older people with substance problems. *European Geriatric Medicine*, **2** (4), 212–236.

NHSLA (2010) *NHSLA Risk Management Standards for Acute Trusts, Primary Care Trusts and Independent Sector Providers of NHS Care.* NHS Litigation Authority, London.

Northway, R., Davies, R., Jenkins, R. & Mansell, I. (2004) *Abuse of Adults with Learning Disabilities: An Examination of Policy, Practice and Educational Implications in Wales,* University of Glamorgan, Pontypridd.

Nursing Standard (2012) Lone workers face ongoing safety risk. *Nursing Standard*, **26** (19), 8.

O'Connell, H. (2003) Alcohol use disorders in elderly people – redefining an age old problem in old age. *British Medical Journal*, **327** (7416), 664–667.

O'Keefe, M., Hills, A., Doyle, M., *et al.* (2007) *UK Study of Abuse and Neglect of Older People: Prevalence Survey Report.* DH, London.

Owens, L., Gilmore, I.T. & Pirmohamed, M. (2000) General practice nurses' knowledge of alcohol use and misuse: A questionnaire survey. *Alcohol and Alcoholism*, **35** (3), 259–262.

Parmar, A., Sampson, A., Diamond, A., Great Britain. Home Office. Research, Development and Statistics Directorate (2005) *Tackling Domestic Violence : Providing Advocacy and Support to Survivors from Black and Other Minority Ethnic Communities.* Home Office, London.

Pearlman, D.N., Zierler, S., Gjelsvik, A. & Verhoek-Oftedahl, W. (2003) Neighborhood environment, racial position, and risk of police-reported domestic violence: a contextual analysis. *Public Health Reports*, **118** (1), 44.

Peckover, S. & Chidlaw, R.G. (2007) Too frightened to care? Accounts by district nurses working with clients who misuse substances. *Health & Social Care in the Community*, **15** (3), 238–245.

Peralta, R.L., Tuttle, L.A. & Steele, J.L. (2010) At the intersection of interpersonal violence, masculinity, and alcohol use: The experiences of heterosexual male perpetrators of intimate partner violence. *Violence Against Women*, **16** (4), 387–409.

Phillips, P. & Johnson, S. (2003) Drug and alcohol misuse among in-patients with psychotic illnesses in three inner-London psychiatric units. *Psychiatric Bulletin*, **27** (6), 217–220.

Plant, M. & Thornton, C. (2002) People and places: Some factors in the alcohol-violence link. *Journal of Substance Use*, **7** (4), 207–213.

Ramsay, J. (2009) Safeguarding vulnerable adults. *Nursing Management*, **16** (4), 24–29.

Reeves, S., Goldman, J., Gilbert, J., *et al.* (2011) A scoping review to improve conceptual clarity of interprofessional interventions. *Journal of interprofessional care*, **25** (3), 167–174.

Reid, M.C. & Anderson, P.A. (1997) Geriatric Substance Use Disorders. *Medical Clinics of North America*, **81** (4), 999–1016..

Resnick, B., Perry, D., Applebaum, G., *et al.* (2003) The impact of alcohol use in community-dwelling older adults. *Journal of Community Health Nursing*, **20** (3), 135–145.

Rose, D., Trevillion, K., Woodall, A., Morgan, C., Feder, G. & Howard, L. (2011) Barriers and facilitators of disclosures of domestic violence by mental health service users: qualitative study. *The British Journal of Psychiatry*, **198** (3), 189–194.

Royal College of Nursing (2000) *Domestic Violence: Guidance for Nurses*. RCN, London.

Spencer-Lane, T. (2011) Reforming the legal framework for adult safeguarding: The Law Commission's final recommendations on adult social care. *The Journal of Adult Protection*, **13** (5), 275–284.

Stead, M. & Stradling, R. (2010) The role of schools in drug education and wider substance misuse prevention. In: *Promoting Health and Well-Being Through Schools* (eds P. Aggleton, C. Dennison & I. Warwick), pp. 84–98. Routledge, London.

The NHS Information Centre, Lifestyles Statistics (2011a) *Statistics on Alcohol: England, 2011*. DH, London.

The NHS Information Centre, Lifestyles Statistics (2011b) *Statistics on Drug Misuse: England, 2010*. DH, London.

Thomas, L. (2008) Women need help to escape domestic violence. *Nursing Standard*, **22** (38), 25.

Walby, S., Allen, J. & Britain, G. (2004) *Domestic Violence, Sexual Assault and Stalking: Findings from the British Crime Survey*. Home Office Research, Development and Statistics Directorate, London.

Weaver, T., Charles, V., Madden, P. & Renton, A. (2002) *Co-morbidity of Substance Misuse and Mental Illness Collaborative Study (COSMIC)*, DH, London.

Wilhelmsson, S. & Lindberg, M. (2009) Health promotion: Facilitators and barriers perceived by district nurses. *International Journal of Nursing Practice*, **15** (3), 156–163.

Williams, S. (2011) Safeguarding adults at risk in the NHS through inter-agency working. *The Journal of Adult Protection*, **13** (2), 100–113.

17

End-of-life Care

Michelle Boot, Karen Harrison-White and Jayne Gwyther

Faculty of Society and Health, Buckinghamshire New University, Uxbridge, UK

Radical changes in science and society in the last 100 years have had a significant impact on both our experience and perception of dying. A hundred years ago, the commonest cause of death was infectious or respiratory disease and life expectancy was below 50 years old. Today, most of us die from chronic illnesses such as cancer or heart failure and can expect to live for about 80 years (Dunnel 2008).

Whereas 100 years ago, people who were dying were cared for at home usually after a relatively short illness; nowadays most people dying from a chronic illness will experience a slow deterioration, perhaps over a number of years. Although it is usually possible to predict that someone is in the final stages of their life, the majority of people will die in hospital, often undergoing life-sustaining treatments (DH 2008a).

As a scientific model of health care has become dominant and death has moved from the home into the hospital setting, the postponement of death and removal of dying from the community setting has led to a society that has lost the ability to engage with the dying process and to accept this as part of the cycle of life (Aries 1981). As a consequence of living longer and the institutionalisation of death, people have lost their ability to talk about dying and to think ahead about their own death (DH 2008a). The significance of this is such that the National Council for Palliative Care (NCPC 2009a) set up the 'Dying Matters Coalition', which encourages the public to think about their own deaths, to talk about their wishes and to address societal problems relating to death avoidance.

Despite the advances in medicine and health care, many people dying in the United Kingdom do not receive optimal care at the end of their lives. To try to address current

Community and Public Health Nursing, Fifth Edition. Edited by David Sines, Sharon Aldridge-Bent, Agnes Fanning, Penny Farrelly, Kate Potter and Jane Wright.
© 2013 John Wiley & Sons, Ltd. Published 2013 by John Wiley & Sons, Ltd.

discrepancies and inadequacies in care, the Government has developed the 'End-of-Life Care Strategy' (DH 2008a). This strategy recognises that many people are experiencing unnecessary suffering at the end of their lives and are not living out their final days in a place of their choice. It emphasises that people's needs, priorities and preferences should be identified, respected and acted upon, enabling more people to die where they choose and the importance of coordinated care being available to them 24/7.

This strategy describes a good death as 'being treated as an individual with dignity and respect, being without pain and other symptoms and being in familiar surroundings in the company of close family and/or friends' (DH 2008a, p. 9). The absence of suffering and presence of relational support are key characteristics of a good death. 'A good death' is, however, a nebulous and fluid concept (Watts 2012), and it remains important not to lose sight of the uniqueness of death to each person and family (Haig 2009). Within the Western world, achieving a good death for all has become a social and political priority (Ellershaw *et al.* 2010).

Although the majority of people die in hospital, most people express a preference to die in the home setting. A key aim of the 'End-of-Life Care Strategy' is to increase the number of people dying in the community (DH 2008a). This will not only increase the numbers of people able to die in a place of their choice but also prove economically desirable, as high-quality care in the community is as, if not sometimes more, cost effective than providing hospital care (DH 2010a).

Whole systems approach

The need for a coordinated approach to the commissioning and delivery of end-of-life care is a core tenant of the 'End-of-Life Care Strategy'. Although progress has been made since 2008, there is still much to do to foster the full engagement of primary care professionals in end-of-life care – too many patients are still being needlessly admitted to hospital (DH 2010a). The redesign of end-of-life care services, using a whole systems approach involving both stakeholders and providers, is ongoing nationally, with organisations being encouraged to share best practice, but with the recognition that service configuration needs to be responsive to local needs (DH 2010a; Marie Curie Cancer Care 2012).

In terms of the care delivery, the most developed coordinated model is the Gold Standards Framework (GSF). The GSF was developed within the primary care setting in response to a desire to improve practice and support a multi-agency team towards providing the highest-quality care for patients in the last stages of life (Thomas 2003).

The framework uses a number of different tools to build a framework through which to deliver care. It is not prescriptive and can be customised to meet local need and allows for a step-by-step introduction. It consists of *three core processes*:

Identify – people who are likely to be approaching the last months of their lives. These patients are placed on a register of patients, which the primary care team uses as a tool to monitor them and to discuss and plan their care. The register is used in conjunction with a monthly meeting of all the relevant community health-care professionals (HCPs).

Assess – once patients have been identified, a holistic assessment of their needs is made. This can be accomplished by using any holistic assessment tool.

Plan – early identification and holistic assessment of patients enables the primary care team to plan proactively to meet the patient's needs and preferences for care. The patient and family are empowered to become active members of the team, and opportunities for them to exercise autonomy and control are maximised (Thomas 2003). The GSF flags up the need for advance care planning (ACP), which is a process that empowers the patient to plan for future care and to express their preferences for future place of care.

The three processes are supported by seven tasks, which the community team, working together, utilise to deliver patient-centred care.

Communication
Coordination
Control of symptoms
Continuity of out-of-hours care
Continuity of learning
Carer support
Care in the dying phase

Community nurses play a central role in caring for the dying. The GSF is a framework that they can utilise to get to know patients at an early stage, discuss their preferences with them and reduce the likelihood of a crisis occurring (Barnes *et al.* 2010). The key strength of the GSF is that if it is implemented effectively, it improves organisational systems, communication and competence and reduces hospital admissions (Hansford & Meehan 2007).

Effective implementation is fundamental to improving the quality of patient care. Thomas (2003) suggests that a 'step change' implementation is desirable: firstly, setting up a register of patients and meeting to coordinate care; secondly, focusing on symptom control, out-of-hours care and the learning needs of the primary care team; and finally, moving on to carer support and care in the last days of life. Leadership, workforce development, communications training and resources are all fundamental to the success of the GSF in improving the patient and family care (Reynolds & Croft 2010).

The GSF alone will not improve end-of-life care (Hansford & Meehan 2007). A key issue for HCPs is not to lose sight of the fact that it is only a framework and that it will only improve the quality of care if the HCPs are committed to working together to improve communication, coordination and care; although education of staff is identified as a 'second stage' criteria in the GSF 'step changes', it is so fundamental to the success of end-of-life care that it may need to be at the forefront of organisational developments.

A systematic review of research studies exploring the effectiveness of the framework concluded that it had potential to improve end-of-life care; there is evidence of improved care regarding equity, access and responsiveness of service and some evidence of improved system management (Shaw *et al.* 2010). This systematic review identifies that many organisations adopting the GSF do not develop beyond the initial step and cites the workload of coordination as being one of the barriers to adoption of a fuller service; this points to the challenge facing community professionals, how to resource the development of end-of-life care services.

An emerging service delivery system, 'Co-ordinate My Care', is currently being developed across London to improve the coordination and delivery of end-of-life care. Initially the project will focus on developing an electronic register of end-of-life care patients that will be available to all community employees and will enhance continuity of care, particularly 'out of hours' (including the Ambulance Service), and enable more people to die in a place of their choice (Smith and Riley 2011).

Assessment: The foundation to providing good care

Assessment of patients' holistic care needs is recognised as a key component to the delivery of both quality care and choice (NICE 2004; DH 2008a). Community nurses universally value their role as palliative care providers (Luker 2000), but there is evidence that they find it difficult to move beyond physical care and chatting to patients to more meaningful conversation (Griffiths *et al.* 2007). The use of assessment tools is an intrinsic part of the community HCPs' role; however, there are specific tools that have been developed within the cancer and palliative care specialties, which facilitate the exploration of holistic needs. The dynamic nature of patient's needs means that monitoring of needs and responsive to care interventions should be carried out over the course of a person's illness (Richardson *et al.* 2007).

A number of assessment tools have been developed within the cancer and palliative care settings, which aim to facilitate assessment along the patient's disease trajectory; the 'Sheffield Profile for Assessment and Referral for Care' (SPARC) assessment tool will be explored as the concept at the heart of this patient-centred assessment tool is to begin a conversation that has the patient's concerns at the centre (Nottingham Trent Cancer Network (NTCN) 2009). It models the range of issues to be assessed, moves away from the biomedical model of care and offers a vehicle that facilitates effective communication. It enables people to identify areas of concern and to set the agenda in terms of what is their priority. The design of the questionnaire also demonstrates to the patient that community practitioners are interested in all aspects of their lives and not just the particular problem for which they have been referred. Assessment tools should act as a bridge between the practitioner and the patient and foster a sense of partnership, which enables negotiated care planning (Richardson *et al.* 2007).

The SPARC tool aims to ask the following: 'what is concerning you the most?' The questionnaire helps the patient to reflect on this question (NTCN 2009). Once they have completed the assessment, the community practitioner can then identify what are the patient's main concerns and can explore these areas further. There are three aspects to the assessment: the completion of the SPARC questionnaire; conversation; action plan.

For a full version of the SPARC assessment tool, go to: www.ncsi.org.uk/what-we-are-doing/assessment-care-planning/screening-and-assessment-tools/

A review of assessment tools designed for the cancer and palliative care setting concludes that there is a need for continued evaluation regarding outcome measures and a recognition that assessment alone does not lead to improved patient outcomes (Richardson *et al.* 2007).

Symptom management

Assessment is fundamental to successful symptom management, but not just physical assessment. If symptoms are to be effectively managed, a holistic framework of assessment and care is required, as symptoms have both a physical and psychological component (Twycross *et al.* 2009).

Research evidence suggests that the symptom burden increases in end-stage disease. There is a high prevalence of all symptoms with fatigue, breathlessness and pain being the most frequently reported (Solano *et al.* 2006).

Each symptom needs to be evaluated in terms of the impact on the patient, the likely cause, the underlying pathology and the treatment tried (Twycross *et al.* 2009). In the last weeks and days of life, it may not be appropriate to expose the patient to investigations and interventions as the burdensomeness of these to the patient is likely to outweigh any benefits gained. However, all new symptoms and the management of symptoms require medical assessment and a team approach at all times. This team approach can be challenging in the community if lines of communication have not already been established across teams. The ability of primary care teams to work together to respond to changing circumstances and to be able to liaise with specialists within the tertiary setting is an important component to successful symptom management.

The anticipation of symptoms in the last days of life and the prescribing of anticipatory drugs is a good practice endorsed by integrated care pathways, as this reduces the likelihood of delays in prescribing. Anticipatory prescribing for five key symptoms is recommended: pain, restlessness, respiratory tract secretions, nausea and vomiting and dyspnoea.

Medicines should be given only when needed, following assessment, at the right time and just enough to relieve the symptom (Marie Curie Palliative Care Institute 2010).

Beyond the management of physical symptoms

In endeavouring to meet holistic needs, there is an ongoing search for a definition of the non-physical dimensions. Within our rich multicultural society, the concept of 'transcultural spirituality' may be a more relevant concept (Holloway 2006), as this recognises the weaving together of these dimensions – although we identify psychosocial and spiritual dimensions, it is not possible to understand a person by exploring these dimensions separately. Indeed, all aspects of personhood need to be considered, as it is not possible to understand a person without recognising their culture and ethnicity (Oliviere 2002). More recently, the sexual orientation for gay and lesbian people with regard to end-of-life care has also been highlighted as an important aspect of a person's identity that is often overlooked in the delivery of end-of-life care (Ward *et al.* 2010).

Community nurses have identified 'knowing patients' as an essential component to the provision of high-quality palliative care, with early contact time spent with the patient and the provision of more than just physical care, being vehicles that establish this therapeutic relationship (Luker *et al.* 2000). However, district nurses have reported that they find it difficult to explain their role and report uncertainty about whether to explore psychological concerns early on (Griffiths *et al.* 2007). This confidence in assessing and managing physical and practical problems, rather than considering psychological and particularly spiritual aspects of care, is partly due to time constraints imposed in practice and partly due to inadequate exposure to training in this area (Hermann 2006).

Exploring what is important to individuals needs to take place within the context of a therapeutic relationship (Luker *et al.* 2000). The community setting is an ideal place to do this, but it requires time and that can be challenging. A significant threat to improving holistic care is the configuration of community services and changes in community nurses' roles (Luker *et al.* 2000). The ability of community nurses to build relationship is a significant measure regarding the quality of end-of-life care. Service developments such as 'whole systems approaches' and frameworks such as the GSF are useful tools in guiding service development and delivery. However, without educating and training nurses regarding communication and how to develop therapeutic relationships and, of equal importance, time to take on this role, there is a risk that the existing service structures will limit their ability to deliver quality end-of-life care.

It seems that spiritual care often amounts to a symbolic acknowledgement late on in the dying trajectory a recent report to the Department of Health identified that the development of spiritual care at the end of life needs further research to gain understanding of the experience and appropriate therapeutic responses (Holloway *et al.* 2010).

Advance care planning

A core tenant of the 'End-of-Life Care Strategy' is the notion that people should be involved in their care planning and that care should be tailored to meet their individual needs and choices. This principle is supported by the Government white paper

'Equity and excellence in the NHS'. People should not be passive recipients of care but should be actively involved in making choices and planning their own care (DH 2010b). As the majority of deaths relate to chronic disease, this gives opportunity to involve many people in planning the care they would like to receive at the end of their lives.

The principle of patient choice is enshrined in law in the Mental Capacity Act (Department of Justice 2005). This Act establishes not only the patient's right to be involved in decision making but the duty of community practitioners to ensure that patients are actively facilitated to exercise this right to their full capacity through education and support.

ACP is the framework that has been developed to help a person with a life-limiting disease to plan for their future care needs. The purpose of ACP is to develop a care plan for those facing divergent options as their disease accelerates (Sawicki *et al.* 2008). It is a process of communication that helps individuals to understand their choices for future health care and reflects on personal goals, values and religious and cultural beliefs (Respecting Choices Programme (RCP) 2010). This process is a key characteristic of the palliative care philosophy (Gott *et al.* 2009).

ACP includes a discussion with the patient regarding their choices and preferences for care. It is different from the usual care planning process as it is anticipated that the plan of care being developed will be initiated in the future at a time when the individual's condition is deteriorating. For a number of individuals, the plan will be initiated at a time when they lack the capacity to be involved in decision making regarding their care needs and where they would like to be cared for (Dimond 2009).

Rigid and prescriptive approaches to introducing ACP are likely to be harmful to patients (Randall & Downie 2010). ACP is not a one-off discussion but usually developed over a period of time as the community practitioner builds a relationship with the patient (Ratner *et al.* 2001). It is a voluntary process, and practitioners need to ensure that they facilitate this process without bringing any pressure to bear on the individual (DH 2008b; Randall & Downie 2010).

Advance statement/Preferred priorities for care

An advance statement (AS) is the documented record of the individual's plan of care. It can include information about where the individual would like to be cared for, what they would like to happen and who they would like to be present and involved in their care. An AS does not have to be made, although it is helpful to record patient preferences and, with the patient's permission, to share these with organisations involved in their care. The Preferred Priorities for Care is one of the documents that has been designed to facilitate the discussion and record patient's wishes (NHS 2012a) although other tools are available, for example, from the GSF toolkit. It is important that patients understand that if they lose capacity, the documented wishes will be used to help make decisions regarding appropriate care.

This record of the individual's preferences and choices does not guarantee that their requests will be met, as resource issues and prioritisation remain factors in access to care at the end of life as in all areas of the NHS care (George & Dimond 2009). There is evidence that clinical nurse specialists in palliative care find themselves facing an ethical dilemma when they are exploring patient preference, given that in reality it is unlikely that their preferences will be met (Simon *et al.* 2008; Boot 2010; Minto & Strickland 2011).

Many community practitioners find introducing the concept of ACP challenging (Gott *et al.* 2009; Horne *et al.* 2009), and it appears easier or more difficult according to the patient's diagnosis, for example, it is easier to introduce the concept to a patient with lung cancer than to a patient with COPD (Crawford 2010; Minto & Strickland 2011). Collaborative working influences the success of implementing advanced care plans, and as such there needs to be a clear agreement regarding who will lead the discussion with other members of the team, with everyone involved then supporting the implementation of the plan of care.

The importance of relationship building and engagement with a patient over time is supported by a number of studies exploring patients' and carers' perceptions. These indicate that the person who conducts the discussion should have excellent communication skills, accurate information and the time to talk through issues raised (Ratner *et al.* 2001; Barnes *et al.* 2007; Horne *et al.* 2006). Community practitioners engaged in facilitating ACP have to balance the need to offer the patient and opportunity to engage with their plan with the risk of harming the patient by introducing an unwanted discussion (Boot 2010). Training needs to be followed up with ongoing supervision as well as communication training programmes (Weiner 2006).

Advanced decisions to refuse treatment (ADRT)

Some people have strong views regarding treatment that they would not want to receive and feel the need to document this. An advanced decisions to refuse treatment (ADRT) is a legally binding document that records treatments that an individual does not wish to receive, that is, treatments that they decide in advance that they do not wish to receive once they have lost the capacity to withhold their consent in person. The ADRT needs to be very specific, to include a statement acknowledging that the individual withholds consent to a treatment even if 'their lives are at risk', and it must be signed and witnessed (DH 2008b). If a person indicates that they wish to make an ADRT, they should have the opportunity to discuss treatment options with one of the doctors caring for them and will need help to ensure that the wording of the document is unambiguous and legally binding (Saunders *et al.* 2006).

Assisted suicide

Within the context of assessment and ACP, it is possible that some patients will raise the issue of wanting to explore the issue of assisted suicide. This chapter identifies the importance of developing a therapeutic relationship with the patient, and such a relationship allows the community practitioner to explore the underlying issues that have led the patient to raise this issue, which then enables care to be directed towards ameliorating suffering and supporting the patient by listening to their fears (Kelly & Varghese 2006).

Do not attempt resuscitation orders

Although cardiopulmonary resuscitation (CPR) is rarely appropriate for patients in the context of end-of-life care, there are circumstances in the last months of life when CPR may be successful. The guidelines jointly issued by the British Medical Association, the Resuscitation Council and the Royal College of Nursing state that involving people in discussions regarding CPR is a good practice and a key aspect of ACP (Resuscitation Council UK 2007).

Discussing CPR with patients is ethically interesting, as it is the only treatment that patients are asked to consider in advance and to have their wishes documented (Randall & Downie 2010). Patients have the right to decline involvement with any such discussions. Such discussions need to be approached sensitively within the context of an informed conversation regarding the patient's wishes.

The focus on ensuring 'Do Not Attempt Resuscitation' (DNAR) orders in the home care setting is fairly new, and evidence regarding how patients and carers experience this and how community practitioners manage the process and the challenges is still to be explored. It has been suggested that patients and relatives may be confused regarding which interventions will not be carried out and that involvement in decision making in the context of end-of-life care can be confusing and can magnify guilt and increase distress (Strecher 2008).

Randall and Downie (2010) suggest that the presumption in favour of CPR, which then leads to the need for a DNAR order and the need to discuss CPR with many people who are unlikely to benefit from it, may need to be challenged. As evidence emerges regarding how patients and families feel at having to deal with CPR discussions and documentation, it may be that a new paradigm needs to be explored. Within the USA, a campaign to adopt a philosophy of 'Allowing Natural Death' (AND) within the end-of-life care context aims to shift the focus from DNAR to exploring which interventions will be offered in terms of palliative care and comfort initiative, thereby removing the burden of an often inappropriate and burdensome discussion from a patient and family (Strecher 2008).

As things currently stand, from an organisational point of view, DNAR orders need to be readily available and easily identifiable to all community practitioners visiting the home. Ambulance services also need to be informed of the existence of an order at a particular address. Practitioners need to develop confidence in facilitating discussions about CPR with patients.

Care in the last days of life

Determining an individual's prognosis is challenging, and the predictive aspect of prognosis is widely variable; the challenge is being able to predict when the dying process begins. The key issues identified when diagnosing dying are diagnosis performance status, disease progression and symptom burden (Haig 2009). However, the ability of practitioners to recognise dying is poor, and the uncertainty around prognosis needs to be acknowledged, not only within the multidisciplinary team, but also with the patient (Murtagh *et al.* 2004).

Diagnosing the dying phase needs team agreement so that a cohesive management approach is achieved, avoiding inappropriate interventions and ensuring consistency with communication with the patient and family (Haig 2009). In an ideal scenario, the patient will be referred to the primary care team in a timely manner so that practitioners have time to get to know the patient and to facilitate the planning for their last days. Optimism regarding survival can result in missed opportunities to plan appropriate care (Murtagh *et al.* 2004) since when patients are referred late, the primary healthcare team may be left scrambling to assess their needs, control symptoms and prepare and support the families.

Regardless of the journey to the dying phase, integrated care pathways for the last days of life offer a framework for ensuring that the holistic care needs of the patient and families are met. However, in situations where the community practitioners have not had time to establish a relationship with the patient, the effectiveness of an integrated pathway in delivering high-quality care may be limited (Veerbeek *et al.* 2008). This underlines the importance of end-of-life care being delivered early in the trajectory.

The Liverpool Care Pathway (LCP), was identified within the 'End-of-Life-Care Strategy' (DoH 2008a) as an example of the standard that is expected to be adopted in the last days of life, however following concerns regarding how the pathway was implemented in some areas a decision has been made to phase out the use of this pathway, however the principles of good palliative care on which it is based must be met these include: *Sensitive communication; Holistic assessment; Appropriate interventions at the end of life; Care for the deceased and the family after death.*

When a patient enters the dying phase a review of management of their care should be undertaken, which includes a review of medication. The appropriateness of artificial nutrition and artificial hydration should be assessed separately as the benefits and burdens are different (BMA 2007). Artificial nutrition and hydration during the dying phase may be burdensome to the patient in terms of administration or increase the risk lead of pulmonary oedema. All decisions regarding the withdrawal of treatment must be made on an individual basis (BMA 2007) and it is very important that families are supported and understand the rationale for these decisions, particularly regarding fluids as this is a very emotive issue.

The need for health care professionals to communicate effectively with families about the decision making process and the rationale for decisions during the dying phase; explaining the focus on appropriate care delivery and quality of life in the last days are key issues (Chapman 2009; Hockley 2009). Further training focusing on difficult communication around end-of-life care has already been highlighted as a key area of need (NHS 2012b).

Models of interdisciplinary working: The road to successful end-of-life care

Primary care providers face a challenge in meeting the end-of-life care needs along-side their other responsibilities. The central role primary care has in providing successful palliative care/end-of-life care is well recognised; however, the multi-plicity and complexity of providing holistic care at the end of life across a range of disease trajectories is such that it cannot be provided by one provider in isolation (Howell 2007). Models of cohesive working have been developed across a number of services where the focus of care is on need and not on diagnosis (Daley *et al.* 2006; Bourke *et al.* 2009). Within palliative care, the importance of interdisciplinary working is recognised, and this needs to be mirrored in the primary care setting. Care pathways can support the process of identifying lead roles along the trajectory (Brown & Sutton 2009), and there are models of care provision where specialist palliative care nurses work alongside specialist nurses (Daley *et al.* 2006; Chadwick & Russell 2012).

Whilst knowledge and skills are more readily identified as core requisites to delivering quality end-of-life care (DH 2008a), the need to address the potential barriers to collaborative working is rarely recognised and poses a potential threat to both the process and outcomes of care. Such barriers include organisational and professional cultural differences, together with finance challenges (Walsh *et al.* 2006).

Community nurses: The lynchpins of successful end-of-life care in the community

Community nurses have been described as the lynchpins of palliative care in the community (Kennedy 2005). One of the key challenges for community nurses is their hectic work schedules. Although community nurses are central to the provision of palliative care in the community setting, the immense satisfaction they feel is often tempered by stress and emotional upset as they struggle to balance the demands of caring for dying patients with their routine work (Burt *et al.* 2008). The importance of getting to know patients is a key element to delivering high-quality care at the end of life (Luker *et al.* 2000), but without empowering community nurses to spend time with patients, the quality of end-of-life care will be limited. Further research is needed to explore how community nurses manage this emotional labour (Burt *et al.* 2008) – the role of supervision is identified as a core concept in developing skills in communication and emotional intelligence with regard to end-of-life care (Weiner 2006; Burt *et al.* 2008).

Death of a child

Childhood malignancies are rare cancers (Moules & Ramsey 2008). In 2006–2009, an average of 1550 children per year in the United Kingdom were diagnosed with cancer, with an average of 260 childhood deaths from cancer in the United Kingdom between 2007 and 2009 (Cancer Research UK 2010). Leukaemia is the most common cancer of children of all ages accounting for 35.4% of all childhood cancers (NICE 2005). The acute leukaemias comprise over half of the leukaemias seen in clinical practice with 80% of leukaemias being of the acute lymphoblastic type. The prognosis of acute leukaemia in children has been greatly improved by the use of chemotherapy, radiotherapy, better supportive therapy and the development of specialist paediatric oncology units (Moules & Ramsey 2008).

Over recent years the care of children and young people with life-limiting illnesses has evolved as a specialist sphere of practice. It is imperative to recognise that palliative care services for children are organised differently than that of adult palliative care mainly due to the early involvement of the palliative care team and the often prolonged period of time this occurs over (Glasper & Richardson 2006). The need for a multi-agency approach is essential in the provision of seamless care to the child and family (ACT 2004). This approach must encompass a partnership centred around the individual needs of the child and family with each team member adopting sound communication skills that encompass a shared understanding of the goals of each individual care plan (Glasper & Richardson 2006).

The Department of Health (England) commissioned ACT (Association for Children with Life-Threatening and Terminal Conditions and their Families) to produce an inclusive multi-agency/multi-professional care pathway to supplement the Department of Health's 'National Service Framework' (NSF) for Children, Young People and Maternity Services 2004 guidance (Department for Education and skills 2004). The resulting pathway endorsed five key standards, of which one (Standard 5) stated that each child and family should be supported to decide on an end-of-life plan and should be offered the care and support to realise this goal as far as possible. The ACT (2004) care pathway advocates that bereavement care should be provided for the whole family as an ongoing process from diagnosis, with clear documentation and parent-held records used to facilitate the process.

The document *Decisions Relating to Cardiopulmonary Resuscitation – A Joint Statement from the British Medical Association, the Resuscitation Council (UK) and the Royal College of Nursing* (2007) identifies the ethical and legal considerations that should inform decisions relating to resuscitation. This document relates to both adults and children. Within the document, it is emphasised that ACP including decisions relating to resuscitation status is a key part of good clinical care for people who may be at risk of cardiorespiratory arrest. Inappropriate CPR could potentially expose people to an undignified death and prolong suffering (Fraser *et al.* 2010). With regard to CPR decisions, children and young people over 16 years are presumed to have the mental capacity to make decisions for themselves, unless proven to the contrary (DH 2001).

End-of-life planning is still often poorly achieved perhaps due to the difficulty in predicting the end of life and the difficulty of 'raising the issue' with the child and family (Fraser *et al.* 2010). Professionals working with children must be aware of the national policy related to palliative care and adhere to their professional responsibilities to ensure that the best possible care is given.

Dementia

Around 800 000 people in the United Kingdom have dementia, and this figure is projected to rise as the population of elderly grows (Luengo-Fernandez *et al.* 2010). Evidence suggests that the care needs of these patients are both poorly recognised and poorly met at a national level (Marie Curie Cancer Relief 2009). The majority of these patients are cared for and die within the care home setting (Simon *et al.* 2011), but significant numbers are admitted to hospital in the last year of life (NCPC 2009b); often this seems to be the only option available to the carers and emergency response teams (Marie Curie Cancer Relief 2009). Attention is being given to address this situation; there are both moral and economic drivers to improving care for people with dementia (Fuller 2012).

A key challenge is managing this group of patients in the community. Evidence suggests that education regarding end-of-life care in the care home setting and coordination of care with a community practitioner leading on dementia care is effective at improving care (Ashton *et al.* 2009). As with other chronic conditions, coordinated models of working are likely to be the best frameworks for care provisions, with cohesion of service provision between general community nurses, palliative care providers and mental health professions.

Symptom management for people with dementia is complex, with pain often being unrecognised and undertreated. Carers need to be alert to the severe distress that some people exhibit, as this is an indication for treatment; the DisDAT assessment tool has been developed to facilitate the assessment of distress in people with dementia (Regnard *et al.* 2007). This tool relies on staff getting to know the individual and recording observations of behavioural responses, such as when they are content, so that this can be used as a baseline. The record can be used to record subtle changes in behaviour and provides useful information when transferring people between care settings. Community practitioners need to work with families and care staff to build up a picture of the person's 'language' of distress.

ACP for people with dementia needs to take place early on whilst they still have language and cognition (Chapman 2011). Research regarding the ACP process with people with dementia is lacking. One research study exploring its use with carers of severely demented patients in an acute unit found that, even with intensive support from a nurse specialist, few relatives wanted to complete an ACP. This indicates a need for further research into their use (Sampson *et al.* 2010) and suggests that there will also be enormous challenges facing their implementation in community settings for people with dementia.

Care of the bereaved

Bereavement is recognised as a normal life process that the majority of people cope with by using their own inner resources, with support from their social network (Machin 2009). Most people have the ability to continue with a life that is meaningful and have the resilience to ensure that they adapt to the change in their circumstances (Monroe & Oliviere 2007). This concept of resilience is recognised within bereavement as an important marker of people's ability to cope (Machin 2009). The challenge for HCP is to assess effectively which of the bereaved do not have the resilience to adapt and to ensure this minority group get specialist support.

The 'End-of-Life Care Strategy' (2008a) identifies that bereavement assessment should be carried out for all bereaved carers, but this is not without controversy as the evidence for effective assessment is weak and there is an ethical tension where carrying out assessments is concerned, given that it has been identified that the majority of people will have no need for intervention (Randall & Downie 2010). Although the need to target the resources of bereavement services to the minority who need them supports the concept of assessment, bereavement assessment tools fail to identify who is 'at risk', perhaps partly due to a time pressure tick-box approach to assessment (Relf *et al.* 2008).

A new paradigm of assessment based on conversation and relationship has been developed, which aims to identify how relatives are coping in the pre- and post-bereavement period. This assessment tool requires community practitioners to undergo training in communications skills and a commitment of time by organisations to ensure that it can be implemented effectively (Relf *et al.* 2008). The fundamental success of assessment rests on the community practitioner having time to establish a meaningful relationship and to listen to the story of how the carer is coping.

One of the challenges of bereavement assessment is that the practitioner may not necessarily meet all of the key family members and it is possible that vulnerable individuals will be overlooked (Relf *et al.* 2008). The use of written information made available to the wider family explaining likely emotions and where to seek help is recommended (Relf *et al.* 2008).

Community practitioners also need to consider their own needs to explore and express their own emotional needs that caring for the dying will engender in them. There is evidence that opportunities to debrief are helpful in reducing burnout and fostering coping strategies, but these are perhaps more likely to be available to specialist palliative care teams (Lobb *et al.* 2010). The reactions to death experienced by practitioners are ubiquitous, and all team members should have optimal training in coping strategies (Danieli 2006). This is a challenge in a time of financial constraints and time pressures but in the long term is likely to lead to an emotionally healthy and effective workforce.

Conclusion

This chapter has identified the sociological perspectives of death and dying at the beginning of the twenty-first century. Science has enabled us to live much longer, but this raises challenges regarding our experience of death or ability to engage with it, and it poses challenges for community practitioners regarding the development of both paradigms and a skilled workforce, which enable large numbers of people with chronic disease both to be cared for and to die in their community setting.

Government strategy has identified the problems and mechanisms through which to meet and managed these. Systems approaches, frameworks, pathways, assessment tools, care planning and multi-organisational models all have a part to play in building a structure from within which quality care can be delivered. Such structures in themselves may facilitate practitioners to be able to deliver care, but the fundamental ingredient is a skilled workforce able to develop a therapeutic relationship with patients; to do this they need knowledge, skills and time. The most important skills community practitioners need are advanced communications skills; these are most likely to be fostered through simulation training and supervision.

A serious threat to the delivery of end-of-life care is the increasing workload within the community setting, particularly if there is a delay in resources being redirected to the primary care setting. As services are developed, there needs to be a culture of empowering community nurses to be end-of-life champions and a valuing of the time that is required to deliver the quality of end-of-life care.

It is when humanity faces challenges that creativity and ingenuity appears to flourish. It is possible that in rising to the 'end-of-life care challenges', the community practitioners will develop new paradigms to inform innovative and responsive care practice.

Case study

Frank is a 73-year-old retired postman who was diagnosed with COPD 5 years ago and who is already known to you. You visit him after his discharge from hospital, to where he was admitted to the acute respiratory ward to be treated for an acute chest infection and to receive BIPAP.

Frank greets you with 'Well I am not going in there again – that was a terrible experience'.

Consider how you would use this opening to facilitate a conversation regarding ACP.

What symptoms would you anticipate that Frank might experience?

How will the GSF help you to manage his care? Which other HCPs would you want to liaise with and who would lead on his care?

What critical junctures will you watch for that may signify that Frank is entering the dying phase?

Which anticipatory drugs would you want the GP to prescribe?

References

Aries, P. (1981) *The Hour of Our Death*. Penguin Books, London.

Association for Children with Life-threatening and Terminal Conditions and their Families. (ACT) (2004) *Integrated Multi-Agency Care Pathways for Children with Life-Threatening and Life-Limiting Illness*, ACT, Bristol.

Ashton, S., McClellon, B. & Roe, B. (2009) An end-of-life initiative for people with dementia. *European Journal of Pallaitive Care*, 16 (5), 240–243.

Barnes, K., Jones, L., Tookman, A. & King, M. (2007) Acceptability of an advance care planning interview schedule: A focus group study. *Palliative Medicine*, 21, 23–28.

Barnes, B., Roderick, S. & Arnold, S. (2010) Improving integrated team working to support people to die in the place of their choice. *Nursing Times*, 106 (32), 14–16.

Boot, M. (2010) *What Challenges do Clinical Nurse Specialists Experience when Facilitating Advance Care Planning*, Unpublished Dissertation University of Bedfordshire.

Bourke, S., Doe, S., Gascoinge, K., *et al.* (2009) An integrated model of provision of palliative care to patients with cystic fibrosis. *Palliative Medicine*, 23, 512–517.

British Medical Association (BMA) (2007) *Withholding and Withdrawing Life-Prolonging Medical Treatment: Guidance for Decision Making*, 3rd edn. BMA, London.

Brown, J. & Sutton, L. (2009) A neuro care pathway for meeting the palliative care needs of people with life-limiting neuro conditions. *International Journal of Palliative Nursing*, 15 (3), 120–127.

Burt, J., Shipman, C., Addington-Hall, J. & White, P. (2008) Nursing the dying within generalist case. A focus group study of district nurses. *Journal of Nursing studies*, 45, 1470–1478.

Cancer Research UK, (2010) Children's Cancers. Available from http://www.cancerresearchuk. org/home/?gclid=COS145_pqLMCFXDLtAodLVwAww. Accessed on 30th October 2012.

Chadwick, S. & Russell, S. (2012) Providing palliative care in advanced respiratory disease- the experience of one hospice. *European Journal of Palliative Care*, 19 (3), 110–112.

Chapman, S. (2009) The LCP 'tick box' approach not encouraged. *International Journal of Palliative Nursing*, 15 (9), 420–421.

Chapman, S. (2011) End-of-life care for people with dementia should be discussed early. *British Journal of Neuroscience Nursing*, 7 (1), 461.

Constini, M. & Linder, U. (2012) A European perspective on the last days of life. *European Journal of Palliative Care*, 19 (4), 175–177.

Crawford, A. (2010) Respiratory practitioners experiences of end-of-life discussions in COPD. *British Journal of Nursing*, 19 (8), 1164–1169.

Daley, A., Matthew, C. & Williams, S. (2006) Heart failure and palliative care services working in partnership report of a new model of care. *Palliative Medicine*, 20 (6), 593–601.

Danieli, Y. (2006) A group intervention to process and examine countertransference near the End-of-Life. In: *When Professionals Weep: Emotional and Countertransference Response in End-of-Life Care*. R. Katz & T. Johnson (Eds) Routledge, London.

Department of Health (DH) (2001) *Seeking Consent: Working with Children*. DH, London.

Department for Education and skills (2004) *The National Service Framework (NSF) for Children, Young People and Maternity Services*. DH, London.

DH (2010a) *End of Life Strategy Second Annual Report*. London DH.

DH (2010b) *Equity and Excellence*: Liberating the NHS. DH, London.

DH (2008a) *End of Life Strategy Promoting High Quality Care for all Adults at the End of Life*. DH, London.

DH (2008b) *Advance Care Planning: A guide for health and social care staff*. DH, London.

Department of Justice (2005) *The Mental Capacity Act* www.justice.gov.uk/protecting-the-vulnerable/mental-capacity-act. Accessed 22 11 12.

Dimond, B. (2009) Understanding Advance Decisions, mental capacity and proxy decision making in medical treatment. *International Journal of Palliative Nursing*, 15 (5), 212–213.

Dunnel, K. (2008) *Aging and Mortality in the UK. National Statistician's Annual Article on Populations*. National Office of Statistics.

Ellershaw, J., Dewar, S. & Murphy, D. (2010) Achieving a good death for all. *British Medical Journal (Clinical Research Edition)* 341 (September 25), 656–658.

Fraser, J., Harris, N., Berringer, A.J. & Finlay, F. (2010) Advanced care planning in children with life-limiting conditions – the Wishes Document. *Archives of Disease in Childhood*, 95, 79–82.

Fuller, A. (2012) Rising to the dementia challenge. *British Journal of Neuroscience Nursing*, 8 (3), 115.

George, R. & Dimond, B. (2009) Ethics and the Law. When an Advanced Care Plan is overruled. *End of Life Care*, 3 (3), 36–46.

Glasper, A. & Richardson, J. (2006) *A text book of children's and young people's nursing*. Churchill Livingstone, London.

Gott, M., Gardiner, C., Small, N., *et al.* (2009) Barriers to Advance Care Planning In Chronic Obstructive Airways Disease. *Palliative Medicine*, 23, 642–648.

Griffiths, J., Ewing, J., Rogers, M., *et al.* (2007) Supporting Cancer Patients with Palliative Care Needs District Nurses' Role Perceptions. *Cancer Nursing*, 30 (2), 156–59.

Haig, S. (2009) Diagnosing dying: symptoms and signs of end stage disease. *End of Life Care*, 3 (4), 8–13.

Hansford, P. & Meehan, H. (2007) Gold Standards Framework Improving Community Care. *End of Life Care*, 1 (3), 56–61.

Hermann, C. (2006) Developing and testing of the spiritual needs inventory for patients near the end of life. *Oncology Nursing Forum*, 33 (4), 737–45.

Hockley, J. (2009) Debating issues around death and dying in general settings. *End of Life Care*, 3 (4), 1754–69.

Holloway, M. (2006) Death the great leveller? Towards a transcultural spirituality of dying and bereavement. *Journal of Clinical Nursing*, Special Issue. Spirituality, 15 (7), 833–839.

Holloway, M., Adamson, S., McSherry, W. & Swinton, J. (2010) *Spiritual care at the end of life – a systematic review of the literature*, Crown.

Horne G., Seymour, J. & Shepherd, K. (2006) Advance Care Planning for patient with inoperable lung cancer. *International Journal of Palliative Nursing*, 12 (4) 172–178.

Horne, G., Seymour, J. & Payne, S. (2009) ACP: Evidence and implications for practice. *End of Life Care*, [3] 1, 58–68.

Howell, D. (2007) Comprehensive palliative home care: a need for integrated models of primary and specialist care. *International Journal of Palliative Nursing*, 13 (2), 54–55.

Janssen, D., Sprat, M. & Wouters, E. (2008) Daily symptom burden in end-stage chronic organ failure: A systematic review. *Pallaitive Medicine*, 22, 938–948.

Kennedy, C. (2005) District Nursing support for patients with cancer requiring palliative care. *British Journal of community nursing*, 10 (12), 566–74.

Kelly B. & Varghese F. (2006) The seduction of autonomy: countertransference and Assisted Suicide . In *When Professionals Weep: Emotional and countertransference response in End-of-life care* (eds R. Katz & T. Johnson). Routledge, London.

Lobb, E., Oldham, L., Vojkovic, S., *et al.* (2010) The workplace support needs of community palliative care nurses after the death of a patient. *Journal of Hospice and Palliative Nursing*, 12 (4), 225–233.

Luengo-Fernandes, R., Leal, J. & Gray, A. (2010) *Dementia. The economic burden of dementia and associated research finding in the United Kingdom*. University of Oxford, Oxford.

Luker, K. (2000) Are we meeting patients' needs? Oncology Nursing Today, 5 (1), 13–15.

Luker, K., Austin, L. & Caress, A. (2000) The importance of 'knowing the patient' Community nurses' constructions of quality in providing palliative care. *Journal of Advanced Nursing*, 31 (4), 775–782.

Machin L (2009) *Working with loss and grief: A new model for practitioners*. London Sage.

Marie Curie Cancer Care (2010) End-of-life Care for people with dementia. http://www.mariecurie. org.uk/Documents/HEALTHCARE-PROFESSIONALS/Innovation/project-report-0210.pdf Accessed on 21 November 2012.

Marie Curie Cancer Care (2012) *Delivering Choice Programme*. http://www.mariecurie.org.uk/ en-gb/healthcare-professionals/innovation/Delivering-Choice-Programme/. Accessed on 21 November 2012.

Minto F. & Strickland K. (2011) Anticipating emotion: a qualitative study of advance care planning in the community setting. *International Journal of Palliative Nursing*, 17 (6), 278–289.

Monroe, B. & Oliviere, D. (2007) Introduction: *unlocking resilience in palliative care*. In: *Resilience in Palliative Care; Achievement in Adversity* (eds B. Monroe, D. Oliviere). OUP, Oxford.

Moules, T. & Ramsey, J. (2008) *The textbook of Children's and Young People's Nursing*. Blackwell, Oxford.

Murtagh, M., Preston, M. & Higginson, I. (2004) Patterns of dying: palliative care for non-malignant disease. *Clinical Medicine*, 4 (1), 39–44.

National Council for Palliative Care (NCPC) (2009a) *Dying matters*. http://www.dyingmatters. org/overview/about-us. Accessed on 22 November 2012.

National Council for Palliative Care (NCPC) (2009b) *Out of the Shadows. End-of-life Care for people with dementia*. NCPC, London.

National Institute for Health and Clinical Excellence (NICE) (2004) *Improving palliative and supportive care for adults*, National Institute for Health and Clinical Excellence, London.

National Institute for Health and Clinical Excellence (NICE) (2005) *Healthcare services for children and young people with cancer*, NICE, London.

NHS (2012a) *Preferred Priorities for Care* http://www.endoflifecareforadults.nhs.uk/tools/core-tools/preferredprioritiesforcare. Accessed on 21 November 2012.

NHS (2012b) *Learning from peoples' experiences of last days of life*. http://www.endoflifecare-foradults.nhs.uk/news/all/learning-from-peoples-experience-of-last-days-of-life. Accessed on 21 November 2012.

NHS (2012c) Consultant Nurses Respond to negative media coverage. http://www.endoflifecare-foradults.nhs.uk/news/all/consultant-nurses-respond-to-negative-media-coverage-of-care-in-the-last-days-of-life. Accessed on 21 November 2012.

Nottingham Trent Cancer Network (NTCN) (2009) *Holistic needs Assessment Process*. NTCN.

Oliviere, D. (2002) Learning in palliative care: stories from and for my journey. In: *Journey into palliative care roots and reflections* (ed. Mason, C.). pp. 99–118. Jessica Kinsley, London.

Randall, F. & Downie, S .(2010) *End-of-life Care Consensus and Controversy*. OUP, Oxford.

Ratner, E., Norlander, L. & Kerstin, M. (2001) Death at home following a targeted Advance Care Planning process at home The kitchen table discussion. *American Journal of the Geriatric Society*, 49, 778–781.

Relf, M., Machin, L. & Archer, N. (2008) *Guidance for bereavement needs assessment in palliative care*, Help the Hospices, London.

Regnard, C., Reynalds, I., Watson, B., Matthews, D., Gibson, L. & Clarke, C. (2007) Understanding distress in people with severe communications difficulties. Developing and assessing the Disability Distress Assessment Tool (Disdat). *Journal of Intellectual Disability Research*, 51 (4), 277–92.

Respecting Choice Programme (RCP) (2010). Advance Care Planning a system that works. http://respectingchoice.org. Accessed on 25 August 2010.

Resuscitation Council UK (2007) *Decisions relating to cardiopulmonary resuscitation*. Available from www.resus.org.uk/pages/knar/htm. Accessed on 22 November 2012.

Reynolds, J. & Croft, S. (2010) How to implement the GSF to ensure continuity of care. *Nursing Times*, 106 (32), 10–12.

Richardson, A., Medina, J., Brown, V. & Sitzia, J. (2007) Patients needs assessment in cancer care: a review of assessment tools. *Supportive Care in Cancer*, 15 (10), 1125–1144.

Sampson, E., Jones, L., Thune-Boyle, I., *et al.* (2010) Palliative assessment of advance care planning in severe dementia. An exploratory RCT of a complex intervention. *Palliative Medicine*, 25 (3), 197–209.

Saunders, C., Seymour, J., Clarke, A., Gott, M. & Welton, M. (2006) Development of a peer education programme for advance end of life care planning. *International Journal of Palliative Nursing*, 12 (5), 214–223.

Sawicki, G., Dill, E., Asher, D., Sellers, D. & Robinson, W. (2008) Advance care planning in adults with cystic fibrosis. *Journal of Palliative Medicine*, 11 (8), 1135–1141.

Simon, W., Haney, C.A. & Buenteo, R. (2011) The Postmodernization of Death and Dying. *Symbolic Interactionism*, 16 (4), 411–426.

Simon, J., Murray, A. & Raffin, S. (2008) Facilitated advance care planning: What is the patient experience? *Journal of Palliative Care*, 24 (4), 256–264.

Shaw, K., Clifford, C., Thomas, K. & Meehan, H. (2010) Review: improving end-of-life care: a critical review of the GSF in primary care. *Pallaitive Medicine*, 24 (3), 317–329.

Smith, C. & Riley, J. (2011) There IT goes again. *BMJ*, 243, 5317. Available from www.bmj.com/content/34/bmj.d5317. Accessed on 9 November 2012.

Solano, J., Gomes, B. & Higginson, I. (2006) A comparison of symptom prevalence in far advanced cancer, Aids, HD, COPD and Renal disease. *Journal of pain and symptom management*, 31, 58–69.

Strecher, J. (2008) 'Allow natural death' vs 'Do not Resuscitate'. *American Journal of Nursing*, **108** (7), 11.

Thomas, K. (2003) *Caring for the Dying at Home Companions on the Journey*, Radcliffe Medical Press, Abingdon.

Twycross, R., Wilcock, A. & Stark Toller, C. (2009) *Symptom Management in Advanced Cancer.* pallaitivedrugs.com.uk, London.

Veerbeek, L., van Zuylen, L., Swart, S., Vogel-Voogt, E., van der Rijt, C. & van der Heide, A. (2008) The effect of the Liverpool Care Pathway for the dying: a multi-centre study. *Palliative Medicine*, 22, 146–151.

Walsh, C., Caress, A., Chew-Graham, C. & Todd, C. (2006) Evaluating partnership working lessons for palliative care. *European Journal of Cancer Care*, 16, 48–54.

Ward, R., Pugh, S. & Price, E. (2010) *Don't Look Back? Improving Health and Social Care Service Delivery for Older LGB Users.* Equality and Human Rights Commission, Manchester.

Watts, T. (2012) End-of-life care pathway as tools to promote and support a good death: A critical commentary. *European Journal of Cancer Care*, 21, 20–30.

Weiner, J. (2006) Emotional barriers to discussing Advance Directives: Practical training solutions. In: *When Professionals Weep: Emotional and countertransference response in End-of-life care* (eds R. Katz & T. Johnson). Routledge, London.

18

Interprofessional Learning and Teaching for Collaborative Practice Community

Sharon Aldridge Bent[1] and Ruth Clemow[2]

[1]Faculty of Society and Health, Buckinghamshire New University, High Wycombe, UK
[2]Faculty Health and Social Care, Buckinghamshire New University, Uxbridge, UK

Introduction

This chapter will provide a rationale for inter-professional learning and teaching in the community within the context of a plethora of complex changes in health and social care provision as a consequence of policy changes and emerging pedagogic evidence that supports and builds collaborative practice. Notions of competence, capability and health literacy will be examined and the structures that support the development of these in the learner, whether at preregistration or as part of the professionals' own continuing professional development. Signposting to principles and practice of IPE will be shown.

Inter-professional education and collaborative practice

Nationally, and to some extent internationally, calls for a flexible workforce and creative ways of working, along with a shift of emphasis from institutional to community-based health, social care and judicial services, may have led to increased role ambiguity and concerns about accountability within professions. However, a plethora of IPE initiatives have been developed and reported showing benefits on a number of levels and

Community and Public Health Nursing, Fifth Edition. Edited by David Sines,
Sharon Aldridge-Bent, Agnes Fanning, Penny Farrelly, Kate Potter and Jane Wright.
© 2013 John Wiley & Sons, Ltd. Published 2013 by John Wiley & Sons, Ltd.

duration, namely, to the individual and teams, showing a potential for impact on the service provided to patients, people and carers. In his review of UK IPE of a 30-year period, Barr (2007) proposed that with emerging evaluative evidence, foundations have been laid whereby governments could incorporate IPE into its health and social care modernisation strategies. Through his international review, Vyt (2009) reiterated the need for 'synergy between education and society'. The contribution of IPE with an emphasis on improving professional education in order to improve ways of working is apparent, although far from exclusive to inter-professional learning as a concept.

The White Paper *Equity and Excellence: Liberating the NHS* (DH 2010) sets out how the UK Government will:

- Put patients at the heart of everything the NHS does;
- Focus on continuously improving those things that really matter to patients – the outcome of their healthcare;
- Empower and liberate clinicians to innovate, with the freedom to focus on improving healthcare services.

Many of the changes proposed in this White Paper required primary legislation, including the creation of a Public Health Service, with a lead role on public health evidence and analysis and the transfer of local health improvement functions to local authorities. It is envisaged that this will result in significant and complex changes to the way professionals in the community work and whom they work with. At the local level, this calls for practitioners and educators to refocus on how evidence-based collaborative practice, as well as how learning and teaching in the community, can be achieved and delivered whilst ensuring that the public and patients remain at the centre of care.

Key implications for professions have also impacted as a result of the changes associated with regulation of health and care professionals; for example, the shift of Social Worker regulation from the General Social Care Council (GSCC) to the Health and Care Professions Council (HCPC) in 2012 further influences the drive for embedding opportunities and outcomes of collaborative practice in the curriculum between health and social care practitioners. Furthermore, professional colleges and associations, as well as other regulatory bodies, have adopted team or inter-professional working and learning to inform collaborative practice, within their standards for education (2012; NMC 2008a, 2010).

Effective collaboration involves the structure, processes and culture of health and social care. The World Health Organisation (WHO 2010) *Framework for action on interprofessional education and collaborative practice* highlights the current status of inter-professional collaboration around the world and identifies the mechanisms that shape successful collaborative teamwork and outlines a series of action items that policymakers can apply within their local health system (http://www.who.int/hrh/resources/framework_action/en/index.html).

The term *inter-professional* indicates a level of working together or collaboratively, in the case of healthcare – with the aim of improving the quality of patient care. Whilst *multi-professional* implies that there are two or more professions involved, although not necessarily working collaboratively. Conversely, the notion of working in *silos*, whether in multi-disciplinary teams or not, portrays negative connotations in managing the care needs of people in community settings, resulting in a failure in effective care provision and poor communication between professionals that can lead to significant system failures. The metaphor *silo* that is used here indicates a self-contained, protective entity or 'storage container' from where 'missiles' can be launched for self-protection. This perceptibly dramatises the opposing construct of collaborative practice. In 2008, McGregor wrote:

Various professionals, such as health visitors, school nurses, district nurses, general practice nurses working in community settings do not hold the same professional identify and therefore can have their own professional agendas. Add an increasing range of other professionals, people and organisations who are involved in the delivery of health and social care in the community to the mix, then it is not difficult to perceive how even with the best interests at heart, such complexity can lead to self-protection of professional identity and discordant practice. Increasingly, through policy development, the importance of adopting new ways of working and enacting innovative processes to support inter-professional collaboration is emphasised (DH 2011).

Based on extensive and longitudinal research, Goleman (1995) proposed that beyond the use of the 'intelligence quotient' (IQ), the competences associated with EI should also be assessed in order to determine whether employees will perform successfully as effective team members. He presents his thesis in two themes:

1. Personal competence – those competencies that determine how people manage themselves, to include self-awareness, self-regulation and motivation
2. Social competence – those competencies that determine how people handle relationships, to include empathy and social skills

Reports of poor nursing care have sometimes been associated with the quality of professional education. In response to these claims in early 2012, the Royal College of Nursing commissioned Lord Willis to undertake an independent inquiry (April 2012) into what excellent nursing in the United Kingdom should look like and how it should be delivered. Willis observed that:

Nursing is an incredibly self-aware profession, constantly striving to improve and give patients the best possible care (Willis November 2012, p. 67).

Willis indicated that it is imperative that nurses are provided with the right education and skills to equip them in their role. Not only that but consideration needs to be given to what types of support nurses require in their transition from a student to being registered as a nurse and thereafter through their continuing professional development, in order to become what the WHO (2010) describe as being *collaborative practice ready*, in order to meet ever-changing and challenging health needs and service. Two of the several recommendations made by Willis (2012) for pre-registration education included those of significant relevance to community nursing and include:

> Nurses and their organisations must stand up to be counted, to restore professional pride and provide leadership and solutions to the challenges of poor care and a decline in public confidence (p. 68).
> Nursing education should foster professionalism which includes embedding patient safety as its top priority, and respects the dignity and values of service users and their carers.

In considering these recommendations, one might readily note how they allude to a need for a change in culture in healthcare organisations, teams and individual ways of working. The former is perhaps outwith the majority of healthcare professionals' circle of influence, whereas influencing the change in culture in teams and at a personal level is achievable, subject to having the attribute of tenacity and motivation to do so. This will lead to a re-thinking of how learning and teaching for collaborative practice in community settings can be achieved.

Learning theory

Due to the nature of health professional education, much learning takes place in the workplace. Learning through simulation or in practice settings is an essential component for professional registration and integral to learning outcomes in many continuing professional development programmes. Experiential learning (Kolb 1984) applied to the context of patient care and public services has been given much attention elsewhere. However, to summarise for this discussion, 'Experiential Learning Theory' (ELT) is an important theory built from eclectic intellectual origins in the writings of Dewey, Lewin and Piaget. Kolb proposed that a synthesis of Dewey's philosophical pragmatism, Lewin's social psychology and Piaget's cognitive-developmental genetic epistemology forms a unique perspective on learning and development (Kolb 1984). ELT is characterised by the view that a whole system of beliefs must be analysed rather than simply its individual parts and includes a multi-parous model of adult learning, growth and development. Experience plays a central role in the learning process, an emphasis that distinguishes ELT from other learning theories. The term 'experiential' is used therefore to differentiate ELT both from cognitive learning theories, which tend to emphasise cognition over affect, and behavioural learning theories that tend to deny any part that the subjective experience in the learning process might play.

In 1990, Senge proposed that *learning organisations* are:

> where people continually expand their capacity to create the results they truly desire, where new and expansive patterns of thinking are nurtured, where collective aspiration are set free, and where people are continually learning to see the whole together (p. 3).

According to Goodman and Clemow (2010), this proposition indicates that new thinking is nurtured, aspiration is set free and people are continually learning. This might appear aspirational in complex organisations and services as characterised by community-based nursing. However, it is in response to the knowledge that people can adapt to changes and are flexible in ways of working, and support the expertise and talents of those who work in organisations, that they will develop the capacity to survive in an ever-changing environment. It is the converse view to traditional working practices that are left unchallenged. Effective collaboration involves developing the structure, processes and culture of healthcare organisations. Wenger's (1999) work on *communities of practice* underpins this proposition. Collaborative practice is at the heart of the aim of inter-professional learning and teamworking.

The WHO (2010) argues that collaborative practice happens when multiple health workers from different professional backgrounds work together with patients, families, carers and communities to deliver the highest quality of care. It allows health workers to engage any individual whose skills can help achieve local health goals (p. 6). We believe this incorporates multi-agency working, for example, to include local authorities and the judicial services.

Largely, the aims of IPE (DH 2000, 2006; CAIPE 2005, 2007; WHO 2007, 2010) are:

- To prepare and develop professionals who work in teams to manage risk, safeguard vulnerable people and deliver safe and effective plans, support, intervention and care;
- To provide generic learning through learning programmes for all professionals and staff;
- To redesign ways of working in order to address the new ways and contexts in which care is to be delivered.

IPE occurs when students from two or more professions learn about, from and/or with each other to enable effective collaboration and improve health outcomes. The WHO (2010, p. 6) believes that IPE is a necessary step in preparing a *collaborative practice-ready* health workforce that is better able to respond to local health needs. Furthermore that a *collaborative practice-ready* health worker is someone who has learned how to work in an inter-professional team and is competent to do so. Whilst much of community practice is transacted through lone working, effective collaboration is essential to achieve a seam-free people-/patient-focused service.

Barr *et al.* (2005), Barr (2007) and WHO (2010) identified four outcomes of IPE that are complementary, overlapping and correspond in part to each other in purpose, function and time. They are:

1. Preparing individuals for collaborative practice
2. Learning to work in groups or teams
3. Developing services and care improvement
4. Collaborative practice to strengthen health systems and improve health outcomes in populations

It is proposed that the latter two elements could have a transformative effect on organisations and society.

A significant amount of healthcare professional learning occurs in practice settings. Goodman and Clemow (2010) concur with Jarmillo (1996) and Bleakley (2006) in that sociocultural and constructivist learning theories and learning methods that take account of the learning environment should and do include learning about professional and public relationships, about working in teams and understanding the tool required to inform *intelligent practice*. These can then predict and provide an explanation of how learning occurs within and between teams in diverse community health and social care contexts.

Goodman and Clemow (2010) propose that inter-professional learning and teaching includes four important concepts beginning with the letter 'C'. They are communicate, co-ordinate, co-operate and collaborate. WHO (2010) identifies three other concepts in their proposition, that is, that health leaders who choose to contextualise, commit and champion IPE and collaborative practice will contribute movement towards the achievement of international goals. The model of inter-professional learning and teaching that we emphasise for community healthcare practice is supported by the WHO (2010) and the 7 'C's identified earlier. It starts with the consideration of the local health and social care needs of individuals and populations and the provision of inter-professional learning and teaching for the current and future workforce (e.g. in pre-qualifying professional programmes) to enable them to become collaborative practice ready, thus strengthening the healthcare system through workforce change and service improvement, to optimise health services and patient/people outcomes (p. 9).

In 1998, Barr focused on collaborative competences being those necessary for working with others. They included personal role clarity in context of others including the constraints and limitations of one's own practice; respect for the contribution of other professions in working together to plan, deliver and improve contextually relevant care and services through a person-centred approach, acceptance of difference and ambiguities such as autonomy and inter-dependence.

At the outset, the importance of understanding the local context is fundamental to building a collaborative practice-ready workforce. Influences based on new commissioning processes and delivery systems where any qualified provider can have a stake in delivering health services will create potential challenges and competition. However, these changes also provide opportunities for agreeing a local or regional inter-professional strategy and fit well with a quality framework for determining educational outcomes through Health Education England and the Local Education and Training Boards (DH 2011).

According to the WHO (2010, p. 7), a range of mechanisms influence effective IPE and collaborative practice. For the community settings, these include:

- Supportive management processes and practices
- Recognising and supporting champions
- The commitment to change the culture and attitudes of health professionals, workers and agencies

- A resolve to update, enhance and develop existing and new curricula
- Influencing policymakers to legislate for IPE and collaborative practice that eliminate barriers to achieving them

As previously highlighted, in the primary care and community context, a number of influences including new policy and national strategic initiatives are influencing the way in which services are delivered and transformed. As discussed earlier in this chapter, nursing and associated professional roles in the community and primary care are varied and continue to evolve. Whilst nurses make up the majority of health workers nationally and globally, the importance of how they work with people, agencies and other professionals who plan and deliver care is high on the political agenda for governments. Patient-, family- and person-centred care should be the catalyst for all education and learning whether at initial preparation or through continuing professional development. The community healthcare setting cannot be considered in isolation from the patient's overall journey through the health service system, and practitioners must ensure that professionalism embeds patient safety at the heart of all service provision.

The emphasis for both professional and inter-professional learning needs to be on services that support people, whether patients, carers or families to self-care, and thus maintain and manage their own health and conditions effectively. This requires practitioners to be health literate and to promote health literacy amongst others. Health literacy represents the cognitive and social skills that determine the motivation and ability of individuals to gain access to, understand and use information in ways which promote and maintain health. By improving peoples' access to health information and their capacity to use it effectively, health literacy is critical to empowerment (Nutbeam 2000, p. 264).

According to the DH (2009) (http://www.dh.gov.uk/en/Publicationsandstatistics), the gap between those who are empowered to help themselves and those who are not is growing. In an earlier report, Wanless (2004) illuminated the ideal that in order for people to become engaged fully, they needed to be able to make informed choices. There are many influences on what enables successful empowerment in people. One of these factors is a requisite standard of literacy and other skills to permit understanding and action on how to use information to improve health status. The term health literacy therefore implies the ability to receive, seek out, understand and act on information that will support and improve health and self-care. Here lies a challenge to health professionals in their own learning and development in order to support those who receive their care.

According to Polkinghorne (2004), in order to promote health literacy in people, there is a need for an integration of previous personal and cultural learning of imagined scenarios, of responses and action and of emotional reading of possible actions in the situation. In reflective understanding, the practitioner is attuned to the salient features of a specific situation and responsive to the nuanced changes that are occurring during the interchange. It is a decision-making process that adapts to the particular complex situation in which practitioners care and students learn. We believe this also requires the building of professional pride and role modelling for health and effective leadership. Inter-professional conversation that considers the context, real live challenges of people and their lived experience, the services that are involved and required can enable learning within the team environment or lone working context. Learning and teaching in the community requires that the professional and learner need to know the patient's or persons' contextual concerns.

This requires knowledge of the person's unique situational experience including socio-economic disparities, family dynamics, healthcare system barriers, health, illness and the life beliefs that truly matter to them and often influence how they learn, use and integrate healthcare information into their lives (Scheckels 2008). Furthermore, being sensitive to the teaching and learning situation necessitates the acquisition of competences associated with EI (Goleman 1999). In the context of promoting health literacy, Van Manen (1991, p. 125) purports that a tactful or perceptive person has the sensitive ability to interpret inner thoughts, understandings, feelings and desires from a range of indirect clues such as gestures, demeanour, expression and body language. *Tact* or perception in this context consists of the ability to interpret the psychological and social significance of the features of the person and self.

One such example emanates from the Green Paper 'Every Child Matters' (Department of Education 2004) where it was suggested that it should become a requirement that everyone working with children and families should have a common set of skills and knowledge across the following areas:

- Effective communication and engagement with children, young people, parents and carer
- Child and young people development
- Safeguarding and promoting the welfare of the child
- Supporting transition, multi-agency working, sharing information

Using these key indicators as competencies within the professional repertoire can form the focus for personal and team reflection; experiential learning that engage the patient as the expert in their experience; and inter-professional learning through critical incident analysis, for professionals and learners alike. Learning and teaching in this example includes an understanding of the political context. Everyday practice including near-miss events, these can be examined through reflection in and on practice that leads to professional reflexivity, thus learning from the challenges that exist in community settings and make changes to ways of working and to the lives of others.

It is recognised that more recent national initiatives include working with *the Troubled Families Programme* (Goverment UK 2012; www.communities.gov.uk) in the community where multi-agency working continues to be challenged and fraught with difficulty associated with failures in cross-boundary working and sharing of information. This government initiative is accompanied by financial investment for the Troubled Families Programme, within a payment by results scheme for local authorities.

It is known that 120 000 families are the targeted focus of this programme, with the prime minister confirming his intention to 'turn around' these troubled families by the end of 2014. These families are often characterised by the absence of working adults within the family, children who are persistently absent from school and the presence of members of the family who are involved in antisocial behaviour and crime. It is noted that these families frequently have other often long-term problems, which can lead to their children repeating the cycle of disadvantage (p. 1). In approximately one third of the families, there is evidence of child protection problems. Other problems such as domestic violence, relationship breakdown, mental and physical health problems and isolation make it highly challenging for families to start extricating from their problems (p. 1). Not only does this initiative aim to deal with troubled families, but it also seeks to learn about changing the trajectory of families and change the way services are delivered to them. The challenge for the local authority lies in the fact that currently many of these families are not known to them. This appears to be symptomatic of historic ways of working and reluctance, even in the best interest of those involved, to share information across services.

The use of a model such as that developed at Leicester Medical School (Lennox & Anderson 2007) where students engage in professional conversations with patients and other professions to understand different perspectives on the experience of those requiring services and their journey can provide a framework for both learning and professional development in the community setting. The model focuses on ways of teamworking, with a primary focus on the family enabling individuals to be cared for in their local context, including consideration of practices within and across services. It acknowledges that a particular focus might be on individuals in the family who are absent but have significant influence on the behaviours of others in the family and on individuals who are in transition from one service to another. We believe this provides an excellent inter-professional learning opportunity, whereby health, social and judicial practitioners can examine and evaluate a range of issues together for purposes of enhancing collaborative practice. One inter-professional strategy might be to use a process map to consider the experience of individuals in families and the influences that impact on their health, mental and physical well-being, health literacy for empowerment and motivation to self-care.

Elsewhere the reader can explore a range of arguments, assumptions and evidence for IPE (Barr *et al.* 2005) and challenges and opportunities that present for the development, delivery and evaluation (Freeth *et al.* 2005) of principles and models of IPE. Broadly, there is significant emphasis on emphasising core competences and capabilities as desirable assessable outcomes of inter-professional learning and teaching (e.g. see Lennox & Anderson 2007; Kell & Helme 2010).

The merits of 'competence' and 'capability' within inter-professional learning and working have been debated since the 1990s (Berman Brown & McCartney 2003; Vyt 2009). In the context of health and social care education, the notion of competence and its measurements are acknowledged. The GSCC (GSCC 2005) and more recently the HCPC (HCPC 2010) both identify mandatory standards for Social Work degrees and Post Qualifying Frameworks that explicitly link competence to practice. The NMC (2010) Standards for Pre-registration Nursing curriculum also discusses the achievement of competencies to practise as a nurse or midwife. The General Medical Council (GMC) (2007, 2009, 2010) refers to the importance of inter-professional training and practising doctors as a key determinant to meet mandatory competencies.

Competence can be defined as the capacity to deal adequately with a subject or task and to be suitable, fit appropriate and proper. This term describes what individuals know or are able to do in terms of knowledge, skills and attitudes at a particular point in time. Capability describes the extent to which an individual can apply, adapt and synthesise new knowledge from experience and continue to improve his or her performance (Berman Brown & McCartney 2003; Walsh *et al.* 2005). It is also defined as the integration of knowledge, skills, personal qualities and understanding that are used appropriately and effectively (Kilgallon & Thompson 2012). There is also an argument that competence and capability cannot be divided, and Fraser and Greenhalgh (2001) suggest that capability incorporates competence. Their view of capability includes the successful demonstration of tasks, the performance of which evolves as practice changes and that capability rather than competence better reflects and describes the requirements of professionals and professional practice.

Competence and capability within the context of IPE and practice are both important for effective collaboration in health and social care.

Teaching and learning in practice

One of the most important aspects of nursing is the clinical placement and the learning, teaching and assessment that takes place within this setting. A key mechanism for facilitating learning in the healthcare profession of students on practice placements is mentoring (Gopee 2011). Mentorship of all learners is widely implemented and utilised for both pre- and post-registration nursing and other health and social care professions.

Specifically, the NMC (2008a) Standards to Support Learning and Assessment in Practice set out benchmarks and outcomes for mentors, practice teachers and teachers of midwives, nurses and specialist community public health nursing (SCPHN) students. The standards identify a clear framework for the development of nurse teachers into four key stages:

Stage 1 NMC registrant – reflects that all nurses and midwives must meet the defined requirements; in particular 'You must facilitate students and others to develop their competence' (NMC (2008b) *The Code: Standards of conduct, performance and ethics for nurses and midwives* NMC London).

Stage 2 mentor – nurses and midwives can become a mentor when they have successfully achieved all the outcomes of this stage. This qualification is recorded on the local registers for mentors.

BOX 18.1   Eight developmental domains

- Establishing effective working relationships
- Facilitation of learning
- Assessment and accountability
- Evaluation of learning
- Creating an environment for learning
- Context of practice
- Evidence-based practice
- Leadership

Stage 3 practice teacher – identifies the standard for a practice teacher for nursing or SCPHN. To become a practice teacher, further outcomes need to be achieved. This qualification is recorded on a local register of practice teachers.

Stage 4 teacher – to become a teacher upon successful completion of an NMC-approved programme and the all outcomes for this stage have been achieved. This qualification is recorded on the NMC register.

There are five principles that underpin the earlier framework and dictate that the mentor/assessor must:

1. Be on the same part of the register as that which the student is working towards (this is significant with SCPHN)
2. Have developed their knowledge and skills beyond registration
3. Hold a professional qualification equal to or at a higher level than that which the students are working towards
4. Have been prepared for their role and met the NMC outcomes for such
5. Record any NMC-approved teaching qualification on the register

There are eight domains within the framework that provide guidance for applying the underpinning principles (Box 18.1). These have been designed for application within the context of inter-professional learning and working in modern healthcare (NMC 2008a).

Responsibilities for teaching and learning of all members of the team

Team leader

The role of the team leader cannot be underestimated within the learning environment of the clinical setting. In order for learning to be achieved, the team leader has to have a commitment to teaching and learning and have the ability to promote an atmosphere that encourages learning (Ogier 1989). The facilitation of learning cannot be divorced from humane and effective leadership and competent management.

Community practice teacher

All SCPHN students must have a named practice teacher (NMC 2008a). The role of the practice teacher is complex and requires an understanding of a specialist practice. In order to be deemed a qualified practice teacher, an NMC-approved practice teacher programme needs to be undertaken. Practice teacher preparation programmes include at least thirty days of protected learning time during which a trainee supports a student under the supervision of a sign-off practice teacher. Practice teachers are responsible and accountable for organising and co-ordinating the students' learning opportunities, assessing total performance and signing off achievement of proficiency. All SCPHN students must also have a named practice teacher.

In the current climate of staff shortages, the NMC (2011) has issued additional guidance around how to support learning in practice. It has outlined models for supporting more than one student in practice at a time and the application of the NMC Standards to Support Learning and Assessment in Practice (NMC 2008a). It is therefore crucial that practice and educational governance processes and policies need to be robust and transparent to all stakeholders (NMC 2010).

Mentor

According to the NMC, a mentor is 'a mandatory requirement for pre-registration nursing and midwifery students' (NMC 2008a). Mentors are accountable to the NMC for their decision that students are fit for practice and that they have the necessary knowledge, skills and competence to take on the role of registered nurse or midwife. The NMC standard defines a mentor as being a registrant who has successfully completed an accredited mentor preparation programme from an approved higher education institution.

Associate mentor

Associate mentor is the term given to an unqualified mentor that may be looking after a learner in the absence of the main mentor. In an area where there are many students and less qualified mentors, this is an educationally good practice; it also allows the learner to observe different ways of working and to witness a wider range of skills (Walsh 2010).

Learner

The learner is the term given to any person that has identified learning outcomes that may need to be achieved within the clinical setting. Here the person could be a preregistration nurse, a qualified nurse studying a continuing professional development course, a healthcare assistant or a new nurse who is being orientated to a new area of practice.

Sign-off mentor

The NMC (2006) Standards introduced the concept of a 'sign-off' mentor so that final judgements about a student nurse's capacity to practise safely and effectively is made by a mentor who has experience and who has fulfilled additional criteria (Walsh 2010). The additional criteria a 'sign-off' mentor must achieve are:

- Clinical currency and capability in the field of practice that the learner is being assessed;
- A working knowledge of current programme requirements, practice assessment strategies and relevant changes in education and practice for the student they are assessing;
- An understanding of the NMC registration requirements and the contribution they make to the achievement of these requirements;
- An in-depth understanding of their accountability to the NMC for the decisions they must make to pass or fail a student when assessing proficiency requirements at the end of a programme;
- Been supervised on at least three occasions for signing off proficiency by an existing sign-off mentor (NMC 2008a, p. 21).

Mastering mentorship

The move to all graduate nursing profession at the point of registration, the increasing emphasis placed on postgraduate level preregistration nursing and the inclusion of social work into the Health Profession's Council demonstrate new challenges for interprofessional mentorship and practice learning. Additionally increasing political and economic uncertainty of preregistration professional programmes in the context of the reconfiguration of the health and social care workforce and the continuing professional development of qualified health and social care practitioners are also under scrutiny, all combining to suggest that we should recognise the value of a master's level qualification in mentorship (Kilgallon & Thompson 2012). Mastery of professional practice can be defined as demonstrating the ability to make sense of complex and divergent concepts, theories and ideas. It is the ability to make sense of and apply new perspectives and ideas into practice in a unique and innovative way into practice that signifies mastery within a profession (Benner 1984).

It is also important for mentors to extend their thinking by considering themselves as role models in the context of the wider organisation and the development of mentorship for the future (Melincavage 2011). It is also essential that learners feel part of the contribution that they can make to the broader health and social care agenda and develop further understanding of their accountability to their employer.

Health and social care professionals practising within the current challenging economic and political climate need to have developed leadership skills in order to articulate their contributions to the organisation and their profession (George 2003). There is a growing

Table 18.1   The jigsaw model[a]

The policy framework	Effective practice
The Law	Characteristics of risk and assessment
Judicial System	Vulnerability
Policy	Working with risk
Procedures	Early intervention/prevention
Empowering practice	**The future**
Working together	'Bigger Picture'
Inter-/multi-agency working (collaboration)	Strategy
Organisational culture and management	Health and social care policy
Inquiries and serious case reviews	Commissioning

[a]Data from Scragg and Mantel (2011).

need for leadership within mentorship to be recognised that is a shift from the traditional view of leaders being managers. Stanley (2008) highlights the interchangeable nature of nursing management and leadership and notes that there needs to be a distinctive difference drawn between the two roles. This notion of difference would then assist the promotion of congruency between mentorship and leadership, making leadership responsibilities more explicit (Kinnell & Hughes 2010).

Adult safeguarding: an example

This example illustrates a model of inter-professional learning that has been applied within a comparative studies module in safeguarding. The module attracts students from various professions and backgrounds, including policing, psychology, nursing, midwifery, education and social work. The merits of collaboration between agencies when applying safeguarding policies are explored in depth. The framework used is introduced as four jigsaw pieces that each covers an aspect of safeguarding. Alongside the jigsaw, students are introduced to a case study that transcends the lifespan of a fictional vulnerable person. Multi-agency working practices and challenges across professional boundaries are explored, and the importance of sharing information is debated within an online blog. The ultimate goal of the learning framework is for the students to make sense of safeguarding issues from a range of perspectives and to synthesise and evaluate their practice (Table 18.1).

Conclusion

The influence of various government policies, changes to professional standards and emerging pedagogic and practice-based evidence has challenged health and social care professionals, service providers and educators to maintain the standards of practice and to support the development of collaborative practice through workforce change by applying effective educational strategies. The NMC framework confirms the responsibilities that employers, educators and learners have in fulfilling their responsibility in achieving the required standards for practice learning. It has been proposed that professionals working in health and social care (as well as policymakers) can contribute meaningfully towards the achievement of the international goal for IPE and collaborative practice. The principles outlined in the chapter comprise of the 7 'C's: communicate, co-ordinate, co-operate, collaborate, contextualise, commit and champion IPE and collaborative practice. Our model starts with the consideration of the local health and social care needs of individuals and populations and the provision of inter-professional learning and teaching for the current and future workforce to enable them to become 'collaborative practice ready'.

A network of roles exists to support learning and assessment in practice, including mentors and community practice teachers who play a key role in confirming competence of learners in practice settings for registration to ensure fitness for practice and registration with the NMC. IPE best serves the need for collaborative practice and is fundamental when caring for people in community settings, within and across care pathways and when in transition from one service to another. Sound preparation is required to ensure that individuals are adequately prepared for their role; opportunities for ongoing professional development must also be made available.

References

Barr, H. (1998) Competent to collaborate; towards a competency-based model for interprofessional education. *Journal of Interprofessional Care*, 12, 181–188.

Barr, H. (2007) *Interprofessional Education in the United Kingdom: 1966–1997*. Health Sciences and Practice Network of the Higher Education Academy, London.

Barr, H., Koppel, I., Reeves, S., Hammick, M. & Freeth, D. (2005) *Effective Interprofessional Education: Arguments, Assumptions & Evidence*. Blackwell Publishing, Oxford.

Benner, P. (1984) *From Novice to Expert*, Addison-Wesley, London.

Berman Brown, R. & McCartney, S. (2003) Lets have some competence here. *Education and Training*, 45 (1), 7–12.

Bleakley, A. (2006) Broadening conceptions of learning in medical education: the message from teamworking. *Medical Education* 40 (2), 150–157.

CAIPE (2005) *Creating an Interprofessional Workforce: An Education and Training Framework for Health and Social Care in England*. CAIPE, London.

CAIPE (2007) *Creating an Interprofessional Workforce: An Education and Training Framework for Health and Social Care in England*, updated version. CAIPE, London.

Department of Education (2004) *Every Child Matters*, Cm. 5860. British Government, The Stationery Office, London.

Department of Health (DH) (2009) *Promoting Health Literacy, Publications Policy and Guidance*. Available from http://www.dh.gov.uk/en/Publicationsandstatistics. Accessed on 18 December 2012.

DH (2010) *Equity and Excellence: Liberating the NHS*. DH, London.

Fraser, S. & Greenhagh, T. (2001) Coping with complexity: educating for capability. *British Medical Journal*, 323, 799–803.

Freeth, D., Hammick, M., Reeves, S., Koppel, I. & Barr, H. (2005) *Effective Interprofessional Education: Development, Delivery and Evaluation*, Blackwell Publishing, Oxford.

General Medical Council (GMC) (2005) *The Foundation Programme Curriculum.* GMC, London.

General Medical Council (2009) *Tomorrow's Doctors.* GMC, London.

General Medical Council (2010) *Regulating Doctors, Ensuring Good Medical Practice.* GMC, London.

George, B. (2003) *Authentic Leadership: Rediscovering the Secrets to Creating Lasting Value,* Jossey-Bass, San Francisco.

Goleman, D.P. (1995) *Emotional Intelligence. Why It Can Matter More than IQ for Character, Health and Lifelong Achievement.* Bantam Books, New York.

Goleman, D. (1999) Working with Emotional Intelligence, Bloomsbury Publishers PLC, London.

Gopee, N. (2011) *Mentoring and Supervision in Healthcare,* 2nd edn. Sage, London.

Goodman, B. & Clemow, R. (2010) *Nursing and Collaborative Practice,* Learning Matters, Exeter.

Government UK (2012) *The Troubled Families Programme.* Available from www.communities.gov.uk. Accessed on.

GSCC (2005) *Assessment in Social Work: A Guide for Learning and Teaching.* Social Care Institute for Excellence, London.

Health and Care Professions Council (2010) *Continuing Professional Development and Your Registration.* HPC, London.

Health and Care Professions Council (HCPC) (2012) *Standards of Education and Training.* HCPC, London.

Jaramillo, J. (1996) Vyygotsky's sociocultural theory and contributions to the development of constructivist curricula. *Education* 117 (1), 133–140.

Kell, C. & Helme, M. (eds.) (2010) *Interprofessional Education in Wales: Case Studies in Health and Social Care,* Higher Education Academy Health Sciences and Practice Subject Centre, London.

Kilgallon, K. & Thompson, J. (2012) *Mentoring in Nursing and Healthcare – A practical approach.* Wiley-Blackwell, Oxford.

Kinnell, D. & Hughes, P. (2010) *Mentoring Nursing and Healthcare Students,* Sage, London.

Kolb, D.A. (1984) *Experiential Learning: Experience as the Source of Learning and Development,* Prentice-Hall, Upper Saddle River, NJ.

Lennox, A. & Anderson, E. (2007) *The Leicester Model of Interprofessional Education. A Practical Guide for Implementation.* The Higher Education Academy Subject Centre for Medicine, Dentistry and Veterinary Medicine, Newcastle upon Tyne.

Melincavage, S. (2011) Student Nurses' experiences of anxiety in the clinical setting. *Nurse Education Today,* 31, 785–789.

Nursing and Midwifery Council (NMC) (2006) *Standards to Support Learning and Assessment in Practice – NMC Standards for Mentors, Practice Teachers and Teachers.* NMC, London.

NMC (2008a) *Standards to Support Learning and Assessment in Practice.* NMC, London.

NMC (2008b) *The NMC Code.* NMC, London.

NMC (2010) *Standards for Pre-registration Nursing Education.* NMC, London.

NMC (2011) *Standards for Pre-Registration Nursing Education.* NMC, London.

Nutbeam, D. (2000) Health Literacy as a public health goal: a challenge for contemporary health education and communication strategies for the 21st century. *Health Promotion International,* 15 (3), 259–264.

Ogier, M. (1989) *Working and Learning,* Scutari Press, London.

Polkinghorne, D.E. (2004) *Practice and the Human Sciences: The Case for a Judgement-Based Practice of Care.* State University of New York Press, New York.

Scragg, T. & Mantel, A. (2011) *Safeguarding Adults in Social Work,* Learning Matters, Glasgow.

Scheckels, M. (2008) *Understanding the Expertise of Diabetes Educators: A Phenomenological study. Paper presented at the American Association of Diabetes,* Educators, Washington DC.

Stanley, D. (2008) Congruent leadership: values in action. *Journal of Nursing Management*, 16, 519–524.

Van Manen, M. (1991) *The Tact of Teaching: The meaning of Pedagogical Thought*. State University of New York Press, New York.

Vyt, A. (2009) *Exploring Quality Assurance in Interprofessional Education in Health and Social Care*, EIPEN, Vyt and Garant Publishers, London.

Walsh, D. (2010) *The Nurse Mentor's Handbook – Supporting Students in Clinical Practice*. Open University Press, Maidenhead.

Walsh, C., Gordon, F., Marshall, M., Wilson, F. & Hunt, T. (2005) Developing a capability framework for interprofessional education. *Nurse Education in Practice*, 5, 230–237.

Wanless, D. (2004a) *Securing Good Health for the Whole Population*, Final report. Department of health, London.

Wanless, D. (2004b) *Securing good health for the whole population: Final report*. Available from www.dh.gov.uk/en/PublicationsAndStatistics/Publications/PublicationsPolicyAndGuidance/DH_4074426. Accessed on 18 December 2012.

Wenger, E. (1999) *Communities of Practice: Learning, Meaning and Identity*. Cambridge University Press, Cambridge.

Willis, P. (2012) *Willis Commission: Quality with compassion: the future of nursing education*. Available from www.williscommission.org.uk. Accessed on 18 December 2012.

World Health organisation (WHO) (2007) *World Health Organization Study Group on Interprofessional education and Collaborative practice*. WHO Press, Geneva.

WHO (2010) *Framework for action on interprofessional education and collaborative practice*. Available from http://whqlibdoc.who.int/hq/2010/WHO_HRH_HPN_10.3_eng.pdf. Accessed on 7 November 2012.

19

User Involvement, Self-Management and Compliance

Maryam Zonouzi

Peer Exchange, London, UK

The twenty-first century will be the era when community Health Care Nursing comes into its own, working in partnership with patients, their families and communities. The contribution outlined in this chapter rests on the proposition that, for very good reasons, twenty-first-century community healthcare nursing will be holistic and relational, whereby individual practitioners, working as members of multidisciplinary teams, will 'co-produce' health improvement, working and learning with patients/users, their families and friends, informed by the newly legislated PPI system.

As this chapter is being written, the NHS is undergoing one of the largest reforms in more than a generation. *The Health and Social Care act* 2012 proposes to abolish NHS primary care trusts (PCTs) and strategic health authorities (SHAs). Thereafter, £60 to £80 billion of 'commissioning', or health-care funds, would be transferred from the abolished PCTs to several hundred 'Clinical Commissioning Groups' (CCGs), partly run by the general practitioners (GPs) in England. A new public body, *Public Health England*, is planned to be established on 1 April 2013. These reforms include changes to PPI initiatives.

The Health and Social Care Act 2012 places greater emphasis on individual patient influence and choice:

> Patients should be at the heart of everything we do. In Liberating the NHS we set out the Government's ambition to achieve healthcare outcomes that are among the best in the world by involving patients fully in their own care, with decisions made in partnership with clinicians, rather than by clinicians alone: no decision about me, without me (DH 2012, p. 3).

Community and Public Health Nursing, Fifth Edition. Edited by David Sines,
Sharon Aldridge-Bent, Agnes Fanning, Penny Farrelly, Kate Potter and Jane Wright.
© 2013 John Wiley & Sons, Ltd. Published 2013 by John Wiley & Sons, Ltd.

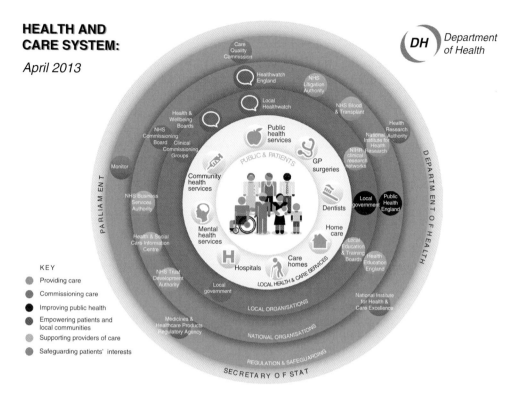

HEALTH AND CARE SYSTEM:

April 2013

KEY

- Providing care
- Commissioning care
- Improving public health
- Empowering patients and local communities
- Supporting providers of care
- Safeguarding patients' interests

Figure 19.1   Model of shared decision-making along the patient pathway (liberating the NHS p. 13)

A model of shared decision-making is proposed all along the patient pathway, giving patients greater involvement in their own care and more say. The Department of Health has developed a diagram to demonstrate to patients, their families and carers the choices that should be available to them all along the pathway (see Fig. 19.1).

The modern PPI system

In the context of PPI, 'patient involvement' is viewed as co-productive, where patients help to define the quality of care and report information on their own health-care experiences, whereas 'public involvement' emphasises the involvement of laypeople as taxpayers who may or may not have special knowledge of the subject under discussion. However, many have struggled with the notion of 'public' involvement in the past. Difficulties have arisen for many reasons primarily to do with there being little in government literature that clearly distinguishes between the involvement of patients and the involvement of the wider public.

There have been several attempts to reform PPI and its value to the NHS and two parliamentary inquiries. In 1974, Community Health Councils (CHCs) were established as arm's-length appointed bodies managed through the then regional offices of the NHS. In 2003, they were replaced by Patient and Public Involvement Forums (PPIFs),

BOX 19.1   Healthwatch England

- The *Health and Social Care Act* 2012 established Healthwatch England to become the national body that enables the collective views of the people who use NHS and social care services to influence national policy, advice and guidance.
- It is a statutory committee of the CQC.
- Healthwatch England will be funded as part of the Department of Health's grant in aid to the CQC and will provide leadership, guidance and support to Local Health Watch organisations.
- Healthwatch England will be able to escalate concerns about health and social care services raised by Local Health Watch to the CQC.
- The Secretary of State for Health will be required to consult Healthwatch England on the mandate for the NHS Commissioning Board.
- Healthwatch England will be required to make an annual report to Parliament.

principally because they were seen as inconsistent in their performance and unrepresentative of local people. PPIFs, supported by a national commission, failed to meet expectations: indeed, they appeared to provoke the same criticisms as did their predecessors, the CHCs. PPIFs were replaced by Local Involvement Networks (LINKs), which had the remit to cover health and social care under the Local Government and Public Involvement in Health Act 2007.

LINKs were intended to differ in three crucial respects from either CHCs or PPIFs: they were contracted through local government and not the NHS; they had a specific brief to be socially inclusive; their role was to report, assiduously, on patient's, user's, and carer's experiences, providing useful and reliable data to trusts, local authorities and the health and social care regulators. Their role was not representative, but enabling and informing, supported by organisations called HOSTs, drawn by competitive tender from the voluntary and community sector in each local authority area. LINKs are now being replaced by Health Watch schemes that will collectively report into Healthwatch England (see Box 19.1), a statutory but autonomous part of the Care Quality Commission (CQC), which has a mandate to provide leadership, advice and support to Local Health Watch Schemes, which are to be funded by local authorities. Like LINKs Local Health Watch schemes encompass both health and social care services (see Box 19.2).

The complexity of the current Health and Social Care system is demonstrated in Fig. 19.1.

The rationale for greater user involvement

The requirement for greater user involvement in Health and Social Care primarily relates to the public funding of national health services. Governments are concerned about delivering 'value for money' and want to appear to have clear justifications for

BOX 19.2   Local Health Watch

Healthwatch will be the new consumer champion for both health and social care. It will exist in two distinct forms – Local Health Watch, at local level, and Healthwatch England, at national level:

- The *Health and Social Care Act* 2012 sets out that Local Health Watch will be established in April 2013. A Local Health Watch will be an independent organisation, able to become the influential and effective voice of the public empowering citizens and communities to influence and challenge how health and social care services are provided within their locality.
- The *Health and Social Care Act* 2012 requires local authorities to have a Local Health Watch organisation in their area and expects them to provide an advocacy service to people who wish to make a complaint about their experience of the local NHS.
- Local Health Watch will have a seat on the new statutory health and well-being boards, ensuring that user experiences are reflected when local needs assessments and strategies are prepared.
- Local Health Watch will enable people to build a picture of where services are doing well and where they can be improved and will alert Healthwatch England to concerns about specific care providers.
- Local Health Watch will provide people with information about their choices; Local Health Watch will provide, or signpost people to, information about local health and care services and how to access them.
- Local Health Watch will provide authoritative, evidence-based feedback to organisations responsible for commissioning or delivering local health and social care services.
- Local Health Watch will establish relationships with local authorities, CCGs, patient representative groups, the local voluntary and community sector and service providers to ensure it is inclusive and truly representative of the community it serves.

The responsibilities relating to PPI under new structures fall under the auspices of a multitude of organisations (see Box 19.3).

public spending they feel this helps to strengthen the public's voice in decisions about the organisation of health and social care and delivery of health services.

More recently, greater calls for patients and public involvement go hand in hand for calls to 'empower' staff working for the health service through 'John Lewis' style cooperatives and mutuals that attempt to break down typical organisational hierarchies and replace them with 'staff-owned' structures.

These reforms go hand in hand with the shift of patient to consumer coupled with the promotion of a patient choice agenda. This redefines the focus of health service

BOX 19.3   Organisations and their responsibilities for PPI

Body	PPI responsibility
NHS Commissioning Board:	To promote PPI.
	To provide guidance for GP Commissioning Consortia in relation to PPI.
GP Commissioning Consortia (GPCC):	To involve the public in their decision making.
	To commission services that are responsive to patients.
Health and Wellbeing Boards:	To perform a comprehensive assessment of local needs.
	To work with GPCC in ensuring that services are responsive to patients.
Local authority:	To commission Local Health Watch
	To commission a health advocacy and complaints service.
	To undertake overview and scrutiny of any planned service changes.
Local HealthWatch:	To provide advocacy and support for individual patients.
	To ensure that patient voices are an integral part of local commissioning.
National HealthWatch:	To support Local HealthWatch.
	To propose CQC investigation of poor services.

provision and reframes healthcare providers as vendors. In this shift from patient to consumer, PPI is 'then presented as the feedback mechanism for the expression of consumer views; an essential component of markets' (Tritter & Macallum 2006).

This presupposes that patients have the necessary information to choose and that their choices change service provision or that their purchasing decisions change the demands of what is provided.

Marinker argues that 'In contemporary Britain, citizenship is confused with consumerism and democracy with marketing. Choice and individualism are elevated to the status of moral imperatives. The consumer is characterised not only by the right to choice but also by entitlement to redress' (1996, p. 13).

A good example of this can be seen by the widespread adoption of the 'personalisation', 'personal budgets in social care' and 'personal health budgets' in the NHS, which 'transforms' 'users' to 'consumers' with their own 'individualised budget'.

Consumerism is currently presented as a mechanism for redressing the power inequality between health professionals and patients. Longley suggests, however, 'The preference for consumerism and individual choice is more about customer relations than any enhanced rights which entail true partnership or power sharing' (1996, p. 147).

Power sharing requires a more nuanced approach than a route to market. Many organisations operating around the patient/user choice agenda believe passionately that greater access to the markets will enrich and empower citizens. However, there is little evidence that providing a route to market correlates to better health or well-being outcomes for the individual or to a better provision of service.

PPI like many things to do with government initiatives sit on a continuum moving from social justice to consumerist models where health and care are seen either as a citizenship rights or individual choice in the markets.

However, the case for most 'patients' such as myself is that I want to understand my rights as a citizen and require clarity on what choices, if any, I do have about my care whether provided for by the NHS, Social Care or private enterprise and that quality of care is viewed as the single highest priority when decisions are made about which service best suits my needs. For me this is more important than being told that I must attend PPI meetings or that my rights are enhanced somehow by PPI initiatives.

Having had the *privilege* of chairing many user involvement initiatives over the past decade, what is clear to me is that perpetuating the myth that PPI enhances citizenship rights is disingenuous. In my personal and professional experience, it neither enhanced our rights as citizens, changed the provision of services nor gave us more choice. At best it acted as a way to legitimise decisions whether good or bad.

As asserted by Ignatieff, It is a symptom of the crisis of citizenship, that most political rhetoric, whether left or right, addresses the electorate not as citizens but as taxpayers or as consumers (1995, p. 71).

The reasons and motivations for governments to 'involve' patients and the public are different than the reasons and justifications for individuals. There may be in many cases a mismatch of motivation. This can lead to frustration for both individuals and those tasked with managing PPI initiatives.

Due to the nature of PPI initiatives needed to be outsourced to 'host bodies' through the local authority at best, each host body will be given between £100 000 and £200 000 locally per year to manage Local Health Watch. This typically pays for two co-ordinators and a number of PPI meetings and sub-meetings throughout the year. Most PPI members are laypeople and act as volunteers. Their scope and reach may seem far reaching, but with increased responsibilities, host bodies and funding authorities will need to be realistic about what they can achieve.

I have witnessed many times lay individuals who have been motivated by improvements in health and social care services. However, I have also witnessed occasions where patient and public involvement has been 'mis-sold' as 'public action', which is defined as activities initiated and controlled by bottom-up groups for purposes determined by them. Conversely, this differs from the concept of 'public involvement', which is about top-down groups that may seek support for decisions already made and consult on issues yet to be decided.

While local Health Watch schemes may feel autonomous, the structures have been mandated from the Government. Healthwatch has been established to take account of views in relation to health and social care, and therefore, the perimeters for discussion and debate have been fixed on service delivery rather than a broader well-being agenda. This forces the discussion towards an over-medicalised narrative rather than a more holistic inclusive conversation like well-being, which is not defined by services. Sadly, like LINKs before, Healthwatch does not represent 'public action' but 'public involvement' and is therefore a top-down manifestation.

One of the major issues with any reform of PPI is that the definition and mechanism for involving the 'public' has never been set out or resolved. Consequently, those involved in PPI initiatives are either those who work in the sector or those who most use its services. Unfortunately, this has the unintended consequence of reinforcing the over-medicalisation of care. A deeply ingrained assumption in our culture is that if you have a 'problem' or a 'need', you get a label. Typically, in the PPI context, labels such as, 'patient', 'users', 'client', 'disabled', 'impaired' and 'sick' are often applied. This separates citizens into categories and groups defined by the service models that have been erected to meet this 'need/problem'.

The major issue with this paradigm is that it takes a one-dimensional approach to the citizen and defines their participation by their 'special needs', 'illness' or 'use of a service,' thus excluding their many purposes, roles, capabilities and aspirations and so on as parents, partners, entrepreneurs and citizens.

I have first-hand experience of how this type of labelling can quash creativity and attempts of co-production. I am a disabled person and therefore a 'service user' in the eyes of my local authority. No matter what other roles I occupy, which include academic researcher, social entrepreneur, software developer, teacher, course developer and e-learning instructor, it was made clear to me that my 'disability' was by far the most useful label I could possess. My 'involvement' and 'participation' was narrowly defined by the services I happen to access, and even then the entry requirement for my involvement was my wheelchair and what organisation I 'represented'.

Any innovation or creativity that I was involved with happened outside or in spite of my relationship with the NHS or social services. It was subsequently my reflection that while the structures that had been erected to 'involve' including LINKs were exclusively interested in listening to stories about the use of services, any suggestions we had for service redesign, innovation or delivering services were seen to be the preserve of 'service providers' and subject to 'tendering'.

The relationship felt one sided as we were there to give our ideas, make suggestions but never to co-produce or co-deliver or benefit in any other way than to be the recipient. It could be argued that 'involvement' will be limited to commenting and scrutinising the status quo until we are able to adopt methodologies that enable us to frame the problem and co-create the solutions.

Sadly, this experience is not just limited to my own experience as noted by Professor Sang where he states:

I recently observed an earnest well-intentioned discussion where a mix of local activists (PPI Forum members, service users, advocates, community development workers), and NHS managers and Clinical Professionals debated the potential structure of their new Local Involvement Networks (LINKs – see below). Whilst they had acknowledged the interim nature of their thinking (as the relevant legislation was then going through the Committee stage in Parliament) they failed to reflect on the assumptions underpinning their discussions, i.e. *The assumption that it was their role to speak for patients' interests and not to enable patients to speak for themselves.*

There was a consequent bias in both the substance and in the process. For example, two women working with asylum seekers and ethnic minority groups struggled to be heard because authority was conceded – by default – to those arguing forcefully about the *representativeness* of the LINKs and how existing vested interests could be reconciled. They did not hear what the women had to say. Indeed, they were modelling the very behaviour (i.e. the traditional paternalist-centralist model of involvement in healthcare) that will continue to undermine the new policy intentions and leave us with a paradigm of involvement that is inequitable, non-inclusive, and anti-participatory (Sines *et al.* 2009, p. 354).

The following section outlines my personal critique of what I believe to be the fundamental problem with current PPI frameworks:

1. Is there a problem? – In most other fields generally if the aim is to improve a service or change a service, we must first seek to involve users in framing the problem. The public sector often fails to apply this basic tenet, and users are expected to evaluate services without understanding if a problem exists with it. This has the unintended outcome of artificially institutionalising people and does not allow them to step outside of the 'patient' role. If the only way people feel involved is through the labels we place on them, then where is the exit points? Stepping up and out of the system is as important as knowing where the entrance is.

2. Do you have the 'power or delegated duty' to make the change? – There is often little clarity on what individuals working in the health service who operate PPI have the 'right' and 'delegated responsibility for'; it is important to be clear about when decisions are made and and when the best opportunity occurs to suggest changes. A willingness of all to work together for change is laudable; however, if the change cannot be realised, it is a wasted opportunity.

3. Appropriate contributions according to the problem – It is also important that involvement is sought not because you have to be seen to be involved but because you have a contribution to make that will help to change the service. That contribution needs to be sought and is as important as recruiting someone for a job. This can take place in an open spiral where the opportunity for users to raise their views is always open but equally time is given to change the service. Instead much time is spent on changing the PPI system itself to move in the direction of prescribed policy changes. As such both PPI and the healthcare system are at the mercy of policy changes set at government level rather than patient led.

4. Open your eyes to the sub-text of people's involvement – The most common complaint I received from commissioners was that meetings always appeared to attract the same ten people. This was often the case and may be the only opportunity they had to get out and meet other people. The problem was one of a lack of social support and isolation

with their desire for social support being continually ignored. Timing of meetings might also be a barrier to attracting greater numbers of users, with service providers and commissioners scheduling events to correspond with their work commitments.

5. Plan the exit – As a social entrepreneur I have pitched to many investors, and one of the questions they will always ask is what your exit plan is. What they mean by this is that they expect you will leave and move onto other things or that you will sell your business. There is an inbuilt mechanism that allows me to move on. However, in PPI there was no exit strategy and no planned route to move beyond certain topics of discussion because the services were static. Therefore, individuals were always carrying their label even though they may have wished to elevate to something else or moved beyond using that service.

6. Evaluate your social impact – The importance of measuring the impact that patient and public engagement has had on service develops and service redesign is essential. It is often difficult to measure how much influence such interventions actually have since problems may not have been clearly defined and required improvements are not always easy to articulate.

7. Don't collude – I know it's difficult to not collude, but it is all too easy to collude with service providers to ensure that users are 'locked into their labels'. This is counterproductive for them, and there is little material benefit for those 'involved'.

The ability for individuals and groups to move towards a more organic 'public action' model involves a genuine power shift away from labels and predefined service models of participation towards a twenty-first-century paradigm based on mutuality, dialogue and a fresh narrative about healthcare. However, this involves understanding firstly how engaged people are and understanding if and how they wish to be involved. A desire by the state to involve 'users' is not the same as genuinely attempting to identify what motivates the individual to take part in something. This requires a process of negotiation and counter-negotiation as a key skill set. These skills typically fall under the role of mediation, negotiation and advocacy rather than project management or event organisation.

However, as local authorities have been mandated to find and fund host organisations to facilitate local Health Watch schemes, it remains to be seen if they will recruit organisations with different approaches and models for speaking up for consumers or if they will engage organisations that are adept at silencing the user voice.

The level of participation is an important measure of the effectiveness of PPI initiatives; however, it is difficult to find precise information on this. 'Most user involvement initiatives require a critical mass of interested people who will stand for election, attend regular meetings and participate in training' (Tritter & McCallum 2006, p. 160).

McCallum and Tritter (2006) looked at attendance levels at PPI initiatives on one North London area; during 1999–2000, they found that more than half of the members attended less than two-thirds of the full meetings and only a third attended more than two-thirds of the meetings of project groups for which they had volunteered. These trends were echoed at higher board levels also.

Engaging local people is crucial for the legitimacy of PPI exercises as they help to reinforce perceptions of local democratic accountability. This has the potential to

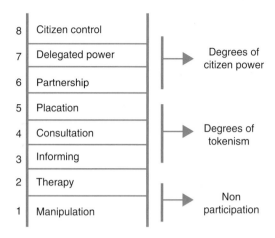

Figure 19.2   Eight levels of citizen participation

increase user and public frustration with the PPI system, as is the case in Sweden where individuals and non-state agencies 'undertake parallel consultation over national health policies and strategies with specific user groups or their representatives' (Tritter & McCallum 2006, p. 160).

The lack of evidence on the effectiveness of PPI may be linked to the fact that 'the key document that continues to shape the theoretical framework for user involvement is Arnstein's 1969 ladder of Citizen Participation'. Critics have argued that this methodology has been applied uncritically and that it may be time to re-evaluate both the methodology and the practice of how PPI is implemented.

Arnstein asserts that citizen participation is citizenship power and produced a ladder with eight levels of participation. The eight types are arranged in a ladder pattern with each rung corresponding to the extent of citizens' power in determining the end product (see Fig. 19.2).

The bottom rungs of the ladder are (1) manipulation and (2) therapy. These two rungs describe the levels of 'non-participation' established to substitute for 'genuine participation' enabling power holders to 'educate' or 'cure' the participants. Rungs 3 and 4 progress to levels of 'tokenism' that allow the 'have-nots' to hear and to have a voice: (3) informing and (4) consultation. These extend to listening exercises; however, individuals lack the power to ensure that their views will be acted upon no changes to the status quo. Rung (5) placation is a higher-level tokenism as the rules allow 'have-nots' to advise; however, the 'power holders' hold the right to decide. Further up the ladder are levels of citizen power with increasing degrees of decision-making clout. Citizens can enter into a (6) partnership that enables them to negotiate and engage in trade-offs with traditional power holders. At the topmost rungs, (7) delegated power and (8) citizen control, have-not citizens obtain the majority of decision-making seats or full managerial power.

They critique Arnstein's claim that citizen participation is a categorical term for citizen power. They argue that user engagement and empowerment are complex phenomena through which individuals formulate meanings and actions that reflect their desired degree of participation in individual and societal decision-making processes.

Additionally, 'power holders' usually themselves employees of state agencies such as the health service are rarely in a position to transfer their workload or responsibility to patients or public, and as such Arnstein's concentration on the delegation of power from officials to users does not lead to citizen control unless authority and responsibility are also delegated.

Critics argue that the processes and methods, in other words 'how' you involve people, are more important than the outcome or 'the act of involvement'. They argue that different user involvement methods need to be applied to secure different levels of involvement from different people and that the aim of user involvement is not solely about user empowerment.

Arnstein sees no relationship between the aims of an involvement exercise and the methods adopted to involve them. As highlighted by my own and others' experience of PPI, Arnstein's critics argue that 'the most important missing rung in Arnstein's ladder associated with methods is the failure to consider the' essential role of users in framing problems and not simply in designing solutions' (Tritter & McCallum 2006, p. 162).

Arnstein's approach conceptualises user involvement activity as a contest between two parties wrestling for control over a finite amount of power. 'This adversarial model seems to exclude opportunities for collaboration and shared decision-making and may simply lead to the creation of a new class of user elite' (Tritter & McCallum 2006, p. 164).

The patient as co-producer

Essentially, this chapter has argued for a much more 'bottom-up' approach to healthcare reform, based on a working partnership between citizens and professionals, enabled by the new system of PPI.

The policy drivers 'talk the talk' of engagement and empowerment, but it is at a local level where creative practitioners are beginning to make a real difference to both the commissioning and provision of care, based on their empathy and ability to work collaboratively with other professionals and with 'clients/service users'.

The normative presumption is that state solutions are always the best and that the state is capable of innovation to support change for individuals. However, change is not something that you can do *for* people; it is something that you do *with* people. This act of working in partnership or co-production is more likely to support transformative change (Needham 2009).

Research has indicated that 'co-production, where it has been happening successfully, has generally been outside nationally funded services that are supposed to achieve this, and usually despite – rather than because of – administrative systems inside public services' (Boyle *et al.*, 2006).

Successful PPI requires health and social care workers to work in co-production. This requires power sharing and individual learning opportunities; this cannot occur without working together with service users to enable them to take on increasing responsibility. Building individual and community capacity is central to this premise. This theme enshrined within the context of the Government's Localism Bill (2010) and through partnership agreements, such as 'Think Local Act Personal, 2010', which support the further devolution of power directly to individuals and communities.

This demonstrates a swing towards service users' active involvement in development and delivery. This shift of policy focus requires further collaboration and social capital and is, in essence, co-production. Co-production recognises and harnesses the expertise of service users in shaping their own care and encourages their involvement in improving and delivering services. It challenges the dominant role of the professional and shifts the service user from the role of a passive recipient to that of a valued participant in the process on an individual and collective level (Needham 2009).

Research suggests that there are three different types of co-production in care services; I see no reason why community health nursing would be any different:

1. Compliance (descriptive) – co-production takes place at the stage of service delivery, as carers and people who use services collaborate to achieve results. People using services make contributions at each stage of service provision, but they are not involved in implementation.
   Weaknesses of the compliance level – despite the acknowledgement that care services cannot be produced without input from the people who use services, the compliance tier offers little opportunity for real change by or for the people who use services because it is about complying with an existing regime.
2. Support (intermediate) – the intermediate level of co-production recognises and values people who come together to co-produce care services. It acknowledges the input and value of service users, utilises existing support networks and improves channels for people to be involved in the shaping of services. It may include new or more involved roles for users in the recruitment and training of professionals and managers. Also it may see responsibilities being shared with the people who use services.
   Weaknesses of the support level – users continue to be supporters rather than controllers or managers of the service. The expertise continues to be situated outside of the users themselves.
3. Transformative – the most effective methods of co-production can transform services and create new relationships between the people who use them and staff. This transformative level of co-production takes 'a whole life focus', incorporating quality of life issues as well as simply clinical or service issues.

At its most effective, co-production can involve the transformation of services. The transformative level of co-production requires a relocation of power and control, through the development of new user-led mechanisms of planning, delivery, management and governance. It involves new structures of delivery to entrench co-production, rather than simply ad hoc opportunities for collaboration. It can be 'a form of citizenship in practice' (Needham 2009, p. 37).

Co-production cannot be realised without support

For co-production to be successful, a number of things need to happen:

- Supporting the building of social capital for all groups in the community: without adequate support, co-production can sideline already marginalised groups as there are limits to the extent that some people can co-produce without support.
- Social exclusion, equality and diversity need to be taken into account to ensure that co-production does not target those who are in a position to be more involved but reaches out in a proactive way to those people who require support to take part.
- Co-production as a means for achieving transformation needs to be sustained; however, this is challenged by the short-term nature of projects and initiatives.
- For co-production to be successful, both staff and service users require access to training. Social care staff require training to share power with service users, and service users need support to fill in skills gaps to be able to contribute.

Being able to take positive risks is essential for both staff and service users as this is essential to the learning and creative process of co-production; this is important in breaking down some of the professional relationships and ensuring staff continuity so that relationships can be built. One way of transforming staff attitudes is through staff taking part in co-productive projects, such as a greater awareness of the contributions of people who use services and their carers and greater recognition of the credibility of service users working as outreach workers (Needham 2009).

However, research has indicated that 'co-production, where it has been happening successfully, has generally been outside nationally funded services that are supposed to achieve this, and usually despite – rather than because of – administrative systems inside public services' (Boyle *et al.* 2006).

This needs to be considered when forging partnerships with non-statutory agencies, voluntary organisations and user-led organisations.

Co-production is not a new delivery mechanism for health and social care services. It is an approach that affirms and supports an active and productive role for people who use services and the value of collaborative relationships in delivering the outcomes negotiated with the person using the service. According to Small (2000), the transition of an individual from passive recipient of services to active subject engaging with services is at the centre of user empowerment.

The development of service user involvement in the voluntary and statutory sectors has stemmed largely from user movements advocating for rights of their members, such as the disability movement (see Rummery & Glendinning 2000 and Ellis 2005; Beresford 2005 for examples).

The aim is to develop a model where the consciousness of users and the wider community is raised, and as a result, the people involved are empowered to make decisions not only about the services they receive but also in their lives as a whole. There is a hope that this in turn will be effective in bringing about change in policy and practice through allowing the voices of those receiving the services to be heard.

Most importantly, the earlier frameworks demonstrate the inherent complexity of human living and the interdependence of the factors that impinge on Health and Wellbeing, positively and negatively. Community nurses are positioned betwixt and between the uncertainty and unpredictability of people's lives, especially those living with long-term conditions and disabilities, and the politicised managerial system that increasingly relies on the mantra of evidence-based choice. In this modern context relationships with patients themselves provide the best data for clinical practice and for influencing decision-making.

This will mean working at a pace that is acceptable to an individual, and understanding that empowerment will mean different things to different people. We should understand what level of support a person needs and offer support that allows them to make informed choices with as much or as little control as they would like to have. Plus we must ensure that those who cannot or do not want to take control have access to adequate person-centred services to help them live the life they want to live.

The stochastic nature of medicine has been recognised since the time of Aristotle and has been conveniently forgotten as medicine has become merchandised (Lerodiakonou 1993). As noted earlier, the inherent complexity addressed by every citizen, as they learn to engage with disease or injury, creates the need for an integrated, dialogic response:

> Science and narrative, the quantitative and the qualitative, are not competitors, but represent a complementary duality. Narrative preserves individuality, distinctiveness, and context, whereas quantitative methods and evidence-based guidelines offer a solid foundation for what is reliably and generally correct (Roberts 2000, p. 440).

Conclusion

Current methods applied for PPI fail to capture the dynamic and iterative process of involvement. Also they fail to recognise the agency of users who have their own methods of involvement and seek out involvement at different times for differing issues. Those issues and interests are likely to be different to the motivations of officials.

The process and reasons for involving patients in decisions about their own care are supported by both patients and health professionals; however, the wider 'public' agenda is less clear as the rights and responsibilities of those taking part are not enshrined or upheld by law. Therefore, their powers cannot be qualified or articulated beyond rhetoric. Furthermore, the lack of effective evaluation of PPI schemes further supports claims that PPI is driven by a top-down desire by governments who feel that PPI acts as an effective lever to rubber stamp decisions.

PPI sets up a system that asserts as fact that 'citizens' demand a 'voice' and must be 'empowered' to 'take control' in decision-making. This sets up professionals and health services as organisations that do not listen or that should listen more. It also wrongly implies that those who work in the health service have the power to change services and sets up a false premise that citizens can through their involvement 'fight' to change the services. This frames the involvement in purely competitive terms, a zero-sum game.

The methods and models of involvement need to be as diverse as the people who are part of our society. There must also be a recognition from government and statutory services that user involvement requires that the structure and process be dynamic and negotiated by users themselves as 'public action' and not 'public involvement'.

This requires less hierarchical structures where needs and problem identification are given equal importance to evaluation of services. Similarly, it is important that the exercise is genuine and conducted when both health service officials, staff and users have the power and influence to effect change.

While continual improvement in service is what is expected, it is not practical or feasible for patients and public to be involved in these exercises as ultimately they are not duties that can be delegated from officials to lay individuals.

In spite of numerous changes to the PPI system, there is little evidence to suggest that the powers of patient or public have been increased. Continual conflation of social justice aims and consumerism within health services act to push the discussion away from the rights of patients as citizens towards the choices they have as purchasers and taxpayers.

By framing PPI within the context of health and care services, the discussion is also locked into a service model that stifles discussion and debate about wider social barriers or the inclusion of other services that both contribute and hinder to the well-being agenda. Furthermore, it acts to label individuals and confines them to narrow roles that are difficult to step up and out of.

Stepping up and out of being passive recipients of services requires officials, staff and participants to become co-producers of healthcare policy and practice at individual and community level.

Acknowledgement

I would like to acknowledge the late Professor Sang's work that imbues this chapter (as presented in the 4th edition of this book).

References

Beresford, P. (2005) 'Service user': regressive or liberatory terminology? *Disability & Society*, 20 (4), 469–77.
Boyle, D., Clark, S. & Burns, S. (2006) *Hidden Work: Co-production by People Outside Paid Employment*. Joseph Rowntree Foundation, York.
Buetow, S. (1998) The scope for the involvement of patients in their consultations with health professionals: rights, responsibilities and preferences of patients. *Journal of Medical Ethics*, 24, 243–247.

Department of Health (DH) (2012) *Liberating the NHS No Decision About Me Without Me*. DH, London.

Ellis, K. (2005) Disability rights in practice: the relationship between human rights and social rights in contemporary social care. *Disability & Society*, 20 (7), 691–704.

Ignatieff, M. (1995). The myth of citizenship. In: *Theorizing citizenship* (ed. R. Beiner). SUNY Press, Albany.

Lerodiakonou, K. (1993) Medicine as a scholastic art. *Lancet*, 341 (8844), 542.

Marinker, M. (ed.) (1996) *Sense and Sensibility in Healthcare*, BMJ Publishing Group, London.

Needham, C. (2009) *Co-Production: An emerging Evidence Base for Adult Social Care Transformation: SCIE Research Briefing 31*. Social Care Institute for Excellence, London.

Roberts, G. (2000) Narrative and severe mental illness: what place do stories have in an evidence-based world. *Advances in Psychiatric Treatment*, 6, 432–441.

Rummery, K. & Glendinning, C. (2000) Access to services as a civil and social rights issue: the role of welfare professionals in regulating access to and commissioning services for disabled and older people under New Labour. *Social Policy and administration*, 34 (5), 529–550.

Small, N. (2000) User Involvement Protocol. Westminster Action Network on Disability, London.

Tritter, J. & McCallum, A. (2006) The snakes and ladders of user involvement: moving beyond Arnstein. *Health Policy*, 76, 156–168.

Index

Note: document titles are printed in italics; page numbers in italics refer to figures; page numbers in bold refer to tables.

Academic Health Science Networks 9
Acheson Report 185
ACP (advance care planning) 290–2, 298
ACS (ambulatory care sensitive)
    conditions 55
ACT (Association for Children with Life-
    Threatening and Terminal Conditions
    and their Families) 297
action research 78
acute care 54
    children, young people and their
        families 119–23
    see also emergency care
ADNE (Association of District Nurse
    Educators) 163
ADRT (advanced decisions to refuse
    treatment) 292
ADSS (Association of Directors of Social
    Services) 274
adult safeguarding 159–60, 271–2
    definitions of abuse 272
    domestic violence 276–9
    inter-professional learning in 318
    legal framework 274–5
    prevalence of abuse 272–3,
        277
    recent guidance 275–6
    responses to abuse concerns 273–4
    substance and alcohol misuse 279–80
'adults at risk' 159, 272
advance care planning (ACP) 290–2, 298
advance statements (AS) 291–2
advanced decisions to refuse treatment
    (ADRT) 292
advanced practitioners 18, 178
    see also specialist community public health
        nurses (SCPHN)
AEC (ambulatory emergency care) 55
Aiming High for Disabled Children 126
alcohol misuse 279–80
Allowing Natural Death (AND) 293

Alternative Provider Medical Services
    (APMS) 172
Alzheimer's Society 44
ambulatory care 54–5
ambulatory care sensitive (ACS)
    conditions 55
ambulatory emergency care (AEC) 55
AND (Allowing Natural Death) 293
antenatal care 101–2
anti-discriminatory practice 225
anti-social behaviour 93–4
any qualified provider (AQP) 5, 39, 246–7
APMS (Alternative Provider Medical
    Services) 172
AS (advance statements) 291–2
Asperger's syndrome 218
Assessing and Investigating their symptoms
    and Referring for support (FAIR) 57
asset-based community development *see*
    capacity building
assistant practitioners 18
assisted suicide 292–3
assistive technology 164
Association for Children with Life-
    Threatening and Terminal Conditions
    and their Families (ACT) 297
Association of Directors of Social Services
    (ADSS) 274
Association of District Nurse Educators
    (ADNE) 163
asthma care 47–8, 123–4, 180
Asthma UK 47, 48
autistic spectrum disorders 218
autonomy, personal 60
Avoid Asthma Attacks campaign 47

behavioural change 142–3
benchmarking of performance 56, 174
bereavement 298–9
Best Interest Assessments (BIA) 275
Best Practice Tariff for diabetes care 124

Community and Public Health Nursing, Fifth Edition. Edited by David Sines,
Sharon Aldridge-Bent, Agnes Fanning, Penny Farrelly, Kate Potter and Jane Wright.
© 2013 John Wiley & Sons, Ltd. Published 2013 by John Wiley & Sons, Ltd.

Beveridge Report 138
BIA (Best Interest Assessments) 275
'Big Society' 24, 246, 262
bioengineering 9
blood pressure monitoring 180–1
British Guidelines on the Management of
    Asthma 180
Buckinghamshire New University
    Centre of Excellence in Tele-Health and
        Assisted Living 40
    'Transition to Community Nursing'
        module 164
burden of disease 2, 38, 135–6

CAF (Common Assessment Framework) 104,
    108
cancer
    in childhood 296
    people with learning disability 228
    screening services 10, 177
capability and competence 313–14
capacity building 27
    see also community development
cardiopulmonary resuscitation (CPR) 293,
    297
'care as communal action' 62, 64
'care as labour' 62, 64
'care closer to home' 2–4, 53–70, 152–3, 247
care homes 55
*Care in Local Communities: A Vision and
    Model for District Nursing* 155–6
'care in the community' 55, 61
care industry 55, 62
care packages 9, 10
Care Quality Commission 23
    Healthwatch 23, 324
    State of Care reports 55, 247
Care Services Improvement Partnership
    (CSIP) 44
career pathways 15
carers 9, 62–3, 164–5, 243
'caring' 61–3
caring relationship 64–5
causes of death 135–6, 227, **228**
CBA (cost benefit analysis) 76
CCGs *see* Clinical Commissioning Groups
    (CCGs)
CCI (Communities Collaborating
    Institute) 37
CCN *see* community children's nursing
    (CCN)
CEA (cost-effectiveness analysis) 76
census information 76–7
Centre for Social Innovation 264
cervical screening 177

Change4life campaign 104
*Changing Behaviour, Improving
    Outcomes* 142
*Child Public Health Outcomes
    Framework* 99
Children Act (2004) 95
children and young people
    effect of domestic violence 278
    emergency and urgent care pathways 120
    end-of-life care 296–7
    health indicators 92–3
    with learning disability 219–20
    in research studies 77, 87
    safeguarding 95, 101, 108–9
    technology dependent 127
    unemployment 93
    well-being 94–6
children and young people services
    Healthy Child Programme (HCP) 97–101
    policy context 95–6
    role of the specialist community public
        health nurse 97
    for young families 101–8
    see also community children's nursing
        (CCN)
Children's National Services Framework 126
Children's Society 110
Choosing Health 23
chronic illness *see* long-term conditions
    (LTC)
chronic obstructive pulmonary disease
    (COPD) 47
CLDN *see* community learning disability
    nurses (CLDN)
Clinical Commissioning Groups (CCGs) 181,
    245, 263–4
    membership 139
    responsibilities 10, 42
*Clinical Governance and Adult
    Safeguarding* 273
Close to Home 153
CMHN *see* community mental health nurses
    (CMHN)
CMHT (community mental health
    teams) 202–3
collaborative practice 306–8, 309–11
commissioning 263–4
    see also Clinical Commissioning Groups
        (CCGs)
Commissioning for Quality and Innovation
    (CQUIN) targets 57, 248, 264
Common Assessment Framework (CAF) 104,
    108
Communities Collaborating Institute
    (CCI) 37

communities of practice 309
community capacity *see* capacity building
community children's nurses
    community care roles 123, 124–5, 129
    professional competences 121, 312
community children's nursing (CCN) 113–34
    acute and short-term conditions 119–23
    continuing care 128
    disabilities and complex conditions 125–7
    history 113–15
    life-limiting and life-threatening
        illness 128–30
    long-term conditions 123–5
    NHS provision 115–19
    technology dependent children 127
community collaboration 37, 40
community context to domestic violence 278
'community' definition 24–5
community development 22–36, 263
    definitions 24–9
    policy context 23–4
    role of community health professionals
        in 29–32
    tackling obesity 46
Community Development Exchange 27
community engagement 25, 28–9
community health practitioners *see*
        community children's nurses;
        community learning disability nurses
        (CLDN); community mental health
        nurses (CMHN); district nurses; health
        visitors; occupational health nurses;
        school nurses; specialist community
        public health nurses (SCPHN)
community learning disability nurses
        (CLDN) 230–6
community learning disability
        nursing 216–40
    see also learning disability
community learning disability services 220–
        4, 233–6
community mental health nurses
        (CMHN) 202–3
    roles and responsibilities 210–13
    therapeutic relationship 205–6, 211
community mental health nursing 201–15
    needs assessment 206–7
    principles of 210–13
    risk assessment and management 212–13
    see also mental health
community mental health teams
        (CMHTs) 202–3
community networks 25
community practice teachers 316
community public health nursing 146–9

community research 78
community-focused care 2–4, 11
Compassion in Practice 161
competences 17, 30–2
    community children's nurses 95, 121
    district nurses 162–3
    general practice nurses 174
    health care assistants (HCAs) 175–6
    for inter-professional working 307, 313–14
    occupational health nurses 186
competition in the NHS 139, 171, 246–7, 262
complex case management 155–7
consumerism in healthcare 4, 14, 23, 326
Co-ordinate My Care 288
COPD (chronic obstructive pulmonary
        disease) 47
co-production (user involvement) 332–5
core competencies *see* competences
cost benefit analysis (CBA) 76
cost utility analysis (CUA) 76
cost-effectiveness analysis (CEA) 76
Council for the Education and Training of
        Health Visitors 97
CPR (cardiopulmonary resuscitation) 293,
        297
CQUIN (Commissioning for Quality and
        Innovation) targets 57, 248, 264
criminal record checks 159
CSIP (Care Services Improvement
        Partnership) 44
CUA (cost utility analysis) 76
cultural influences on health 48–9

DALY (Disability-Adjusted Life Year) 136
Darzi Report 262
data collection methods 79
data management, analysis and
        interpretation 79–81
DCSF *see* Department for Children, Schools
        and Families (DCSF)
DDA (Disability Discrimination Act)
        (1995) 126, 218, 225
definitions of health 58–61, 94–5
Dementia 2012: A National Challenge 44
dementia care 297–8
    hospital admissions 55
    multi-sector working 44–5
demographics 1, 76–7
Department for Children, Schools and
        Families (DCSF)
    Healthy Child Programme 96
    *Working Together to Safeguard
        Children* 104
Deprivation of Liberty Safeguards (DoLS) 275
DESMOND approach for diabetes 177

determinants of health 48–9, 140–1, *144*
Developing the Healthcare Workforce 6
diabetes care 123–4, 124, 177
digital media 83
direct payments 9
Disability Discrimination Act (1995)
    (DDA) 126, 218, 225
Disability-Adjusted Life Year (DALY) 136
disabled children 125–7
disabled people in the workplace 196
DisDAT assessment tool 298
disease patterns across the world 135–6
district nurses 154, 158, 160
    key skills 161–2
    support and supervision 165–6
district nursing 155–7
do not attempt resuscitation (DNAR)
    orders 293
DoLS (Deprivation of Liberty Safeguards) 275
domestic violence 276–9
domiciliary care *see* home care
dressings 178
drugs tests 86
dual diagnosis 280
Dying Matters Coalition 285

Ealing asthma campaign 47–8
early intervention 254
    ambulatory care sensitive (ACS)
        conditions 55
    child safeguarding 101, 110
    public health nursing 147
    respiratory disease 47
early years education 95, 103
e-based systems 6, 10, 83, 164
EBP (evidence-based practice) 72–3
economic influences on health 26, 92–3,
    135–6
    see also health inequalities; poverty
education and training
    of children and young people 95–6
    for community development role 31–2
    community nurses 58, 163
    for dementia treatment and care 44–5
    general practice nurses 175, 178, 180
    government review 6
    nurse teachers 314–15, 316
    Willis Commission 307–8
effectiveness measurement 56, 146, 160,
    253–4
    see also health impact assessments (HIA)
eHealth 6, 10, 83, 164
electronic health-care record 254
ELT (experiential learning theory) 308
emergency care 9, 119, 120

emotional health 94, 104, 109–10
empowerment 311–12
    in care settings **165**
    definition 26–7
    mental health patients 206
End of Life Strategy 286
end-of-life care 285–304
    advance care planning 290–2
    advanced decisions to refuse treatment
        (ADRT) 292
    assisted suicide 292–3
    bereavement 298–9
    children and young people 128–30
    community nurses role 296
    death of a child 296–7
    dementia 297–8
    do not attempt resuscitation (DNAR)
        orders 293
    interdisciplinary working 295–6
    last days of life 294–5
    needs assessment 288–9
    psychological and spiritual aspects 290
    symptom management 289
    whole systems approach 286–8
End-of-Life Care Strategy 286, 290, 299
environmental influences on health 48–9,
    60–1, 136
epilepsy care 123–4
Equality Act (2010) 196
*Equity and Excellence: Liberating the
    NHS* 2, 139, 153, 306
ethical issues
    in research 84–5, 86–7
    in treatment 137
ethics committees 86–7
ethnic minority communities
    domestic violence in 279
    involving 25
    learning disability services 223
    risk factors 75
European Convention on Human Rights 225
evaluation
    clinical educational innovation 80–1
    health impact assessment (HIA) 75–7
    public health interventions 146
    qualitative research 82
    see also effectiveness measurement;
        outcome measurement
Every Child Matters 95, 100, 126
evidence-based practice (EBP) 72–3
experiential learning theory (ELT) 308

FAIR (Assessing and Investigating their
    symptoms and Referring for
    support) 57

Fair Society, Healthy Lives 24, 140–1
family care 62, 63, 101–8
family life 94
Federation for Community Development
    Learning 30
Field report on child poverty 93
Fit for Work Services (FFWS) 190
fitness to work 195–6
Food Futures Strategy for Manchester 46
Foresight Report 45
Foundation Trusts 9, 10
Francis Report 61, 62, 245, 251–2
Friends and Family Test 57, 160, 254
Front Line Care 262
frontier measurement 56
Frontline First Innovation Awards 264

General Medical Council (GMC) 314
General Medical Services contract 171,
    173
general practice 170–4
general practice nurses
    consultations with 178–9
    core skills 174
    education and training 175, 178, 180
    origins 173
    prescribing of drugs 178–9
    roles and functions 176–81
general practice nursing 169–83
    history 172–4
    long-term conditions 179–81
    scheduled care 176–8
    unscheduled care 178–9
*Getting It Right for Children, Young People
    and Families* 43
global comparisons *see* international
    comparisons
Gloucestershire dementia strategy 44–5
GMC (General Medical Council) 314
Gold Standards Framework (GSF) 286–8
government policy *see* public policy
GP Commissioning Consortia (GPCC) 326
    see also Clinical Commissioning Groups
    (CCGs)
GSF (Gold Standards Framework) 286–8
*Guidance on Involving Adult NHS Service
    Users and Carers* 243
Guide to the Right to Provide 262

HCA (health care assistants) 163, 173, 175
HCP (Healthy Child Programme) 97–108
*Health, Work and Wellbeing – Caring for Our
    Future* 189
Health and Care Professions Council
    (HCPC) 306, 313

Health and Safety at Work etc. Act
    (1974) 192, 197
Health and Safety Commission 198
Health and Safety Executive (HSE) 187
Health and Social Care Act (2012) 5, 8, 42,
    139–40, 190
    Healthwatch 23, 325
    individual patient influence and
        choice 322–3
    social innovation 262–3
    see also Clinical Commissioning Groups
        (CCGs)
Health and Social Care Information Centre
    (HSCIC) 154
Health and Wellbeing Boards 42, 145, 326
health as well-being 60, 94–5
health assessment *see* nursing assessment
'health care' 58–61
health care assistants (HCAs) 163, 173, 175
health care needs assessment *see* needs
    assessment
health care providers 10
    any qualified provider (AQP) 5, 39, 246–7
    care industry 55, 62
health concerns 2, 38, 65, 135–6
'health' definitions 58–61, 94–5
health determinants 140–1, *144*
health education 147
Health Education England 6
health impact assessments (HIA) 75–7
health improvements 141, 198
health inequalities 24, 26
    tackling 136–7, 140–1, 185, 190
    see also vulnerable groups
health information 142
health literacy 311
health promotion 41, 137, 141, 142–3
    children 103
    practice nurse role 176
    versus public health 143–4
health protection 141–2, 145–6
    occupational health nurses role 194–5
    practice nurse role 176
Health Protection Agency (HPA) 145
Health Visitor Implementation Plan 25, 30,
    96, 101
health visitors
    in community development work 30–1, 32
    implementation plan 100, 101
    improving emotional health and
        well-being 109–10
    services for families 96, 101–8
Healthwatch 23, 324
Healthy Child Programme (HCP) 97–108
healthy choices 142

Healthy Lives, Healthy People 24, 139
Healthy Schools Initiatives 104
hermeneutic study 77
HIA (health impact assessments) 75–7
High Quality Care for All 42, 248
higher education institutions
    Academic Health Science Networks 9
    Buckinghamshire New University
        Centre of Excellence in Tele-Health and
            Assisted Living 40
        Health and Care Alliance 39
        'Transition to Community Nursing'
            module 164
    Imperial College, London, obesity
        research 46
    Leicester Medical School 313
    Manchester University
        review of technology-dependent
            children 127
    Swansea University, 'Public Health and
        Partnerships in Care' course 39
    training role 38–9
holistic care 286–7, 289, 290
holistic model of health 48, 205, 234
home care 55, 63, 65–8, 151–68
    24 hour provision of care 63
    adult safeguarding 159–60
    complex conditions 155–7
    informal carers 9, 62, 164–5
    leadership in 161
    long-term conditions 154–5
    maximising health and well-being 158
    measuring impact of service 160
    policy context 152–4, 247
    quality and effectiveness of care 160
    support and supervision 165–6
    technology in 164
    therapeutic relationship 158–9
    workforce planning 161–4
    see also district nurses; health visitors
homeless people 81, 260, 265
hospital admissions
    children and young people 119
    dementia 55
hospital facilities 11
hospital nursing 63
hospitals
    average length of stay 56–7
    centralisation and specialisation of
        services 54
    performance measurement 56
    reduction in number of beds 53–4, 55
HPA (Health Protection Agency) 145
HSCIC (Health and Social Care Information
    Centre) 154

HSE (Health and Safety Executive) 187
human resources *see* workforce
Human Rights Act (1998) 87
hypertension care 180–1

ILO (International Labour Organisation) 184
immunisations 102, 103, 104, 105, 177
*Improving Health and Care: The Role of the
    Outcomes Frameworks* 158
income inequality 93
    see also health inequalities; poverty
Independent and Supplementary Nurse
    Prescribing 178
independent living 158
Independent Nurse Prescribers 179
independent providers *see* health care
    providers
inequality *see* economic influences on
    health; health inequalities
informal care 9, 62, 164–5
information technology 10, 83
informed consent 159–60
innovation 9, 40
    in community children's nursing
        (CCN) 121–2
    CQUIN targets 57, 248, 264
    translational research 73–4
    see also social innovation
Innovation, Health and Wealth 40
integrated care 7, 11, 13, 43, 67, 151, 153–4
    see also multi-agency working
Integrated Research Application System
    (IRAS) 84
intensive care 77, 129
interdisciplinary working in end-of-life
    care 295–6
international comparisons
    hospital length of stay 56–7
    patterns of disease 135–6
International Labour Organisation (ILO) 184
internet for research information 83
interpersonal skills 251
inter-professional education (IPE) 305–21
    learning theory 308–14
    responsibilities for teaching and
        learning 315–18
    teaching and learning in practice 314–15
IRAS (Integrated Research Application
    System) 84

joint health and well-being strategies 145
joint sector working *see* multi-sector
    working
Joint Strategic Needs Assessments
    (JSNAs) 23, 145

Kaiser Permanente triangle 154, *155*
Kennedy Review 121, 123–4
King's Fund 138, 151, 246, 254

LAC (looked-after child) 105
Laming Report 95
LAs *see* local authorities (LAs)
Law Commission, *Adult Social Care* 272, 275
LCP (Liverpool Care Pathway) 294–5
leadership 241–6
    community development and capacity
        building 32
    community nurses 161
    effectiveness of delivery 253–4
    front-line staff 247–51, 262
    influencing people 248–9
    policy context 245–7
    qualities 243–4
    styles of 251–3
leading causes of death 2, 135–6
*Leading The Way Through Social
    Enterprise* 262
learning disability 217–20
    demographics 218–19
    health of people with 226–9, 233–4
    and learning difficulty 218
    research 87, 227–8
    see also community learning disability
        nursing
learning disability services *see* community
        learning disability services
learning organisations 308–9
learning theory 308–14
Leicester Medical School 313
leukaemia care 296
Liberating the Talents 155
life expectancy 136
lifestyle-related diseases 9, 137, 280
    see also health promotion
LINK (Local Involvement Networks) 324
Liverpool Care Pathway (LCP) 294–5
Living Well With Dementia 44
local authorities (LAs)
    Health and Wellbeing Boards 42, 43, 190
    public health responsibilities 140, 145, 190
    responsibilities for PPI 326
Local Education and Training Boards 6, 11
Local Healthwatch 325, 327–30
Local Involvement Networks (LINKs) 324
local leaders 25
local needs assessment 23, 65, 140, 145, 147–
        8, 264
Localism Bill (2010) 333
long-term conditions (LTC) 9, 136, 154–5
    chronic care model 66

practice nurse role 179, 179–81
    see also end-of-life care
looked-after child (LAC) 105
Luton dementia care 45

Manchester Alliance for Community Care 46
Manchester tackling obesity 46
Manchester University review of technology-
        dependent children 127
marginalised groups 24, 25
    see also vulnerable groups
marketing of services 160, 326–7
Marmot Review 24, 61, 136–7, 140–1
measurable outcomes *see* outcome
        measurement
measuring effectiveness *see* effectiveness
        measurement
Medical Research Council 46
medical technology 9, 127, 164
MEND (Mind Exercise, Nutrition, Do it) 105
Mental Capacity Act (2005) 274–5, 291
mental health 201–15, 228
    burden of disease 136
    children 104–5
    and domestic violence 277
    institutional care 202
    mothers of young children 102
    needs assessment 206–7
    people with learning disability 228–9
    recovery process 203–4, 207–10
    research 87
    therapeutic relationship 205–6, 211
    see also community mental health nursing
mentoring 314–15, 316–17
Mind Exercise, Nutrition, Do it (MEND) 105
monitoring equipment 164
morbidity 136
mortality 2, 136
MSD (musculoskeletal disorders) 192
multi-agency working 37–52
    end-of-life care 286–8, 297
    examples 43–8
        asthma care 47–8
        dementia 44–5
        obesity prevention 45–6
    home care 152
    inter-professional education (IPE) 309
    key drivers 41–3
    UK context 38–41
    see also integrated care
multi-disciplinary teams 307
multi-method evaluation 79, 80–1
multi-sector working *see* multi-agency
        working
musculoskeletal disorders (MSDs) 192

NaTHNac (National Travel Health Network and Centre) 177–8

National Audit Report, *Tackling Child Obesity: First Steps* 46

National Child Measurement Programme (NCMP) 104

National Council for Palliative Care (NCPC) 285

National Dementia Strategy 44, 45

National Framework For Children And Young People's Continuing Care 128

National Health Service *see* NHS

National Health Service (Primary Care) Act (1997) 172

National Nursing Research Unit 253

National Occupational Standards for Community Development Work 30

National Occupational Standards for the Practice of Public Health 30, 31

National Research Ethics Service (NRES) 86

National Service Framework for Children, Families and Maternity Services 100

National Social Marketing Strategy (NSMS) 142

National Travel Health Network and Centre (NaTHNac) 177–8

NCB (Nuffield Council on Bioethics) 137

NCMP (National Child Measurement Programme) 104

NCPC (National Council for Palliative Care) 285

needs assessment *see* local needs assessment; patient needs assessment

neonatal care 128

Network of Public Health Observatories 148

Newquay Pathfinder pilot project 265

NHS
    community children's nursing (CCN) 115–19, 121
    competition in 139, 171, 246–7, 262
    definition of health 61
    efficiency savings 57
    establishment 138
    productivity trends 56
    quality of care 57
    reforms 2–4, 5, 139–40, 245–7, 268–9
    research passport 85–7
    Safety Thermometer 57
    social innovation and enterprise in 260
    spending increases 56
    Structural Reform Plan 152
    as vendor of services 326
    workforce *see* workforce
    see also Care Quality Commission; Clinical Commissioning Groups

(CCGs); Healthwatch

NHS and Community Care Act 41

NHS at Home: Community Children's Nursing Services 118

NHS Commissioning Board 10, 42, 160, 245, 263–4

NHS Future Forum 139

NHS Innovation Challenge 262, 263

NHS Institute for Innovation and Improvement 262
    exemplars of community children's nursing 122
    High Impact Innovations 40
    measuring the effectiveness of service delivery 253

NHS National Innovation Centre (NIC) 262

NHS Next Stage Review 20

NHS Outcomes Framework 98–9, 124, 142

NHS Plus 196

NHS providers 10

NMC *see* Nursing and Midwifery Council (NMC)

No Health Without Mental Health: Implementation Framework 136

No Longer Afraid: The Safeguard of Older People in Domestic Settings 274

No Secrets 272–4, 275, 276

noise hazards 189, 191, 197

Northern Ireland
    health protection 145
    learning disability services 118, 219, 220, 221–2

NRES (National Research Ethics Service) 86

NSMS (National Social Marketing Strategy) 142

Nuffield Council on Bioethics (NCB) 137

nurse consultants 18

nurse leadership 161

nurse practitioners *see* general practice nurses

nurse teachers 314–16

Nursing and Midwifery Council (NMC)
    Competencies for Entry to the Register 147, 163
    registration as specialist community public health nurse (SCPHN) 186, 198–9
    Standards for Pre-registration Nursing Education 314
    Standards for Specialist Education and Practice 162
    Standards of Proficiency for Specialist Community Public Health Nurses (SCPHN) 97, 148–9
    Standards to Support Learning and Assessment in Practice 314, 316

nursing assessment
  mental health nursing 206–7
  occupational health nurses 195–6
  people with learning disability 234, 236
nursing home care 55

obesity
  prevention 45–6, 103, 105
  research and responses to 45–6
occupational hazards 188–9, 191–3
occupational health nurses 184, 186
  domains of practice 193–8
  education and training 186
  educational role 197–8
  historical perspective 185–9
  public health role 198
occupational health services 189–91, 193, 196
OECD *see* Organisation for Economic
    Co-operation and Development
    (OECD)
Office for National Statistics 76
older people
  abuse and neglect 272–3, 274
  home care 153, 279
  hospital admissions 55–6
  with learning disability 219–20
  primary care 179–80
  residential and nursing home care 55
  substance and alcohol misuse 279–80
Open Door Project 265
Operating Frameworks for the NHS 12
Organisation for Economic Co-operation and
    Development (OECD)
  comparisons of hospital length of stay 56–7
  social innovation 263
organisational learning 308–9
Our Health, Our Care, Our Say 41–2
outcome measurement 140, 254
  community care 160
  community learning disability nursing 236
  public health interventions 146
*Outcomes Strategy for Chronic Obstructive
    Pulmonary Disease (COPD) and
    Asthma* 47
out-of-hours services 173
overweight children 103, 105

PA (participatory appraisal) 78, 80, 81
paediatric nursing *see* community children's
    nursing (CCN)
pain management 289
palliative care *see* end-of-life care
parenting support 102–3
participation *see* user involvement
participatory appraisal (PA) 78, 80, 81

participatory research 78
partnership working 18, 28, 31
  see also inter-professional education (IPE);
    multi-agency working
Pathfinder project 265
Patient and Public Involvement Forums
    (PPIFs) 323–4
patient choice
  advance care planning 291
  along the patient pathway 322–3
  consumerism and citizenship 326–7
  informed consent 159–60
  people with learning disability 225–6
patient engagement 3, 4, 243, 251
patient group direction (PGD) 177
patient information sharing 254
patient involvement *see* public and patient
    involvement (PPI)
patient needs assessment
  end-of-life care 288–9
  mental health patients 206–7
patient-centred care 7, 243
  end-of-life care 287
  people with learning disability 225–6
PCT (Primary Care Trusts) 172, 173
PCTMS (Primary Care Trust Medical
    Services) 172
performance measurement *see* effectiveness
    measurement; outcome measurement
personal budgets 9, 10
personal care 62, 64
Personal Medical Service (PMS) 172
PGD (patient group direction) 177
planning agreements 10
PMS (Personal Medical Service) 172
PMSU (Prime Minister's Strategy Unit),
    *Improving the Life Chances of
    Disabled People* 125–6
policy context 2–13, 245–7
  children and young people services 95–6
  community development 23–4
  home care 152–4, 247
  public health 138–40
  public health interventions 137
political engagement 139
population *see* demographics
poverty
  and domestic violence 278
  link with poor health 26, 92–3, 136–7
  see also vulnerable groups
PPI *see* public and patient involvement (PPI)
PPIF (Patient and Public Involvement
    Forums) 323–4
practice nurses *see* general practice nurses
practice teachers 316

Preferred Priorities for Care 291–2
pregnancy services 101–8
preventable ill health 136, 141, 142
Primary Care, General Practice and the NHS Plan 173
Primary Care Trust Medical Services (PCTMS) 172
Primary Care Trusts (PCT) 172, 173
Prime Minister's Commission of Nursing and Midwifery in England 4, 14
Prime Minister's Strategy Unit (PMSU), *Improving the Life Chances of Disabled People* 125–6
private providers *see* health care providers
private travel health clinics 177
privatisation 39
productivity
    measuring 56–7, 160
    trends in 56
    see also effectiveness measurement; outcome measurement
professional competences *see* competences
professional specialisms *see* specialist community public health nurses (SCPHN)
Protection of Freedoms Act (2012) 159
public and patient involvement (PPI)
    effectiveness 324–32
    Healthwatch 325
    new PPI system 323–4
    organisations and their responsibilities for 326
    partnership and co-production 232–3
    see also community engagement; user engagement
public health
    and care closer to home 65–8
    and community nursing 146–9
    community practitioners' role 15
    versus health promotion 143–4
    health protection 137, 141–2, 145–6
    outcomes framework 140–3
    policy context 138–40
    social marketing 142–3
    social model 145
Public Health England 140
Public Health Framework 146
public health networks 83
public health nursing 135–50
    community nursing and public health 146–9
    health promotion versus public health 143–4
    health protection 144–5
    policy context 138–40

public health outcomes framework 135, 139, 140–3
public health strategies 198
public health teams within local government 32
public involvement *see* public and patient involvement (PPI)
public policy 2–13, 41–2
    critiques 40
publication of research 82

QIPP (Quality, Innovation, Productivity and Prevention) 57, 118
QNI *see* Queen's Nursing Institute (QNI)
Qualified Providers 5, 8, 39
Quality, Innovation, Productivity and Prevention (QIPP) 57, 118
quality adjusted life years (QALYS) 76
Quality and Outcomes Framework (QOF) 173–4, 180
quality of care measurement 57, 253–4
Queen's Nursing Institute (QNI)
    2020 Vision: Focusing on the Future of District Nursing , 247, 264
    Nursing People at Home 153, 154, 161
    Smart New World 161, 164

randomised controlled trials (RCT) 74–5
RCN *see* Royal College of Nursing (RCN)
RCP (Respecting Choices Programme) 291
reciprocity between carer and cared 64
reflective practice 312
refusal of treatment 137
releasing capacity *see* capacity building
research 72–90
    data collection 79
    data management, analysis and interpretation 79–81
    designing the study 73
    ethical issues 84–5, 86–7
    evidence-based practice (EBP) 72–3
    health impact assessment (HIA) 75–7
    methodologies and methods 77
    NHS research passport 85–7
    participatory approaches 78, 81
    presentation and dissemination 82–3
    proposals 83–4
    qualitative 79, 80, 81–2
    randomised controlled trials (RCT) 74–5
    translational research 73–4
    validity, reliability and generalisability 81–2
Research Governance Framework for Health and Social Care 84
residential care homes 55

Respecting Choices Programme (RCP) 291
respiratory disease *see* asthma care
Revitalising Health and Safety 198
RIO system 254
risk assessment
   in community mental health
      nursing 212–13
   domestic violence 278–9
   occupational health 197
Royal College of Nursing (RCN)
   *Domestic Violence: Guidance for
      Nurses* 279
   Frontline First Innovation Awards 264
   *Going Upstream: Nursing's Contribution
      to Public Health* 148
   *Health Visiting and Public Health
      Nursing* 148
   *Nurses as Partners in Delivering Public
      Health* 148
   *Occupational Health Nursing: Career and
      Competence Development* 186
   Pillars of the Community 148
   *Position Statement on the Education and
      Training of Health Care Assistants* 175
Royal College of Paediatrics and Child
   Health, *Facing the Future* 120

safeguarding *see* adult safeguarding; children
   and young people
Safety Thermometer 57
Saving Lives: Our Healthier Nation 198
School Nurse Implementation Plan 97
school nurses
   advocates for children's health and
      well-being 43
   in community development work 30–1
   educating young people about substance
      use 280
   implementation plan 97, 101
   role in improving emotional health and
      well-being 109–10
   services for families 104–5
SCIE (Social Care Institute for
   Excellence) 159, 272
Scotland
   health protection 145
   learning disability services 218, 219, 220–1,
      233
SCPHN *see* specialist community public
   health nurses (SCPHN)
screening services 10, 177
SEAL (Social and Emotional Aspects of
   Learning) 104
*Securing Our Future Health: Taking a Long
   Term View* 138

self-care 64
   mental health patients 209–10
   technology for 164
self-management of health 9–10, 40, 41
service planning 65–6
service quality 57
service users *see* patient-centred care
sexual health advice 107
shared decision-making 2, 322–3, 327, 332–5
Sheffield Profile for Assessment and Referral
   for Care (SPARC) 288–9
'sick role' 59, 61
smoking 137
Social and Emotional Aspects of Learning
   (SEAL) 104
'social capital' definition 25–6
Social Care Institute for Excellence
   (SCIE) 159, 272
social care, integration with
   healthcare 10–11, 42–3, 67–8, 306, 324
Social Care white paper (2012) 7
social enterprise 258, 260, 262
social inclusion/exclusion 24, 26, 225
social influences of health 26, 48–9, 60–1
social innovation 257–70
   approaches to 264–5
   case studies 265–8
   characteristics of a social innovator 260–1
   in commissioning 263–4
   and community health 261–3
   research on 259–60
social marketing 142–3
social services *see* social care
socio-demographic factors 1–2
socio-economic influences on health 135–6
SPARC (Sheffield Profile for Assessment and
   Referral for Care) 288–9
special educational needs 105
specialist clinics 179
specialist community public health nurses
   (SCPHN) 162–3
   community children's nurses 121, 124
   community learning disability nursing 217
   district nurses 162–3
   general practice nurses 172, 174
   occupational health nurses 186
   registration 198–9
   role in community care 18, 97
   see also general practice nurses
specialist treatment centres 9
Sport and Physical Activity Alliance 46
staff resources *see* workforce
'staff-owned' structures 325
standard of living 93
statistical analysis 79–80

stroke services 54
substance misuse 279–80
surveys in research 76–7, 79
sustainable development 49
Swansea University, 'Public Health and
    Partnerships in Care' course 39
symptom management 289

TAC (Team around the Child) 104, 108
Tacking Obesities: Future Choices 45
Tackling Child Obesity: First Steps 46
*Taking a Public Health Approach in the
    Workplace* 198
Targeted Mental Health in Schools
    (TaMHS) 104
targeting of services 25, 40
Team around the Child (TAC) 104, 108
technicians 187
technology 9, 40, 164
    access to services 10
    electronic health-care record 254
    information sharing 83
technology dependent children 127
telehealth 6, 164
therapeutic relationship 158–9, 176
    end-of-life care 290
    mental health nursing 205–6, 211
Torbay model of health and social care 67–8
transformational leadership 161
translational research 73–4
Travax 177–8
travel health advice 177
travel vaccinations 177
treatment room nurse 176
Triple A campaign 47
troubled families 94, 312–13
Troubled Families Programme 312–13

unemployment 93
UNICEF investigation on child well-
    being 94, 110
universal definitions of health 59–61
universities *see* higher education institutions
unpaid care 63–5
user engagement 3, 4, 7, 23
user involvement 28–9, 322–37
    effectiveness 324–32
    modern PPI system 323–4
    see also patient choice

vaccination *see* immunisations
Valuing People 217–18, 221, 222–3
Valuing People Now: The Delivery Plan 223
venous thromboembolism (VTE) 57

Vision and Model for School Nursing 101
VTE (venous thromboembolism) 57
'vulnerable adult' 159, 272
vulnerable groups 48–9
    adults at risk 159, 271–84
    homeless people 81, 260, 265
    occupational health 185
    services for families 102, 102–3
    Troubled Families Programme 312–13

Wales
    community children's nursing 113
    demographics 76–7
    health protection 145
    learning disability services 220, 222
Wanless Report 58, 61, 138, 245
websites for research information 83
well-being 60
    children's 94–6, 109–10
Wellcome Trust 74
whistle-blowing 245
WHO *see* World Health Organization (WHO)
Willis Commission 307–8
Winterbourne Report 245
WIPP (Working in Partnership
    Programme) 175
workforce
    changing roles 15–18, 39
    planning 3, 4–7, 65
        home care 153–4, 161–4
Working For A Healthier Tomorrow 190–1,
    194
Working in Partnership Programme
    (WIPP) 175
Working Together to Safeguard Children 104
workplace hazards *see* occupational hazards
workplace learning *see* inter-professional
    education (IPE)
World Health Organization (WHO)
    Disability-Adjusted Life Year (DALY) 136
    *Framework for Action on Interprofessional
        Education and Collaborative
        Practice* 306, 309
    health definition 60
    health level targets 41
    Occupational Health (OH) services
        recommendations 184
    Ottawa Charter for Health Promotion 139,
        143
wound care 178

Young Foundation 260
young people *see* children and young people
youth unemployment 93